T0184803

DISORDERS OF THE SELF

New Therapeutic Horizons

The Masterson Approach

OTHER WORKS BY
JAMES F. MASTERSON, M.D.

THE EMERGING SELF
A Developmental, Self, and Object Relations Approach to the Treatment
of the Closet Narcissistic Disorder of the Self

COMPARING PSYCHOANALYTIC PSYCHOTHERAPIES
Developmental, Self, and Object Relations • Self Psychology • Short-Term
Dynamic
(with Marian Tolpin, M.D. and Peter E. Sifneos, M.D.)

PSYCHOTHERAPY OF THE DISORDERS OF THE SELF
(with Ralph Klein, M.D.)

THE REAL SELF
A Developmental, Self, and Object Relations Approach

TREATMENT OF THE BORDERLINE ADOLESCENT
A Developmental Approach

THE PSYCHIATRIC DILEMMA OF ADOLESCENCE

COUNTERTRANSFERENCE AND PSYCHOTHERAPEUTIC
TECHNIQUE
Teaching Seminars on Psychotherapy of the Borderline Adult

THE NARCISSISTIC AND BORDERLINE DISORDER
An Integrated Developmental Approach

FROM BORDERLINE ADOLESCENT TO FUNCTIONING ADULT
The Test of Time

PSYCHOTHERAPY OF THE BORDERLINE ADULT
A Developmental Approach

DISORDERS OF THE SELF

New Therapeutic Horizons

The Masterson Approach

Edited by

James F. Masterson, M.D.

and

Ralph Klein, M.D.

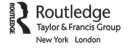

Routledge
Taylor & Francis Group
New York   London

Library of Congress Cataloging-in-Publication Data
Disorders of the self : new therapeutic horizons : the Masterson
approach / edited by James F. Masterson and Ralph Klein.
  p.   cm.
  Includes bibliographical references and index.
  ISBN 0-87630-786-1 (hardcover)
  1. Personality disorders—Treatment.   2. Object relations
(Psychoanalysis)   3. Self psychology.   I. Masterson, James F.
II. Klein, Ralph.
RC554.D57   1995   95-20920
616.8'58—dc20   CIP

First published 1995 by
Brunner/Mazel, Inc.

Published 2013 by Routledge
711 Third Avenue, New York, NY 10017
2 Park Square, Milton Park, Abingdon, Oxfordshire OX14 4RN

First issued in paperback 2015

Routledge is an imprint of the Taylor & Francis Group, an informa business

ISBN 13: 978-1-138-88374-1 (pbk)
ISBN 13: 978-0-87630-786-1 (hbk)

Contents

Contributors

KARLA R. CLARK, Ph.D., received her M.A. from the University of Chicago School of Social Service Administration and her Ph.D. in clinical social work from the California Institute for Clinical Social Work. A Board Certified Diplomate in Clinical Social Work, Dr. Clark served on the faculty of the Masterson Institute (San Francisco) for eight years.

RICHARD E. FISCHER, Ph.D., received his degree in clinical psychology from S.U.N.Y., Buffalo. He was a Post-Doctoral Fellow at the New York Hospital—Cornell Medical Center (Westchester Division) and Psychology Fellow at the Langley Porter Institute, University of California at San Francisco, School of Medicine. Dr. Fischer is a faculty member and supervisor in the Masterson Institute (New York).

DAVID GRUBB, M.D., is a board certified psychiatrist who received his training in psychiatry at the San Francisco General Hospital. He is a member of the clinical faculty in psychiatry at the University of Washington School of Medicine. Dr. Grubb is a graduate of the Masterson Institute (Spokane).

SHIRLEY ZUCKERMAN ISSEL, M.S.W., received her Master's degree in social work from Smith College. She is a graduate of the Masterson Institute (San Francisco).

RALPH KLEIN, M.D., is Clinical Director of the Masterson Institute. He received his training in both pediatrics and psychiatry at New York Hospital–Cornell. He is Assistant Clinical Professor of Psychiatry, Columbia College of Physicians and Surgeons, and is co-editor of *Psychotherapy of the Disorders of the Self: The Masterson Approach* and of this volume.

CANDACE ORCUTT, M.S.S.W., Ph.D., is a Board Certified Diplomate in Clinical Social Work who received her degrees from Columbia University and International University. Dr. Orcutt is a certified psychoanalyst who trained at the New Jersey Institute. She is also a certified clinical hypnotist and member of the American Society of Clinical Hypnosis. Dr. Orcutt is a faculty member and supervisor in the Masterson Institute (New York).

JUDITH PEARSON, Ph.D., received her degree in psychology from Fordham University. She is supervising psychologist, Bronx Psychiatric Center, and Clinical Instructor, Albert Einstein College of Medicine. A graduate of the Masterson Institute, she is a faculty member and supervisor in the Masterson Institute (New York).

BILL ROBBINS, Ph.D., received his degree in clinical psychology from the Professional School of Psychology, San Francisco. Dr. Robbins is a graduate of the Masterson Institute (San Francisco).

KEN SEIDER, Ph.D., received his degree in clinical psychology from the California Graduate School. Dr. Seider, a graduate of the Masterson Institute, is certified in psychoanalytic psychotherapy from the Mount Zion Hospital. He is a faculty member and supervisor in the Masterson Institute (San Francisco).

STEPHEN SILBERSTEIN, M.D., is Associate Clinical Professor of Psychiatry, University of California at Davis, School of Medicine. He is staff psychiatrist at the California Department of Corrections Medical Facility at Vacaville and is a graduate of the Masterson Institute (San Francisco).

BARBARA L. SHORT, Ph.D., received her degree in community psychology at the University of California, San Francisco. Dr. Short is a Fellow and Diplomate of the American Board of Medical Psychologists. She is a graduate of the Masterson Institute (San Francisco).

Preface

The Masterson Approach to the study and treatment of the disorders of the self (formerly the personality disorders) has been carried forward in the past decade by myself and by the continuing efforts of a second generation of clinicians with whom I have worked—first as my students, and subsequently as my colleagues. The initial fruit of that collaboration was presented in *Psychotherapy of the Disorders of the Self* (1989).

My own work has turned in the past number of years to a sharper focus on the self and the elucidation of the closet narcissistic disorder of the self (*The Emerging Self*, 1993).

To retain its vitality and to have continued life, any theory must be so integrated by those who learn it that they are able to use it to explore and extend its horizons. In *Psychotherapy of the Disorders of the Self*, my colleagues demonstrated their mastery of the theory and its clinical application. In the present volume, they now explore and extend the horizons of the theory.

First, the clinical importance of the schizoid disorder of the self was only hinted at in my previous work. The development of the understanding and treatment of the disorder in a developmental, self, and object relations perspective has now advanced rapidly through the efforts of Ralph Klein, Clinical Director of the Masterson Institute. With the publication of this volume, the schizoid disorder of the self takes its place alongside the narcissistic and borderline disorders of the self as a third major dimension of psychopathology.

Second, the vast amount of attention that has been paid to the impact of early physical and sexual abuse on the developing self and the disorders of the self has forced clinicians to refocus once more the dual therapeutic lenses of diagnosis and treatment. How does early physical and sexual trauma affect the development of the self, our view of psychopathology, and our efforts to match therapeutic interventions to this new knowledge? These subjects are introduced and dealt with for the first time in the Masterson Approach by the work of Candace Orcutt, Faculty Member of the Masterson Institute.

Third, the publication of *The Emerging Self* stimulated great interest in refining treatment strategies to address the difficult narcissistic patients, those with closet and devaluing narcissistic disorders of the self. Part III in this volume expands and further develops the ideas that were presented in my previous writings on the diagnosis and treatment of narcissistic pathology.

Fourth, while the Masterson Approach to the disorders of the self largely focuses on the individual, intensive psychotherapy, other treatment strategies have evolved from this basic work; for example, Ken Seider and Candace Orcutt present their work in couples therapy and Richard Fischer presents his work in group therapy. These are slowly growing and becoming an invaluable addition to our therapeutic armamentarium. The complexities of drug therapy and comorbidity and their interactions with psychodynamic forces are presented by David Grubb.

In this volume, all the clinicians continue to listen to patients through the eyes of developmental, self, and object relations theory. From that perspective, they have explored new areas of great clinical importance and added important dimensions to the Masterson Approach. Unquestionably the horizons will continue to expand, and the current state of our understanding will be just one more way station on a complicated and fascinating journey of discovery into the nature of the self and the disorders of the self.

                                                                    J.F.M.

DISORDERS OF THE SELF

New Therapeutic Horizons

The Masterson Approach

PART I

The Self-in-Exile: A Developmental, Self, and Object Relations Approach to the Schizoid Disorder of the Self

In Chapters 1 to 7 on the schizoid disorders of the self, Ralph Klein has combined the work of Fairbairn and Guntrip with the Masterson Approach in a unique way to develop an updated, broader, original, and useful concept of those disorders.

He first traces the history of the concept and then describes the clinical picture. This is followed by a consideration of the contributions of developmental theory reviewing both Mahler and Stern. The intrapsychic structure and prototypical parental relations are described. The last three chap-

1

ters on psychotherapy describe how to establish a therapeutic alliance, shorter-term therapy, and intensive analytic therapy.

The force of his approach is illustrated by the focus throughout on the schizoid dilemma and the schizoid compromise. These concepts are clearly stated theoretically and, even more important, they are beautifully illustrated clinically.

In the last two chapters in this section, Dr. Silberstein and Dr. Short describe further clinical applications of this approach to the schizoid disorder.

J.F.M.

CHAPTER 1

Evolution

Ralph Klein, M.D.

The evolution of the dynamic schizoid concept and the more specific diagnosis of the schizoid personality disorder (henceforth referred to as the schizoid disorder of the self) brings several questions to mind:

1. Is the concept of a schizoid disorder really a valid, discrete, and clinically useful construct, or might it not be equally well subsumed within the other broad dimensions of psychopathology? In that view, the schizoid patient might be considered as having a distancing borderline or a contact-shunning narcissistic disorder. Is the concept of a schizoid disorder, therefore, really needed?
2. Can a useful clinical distinction be made between schizoid as an adjective and schizoid as a noun? While schizoid phenomena and defenses may be present in many persons, is there enough justification to use the concept "schizoid" as a noun and to construct a dimension of pathology? When does a characterological defense shift from being a trait to being a disorder of the self?
3. Should the concept of a schizoid disorder best be restricted to a relatively limited categorical classification, such as is found in the *Diagnostic and Statistical Manual of Mental Disorders* (DSM) or, in fact, is the concept made more useful clinically if it is extended to include contributions from developmental, self, and object relations theory?
4. Further, any review of the concept of schizoid must look at its historical relation to the schizophrenic spectrum disorders, to the phobic character, and to the anxiety disorders, especially social phobia. The fundamental question is whether schizoid disorder should be included in those constructs.

3

These are the questions that clinicians seem most often to pose when presented with an argument in favor of the schizoid disorder as a discrete clinical condition. The ensuing chapters will answer those questions, in order for the diagnosis of schizoid disorder to be justified and for the concept of schizoid to join the other generally accepted disorders of the self— the narcissistic and borderline disorders—as a concept of equal clinical importance.

What does the history of psychiatry teach about the notion of schizoid? There have been several good reviews of the schizoid personality disorder (Akhtar, 1987; Guntrip, 1969; Nannarello, 1953; Seinfeld, 1991). Generally, there have been two separate paths down which this concept has traveled. One path is that of descriptive psychiatry. Its focus is primarily on behavioral, describable, observable symptoms, and its most current and clearest exposition is to be found in the fourth edition of DSM (DSM-IV).

The second path is that of dynamic psychiatry and includes contributions from classic psychoanalysis and object relations theory. This path also includes the exploration of unconscious motivation and character structure. Along the first path, that of descriptive psychiatry, one finds that the notion of schizoid is fundamentally and inevitably linked to the schizophrenic disorder. If it does not directly belong in the group of schizophrenias, the schizoid disorder is at least viewed as a close relative. In fact, this path begins with the observations made at the turn of the century by Emil Kraepelin (1907) that the relatives of patients with dementia praecox had a high incidence of nonpsychotic pathology. He first drew attention to the similarity between the premorbid personalities of patients and the personalities of their relatives.

The path invariably identifies the schizoid patient as being unsociable, quiet, humorless, eccentric, or strange—a group of features that runs "like a scarlet thread through the whole of schizoid characterology" (Kretschmer, 1925). The path of descriptive psychiatry is practically synonymous with this thread.

Although the thread describes part of the story of the schizoid patient, it is far from the whole story. However, the part has far too often been mistaken for the whole and has impeded understanding of the schizoid disorder of the self. In defining the schizoid patient, path 1 has held unquestionable sway in psychiatry, as demonstrated by its central place in the DSM criteria for schizoid personality disorder.

The second path, that of dynamic psychiatry, began with Eugen Bleuler (1924), who, although using the term "schizoid" to describe the same patients whom Kraepelin had identified, added the important observation that the term designated a "natural component of man's personality which directed his attention toward his own inner life and away from the external world." This was a crucial observation. Rather than focusing attention on unusual or strange features, it focused on aspects of character that were universal. The schizoid patient and pathology were no longer, in this view, someone and something set apart. Far greater attention has to be paid clinically to universal components of personality than has to be paid to the strange and unusual. Unhappily for the development of the concept of schizoid, Bleuler's observations were largely left unacknowledged and unused.

The next major figure to contribute to the evolution of the concept of schizoid was Emile Kretschmer (1925). He organized his observations of the schizoid personality into three groups of characteristics. One group included as characteristics unsociable, quiet, reserved, serious, and eccentric. This group is essentially identical to that described by Kraepelin. In a second group were the characteristics timid, shy with feelings, sensitive, nervous, excitable, and fond of nature and books. Kretschmer used the term "hyperaesthetic" (overly sensitive) to describe these characteristics. The third group of characteristics included pliable, kindly, honest, indifferent, and silent. Kretschmer characterized this group as having cold or anesthetic emotional attitudes.

At first glance these three groups of characteristics might seem to describe three very distinct and different clinical entities. However, Kretschmer did not suggest dividing the schizoid personality into three separate groups. In other words, he considered all these characteristics to be simultaneously present in various degrees in all schizoid individuals. What Kretschmer declined to do, the third edition of DSM (DSM-III) proceeded to do by dividing the schizoid diagnosis into the avoidant, the schizoid, and the schizotypal.

Kretschmer had a very different view: "The majority of schizoids are not either over sensitive or cold but they are over sensitive and cold at the same time in quite different relative proportions" (1925, p. 156).

Livesley, West, and Tanney (1985), in reviewing Kretschmer's work concluded: "Different schizoid patients were considered to show these two features to different degrees so that they formed a continuous series. Additionally, schizoid patients were thought to be unstable along these dimensions moving from one to the other. Even those who are at the extremity of insensitivity and coldness have a deep sensitivity. *It is the tension between opposing dimensions that lies at the heart of schizoid pathology. Kretschmer did not suggest division into distinct groups, to do so would be to ignore the essential features of schizoidness*" (italics added).

At this point in the review of the evolution of the concept of schizoid, one can see that the concept has moved beyond the narrow range suggested by the scarlet thread of traditional descriptive psychiatry to include a natural component of personality (Bleuler) and a tension between opposing dimensions that lies at the heart of schizoid pathology (Kretschmer).

But what do these constructs really mean? How can they be integrated into a truly comprehensive picture of the schizoid disorder? For the answers, one must turn to the contributions of Melanie Klein and the British object relations theorists. These sources provide many helpful additions to the understanding of schizoid pathology. At the same time, there are some very harmful and obstructive influences. Perhaps of these two, the more impeding influences prevailed until recently.

MELANIE KLEIN

Much has been misunderstood about the contributions of the British school, particularly the work of Melanie Klein. Her work, while brilliantly contributing to the understanding of character pathology and early intrapsychic structures, had a deleterious effect in the specific arena of understanding schizoid pathology per se and the nature of normative schizoid experience. Klein's concept of schizoid has little, or no applicability to the understanding of schizoid phenomena in general and to the schizoid disorder of the self specifically. For Klein (1946), the concept of schizoid meant splitting. In describing the intrapsychic world of the infant and small child— the preoedipal world—she used splitting to describe one mechanism by which the infant or child tries to organize a whole body of perceptions and internalizations. Splitting, defined as keeping good and bad perceptions and internalizations apart, was, along with projective and introjective techniques, a major tool by which order was brought into the child's chaotic internal world.

Despite the fact that Melanie Klein wrote often about schizoid mechanisms, she was not describing fundamental features of the schizoid personality disorder. Rather, she was mapping out the preoedipal world of the child, which included the mechanism of splitting (schizoid maneuver). Klein's contribution, in other words, was to the study of character pathology generally and not to the understanding of the schizoid disorder of the self specifically (Klein, 1932).

It was primarily the work of two prominent clinicians of the British school—Fairbairn and Guntrip—that was to provide the next giant step toward explicating and integrating the observations that had been made previously by Kraepelin, Bleuler, and Kretschmer.

W. R. D. FAIRBAIRN

W. Ronald D. Fairbairn's contribution (1984) to the understanding of the schizoid condition was intimately connected to the efforts, such as those of Melanie Klein, to delineate character pathology. Fairbairn was not setting out to describe a schizoid personality disorder in the narrow sense, but was trying to describe what he considered to be the essence of character pathology. For Fairbairn, there were essentially three levels of personality organization: the neurotic, the schizoid, and the psychotic. Fairbairn's description of the schizoid is thus very broad. One might reasonably compare this division of pathology to Kernberg's (1975) classification of pathology into neurotic, borderline personality organization, and psychotic. The descriptions are purposely broad because the effort, for Fairbairn as for Kernberg, is to describe a whole range of pathology—character pathology—that runs from the neurotic to the psychotic.

Fairbairn, however, was not describing the same patients as Klein and Kernberg were describing. In Klein's efforts to understand character pathology in terms of early intrapsychic structure formation, she focused attention on those patients who utilized splitting and projective and introjective mechanisms. Klein's work was to focus attention, therefore, on those patients who, as psychiatry developed, would ultimately be diagnosed as *borderline*. Fairbairn focused on particular aspects of the personality that direct a person's attention more toward the inner world than toward the outer world. Therefore, Fairbairn's focus on the preoedipal world and on character moved in the direction of describing those kinds of patients who were subsequently to be identified in clinical psychiatry as *schizoid*. This was a shift in the focus of attention from one phenomenon, projective and splitting techniques, to another phenomenon, a tendency toward focusing on the inner world as opposed to the outer world. The consequence is that different clinical populations are targeted. The problem lies not in the accuracy of the observations that the clinicians made, but in trying to make a part into the whole, to make the phenomenon that each was describing into the nature of character pathology.

For Fairbairn, psychopathology could be organized on three levels: the neurotic, the schizoid, and the psychotic. Fairbairn, as had Bleuler before him, described a schizoid factor that was inherent in the human condition and was manifest in a wide range of normal as well as pathological forms.

The pathological manifestations ranged from schizophrenia and psychopathy at one extreme to the more quietly introverted person at the other. This factor was an attitude of emotional detachment and preoccupation with inner reality that was also associated with an attitude of omnipotence. Fairbairn was emphasizing the schizoid individual's capacity to regulate his or her interpersonal distance and to mobilize self-reliance and self-preservative (omnipotent) defenses as the fundamental ways of organizing the person's internal world and defending against anxiety, conflict, and other traumatic situations that could threaten the self.

The nature of the endopsychic structure (internalized object relationships), according to Fairbairn, revolved around the alternating need for social contact, which was anxiety laden, and the defensive need for distancing associated with seeming indifference and a general overevaluation of the internal world at the expense of the external world. Here Fairbairn delineated four critical and central schizoid themes. First, there is the need to regulate interpersonal distance as a primary focus of concern. Second, the schizoid patient displays the ability to mobilize self-reliant and self-preservative defenses. Third, there is a dynamic, pervasive tension between the need for attachment, which is anxiety laden, and the defensive need for distancing, which is manifest by *seeming* indifference. Fourth, there is a general overevaluation of the internal world at the expense of the external world.

Fairbairn went much beyond these four fundamental themes. His precise description of schizoid mechanisms was presented as a comprehensive description of intrapsychic structure generally and, in essence, a complete object relations theory of character pathology. This is where Fairbairn went astray, in that he moved away from describing a delimited dimension of psychopathology, the schizoid dimension, and suggested that the part was equal to the whole and that his concepts described more broadly the entire range of character pathology lying between the neuroses and psychoses. The following quotation makes this clearer. It is one of Fairbairn's (1984) best-known and most frequently cited observations.

> The great problem of the schizoid individual is how to love without destroying by love . . . the devastating nature of the conflict . . . lies in the fact that if it seems a terrible thing for an individual to destroy his object by hate, it seems a more terrible thing for him to destroy his object by love. It is the great tragedy of the schizoid individual that his love seems to destroy and it is because his love seems so destructive that he experiences such difficulty in directing libido toward the object and outer reality. He be-

comes afraid to love and therefore he erects barriers between his objects and himself.

Although this is a moving portrayal of a person in conflict and in turmoil, it has no more application to a schizoid individual than to one with any other disorder of the self. For every disorder of the self, the nature of attachment is so conditional, dysphoric, and potentially destructive, and is maintained at such a high, perilous, and often destructive cost, that these individuals have a hard time believing that attachments of any nature are truly gratifying and sustaining.

All self disorders find that attachments (relationships) bring with them the experience of dysphoria and actual, or potential, destructiveness. This fact is at the core of the nature of self pathology and helps to define all the disorders of the self. For all self disorders, the conditions of relatedness require the giving up of the development of the real self in favor of the defensive substitution of an impaired, false self. Thus for all self disorders, love (the yearning for relatedness) seems to destroy (both the real self and, by projection, the other). All self disorders experience the barriers between the self and others as a consequence of having to relate through the distortions imposed by the false self. For all self disorders, truly authentic intimate attachments are not possible. For all self disorders, it is not rage or hatred that is most destructive, but the sacrifices and compromises made around the conditions of relatedness that are most devastating to the self.

Thus the unique schizoid conflict is not how to love without destroying by love. That is a conflict generic to all disorders of the self. Rather, the unique schizoid conflict can only be identified by defining the specific conditions of attachment for the schizoid patient that are so destructive to the life of the self and to the interpersonal world of the schizoid. These specific conditions were more clearly targeted by Fairbairn's four fundamental themes than by the more famous observation quoted above.

One additional major contribution by Fairbairn should be mentioned. He added a significant developmental understanding to the genesis of the schizoid disorder when he observed: "In early life they [schizoid patients] gained a conviction whether through apparent indifference or through apparent possessiveness on the part of their mother that their mother did not really love them as persons in their own right" (Fairbairn, 1984, p. 113).

This observation foreshadowed the important focus on maternal emotional availability that became a central theme in the understanding of the borderline disorder of the self (Masterson, 1976) and the narcissistic disorder of the self (Kohut, 1971; Masterson, 1981). But, more specifically, the observation by Fairbairn that the schizoid patient gained a conviction may be literally understood to mean that the schizoid patient consciously acquired a belief in his or her own unlovableness and in the maternal inability to love. The critical difference between the schizoid patient developmentally and those with other self disorders is that the awareness of maternal emotional unavailability is an actual, explicit experience and not a potential, implicit possibility. There is a world of difference developmentally between these two positions. The former leaves little room for hope and little reason to turn to external reality to consummate the yearning for attachment. The latter leaves endless room for hope and countless reasons to continue to turn to external reality to achieve attachment, acknowledgment, affirmation, and approval.

In summary, Fairbairn clearly laid the basis for a comprehensive, developmental, object relations view of the schizoid disorder of the self. His observations went well beyond previous discussions of schizoid pathology, and he sketched out most of the significant arenas to be explored: descriptive, dynamic, and developmental.

HARRY GUNTRIP

Harry Guntrip (1969) was able to rescue the concept of schizoid (factor, pathology, and phenomena) from overinclusiveness (and potential oblivion) by developing Fairbairn's observations into a more precise and exacting description of the schizoid patient. While, like Fairbairn, Guntrip was interested in describing an extensive clinical arena of psychopathology and in focusing on a wide range of patients, he was able to lend a degree of specificity throughout his clinical writings to the concept of schizoid in a number of ways.

First, he developed a very clear set of nine characteristics that he felt distinguished and identified this group of patients (Guntrip, 1969, pp. 41–44). These criteria established a degree of specificity that was previously lacking.

Second, Guntrip focused clinical attention not on the concept of the destructiveness of the schizoid patient's love, but rather on the four fundamental themes described by Fairbairn. In fact, the schizoid patient's pattern of alternately striving to maintain relatedness in order to achieve security, and subsequently needing to break away or distance in order to maintain freedom and independence from the object, was, for Guntrip, at the heart of the schizoid patient's intrapsychic world and defined the *fundamental schizoid dilemma* (or dynamic). Again, it should be stressed that while Guntrip's observations were borrowed from Fairbairn and were not unique, he rescued the concepts from possible oblivion and applied them clinically in a fashion that Fairbairn had not.

Third, in addition to his description of core characteristics and his clear articulation of the schizoid dilemma, Guntrip described the concept of the *schizoid compromise*, which is the schizoid patient's effort to deal with the schizoid dilemma. It is *the* organizing defensive operation for the schizoid patient, and can be defined as all those self functions whose goal is to protect the schizoid patient from the twin dangers of closeness and distance.

Fourth, Guntrip was also clear in describing the importance of fantasy life for the schizoid individual. However, he focused on the defensive, regressive use of fantasy, while generally neglecting the aspect of fantasy that makes it an excellent example of schizoid compromise.

Despite the enormous contribution that Guntrip made to the understanding of the schizoid patient, he left several large areas that required further understanding and elaboration.

1. A fuller, more detailed understanding of developmental issues as they relate to the genesis of the schizoid disorder.
2. A comprehensive description of the internalized object relations units of the schizoid individual. The endopsychic structure proposed by Fairbairn (1984, Chap. 4) is too general and broadly applicable, as evidenced by its use as the starting point for many clinical descriptions of the borderline patient's intrapsychic structure (Kernberg, 1975; Masterson, 1976; Runsley, 1982). It suffers from the problem of overinclusiveness. Guntrip failed to go beyond Fairbairn's observations about intrapsychic structure, and, therefore, his ideas are vague and imprecise in this area.
3. Guntrip's treatment recommendations lack a consistent focus and specificity, and suffer from this vagueness. Therapeutic interventions are not consistently integrated with Guntrip's dynamic understanding and observations. Despite the clarity of his clinical descriptions, the therapist is left with the question, "But what exactly do I do?"

At the time of the publication of Guntrip's work on the schizoid patient in 1969, many other clinicians were focusing their attention on introducing and consolidating their observations on borderline and narcissistic pathology and disorders. Guntrip's work attracted far less attention, and the diagnosis of schizoid seemed doomed to be relegated to the role of neglected stepchild.

Although there has been renewed interest in the schizoid disorder, the existence of this important dimension of psychopathology remains precarious. For appropriate clinical attention to be paid to the schizoid disorder, a comprehensive, developmental, object relations perspective must be clearly described. Such a comprehensive picture, including phenomenology, developmental issues, nature of the intrapsychic structures, and specific treatment approaches, would allow for more precise differential diagnosis, including diagnosis of the schizoid disorder of the self, and for testing of treatment hypotheses in the clinical arena.

REFERENCES

Akhtar, S. (1987). Schizoid personality disorder: A synthesis of developmental, dynamic, and descriptive features. *American Journal of Psychotherapy*, *41*, 499–518.

Bleuler, E. (1924). *Textbook of psychiatry*. New York: Macmillan.

Fairbairn, W. R. D. (1984). *Psychoanalytic studies of the personality*. London: Routledge & Kegan Paul.

Guntrip, H. (1969). *Schizoid phenomena, object relations and the self*. New York: International Universities Press.

Kernberg, O. (1975). *Borderline conditions and pathological narcissism*. New York: Aronson.

Klein, M. (1946). Notes on some schizoid mechanisms. In J. Riviere (Ed.), *Developments in psychoanalysis*. London: Hogarth Press.

Klein, M. (1932). *The psychoanalysis of children*. London: Hogarth Press.

Kohut, H. (1971). *The analysis of the self*. New York: International Universities Press.

Kraepelin, E. (1907). *Clinical psychiatry*. New York: Macmillan.

Kretschmer, E. (1925). *Physique and character*. London: Kegan, Paul, Trench & Trubner.

Livesley, W. J., West, M., & Tanney, A. (1985). Historical comment on DSM-III schizoid and avoidant personality disorders. *American Journal of Psychiatry*, *142*, 1344–1346.

Masterson, J. (1976). *Psychotherapy of the borderline adult: A developmental approach*. New York: Brunner/Mazel.

Masterson, J. (1981). *The narcissistic and borderline disorders*. New York: Brunner/Mazel.

Nannarello, J. J. (1953). Schizoid. *Journal of Nervous and Mental Disease*, *118*, 237–249.

Rinsley, D. B. (1982). *Borderline and other self disorders*. New York: Aronson.

Seinfeld, J. (1991). *The empty core: An object relations approach to psychotherapy of the schizoid personality*. New York: Aronson.

CHAPTER 2

Description

Ralph Klein, M.D.

The schizoid personality disorder has been recognized as a distinct clinical syndrome, in one form or another, since shortly after the turn of the century. The description of schizoid persons initially referred to those nonpsychotic but strange and often isolated individuals who seemed to exist as close relatives of schizophrenics. Later, due to the work of the object relations theorists, the concept evolved and began to denote patients who demonstrated a tendency, often quite marked, toward directing their attention to their own inner worlds and away from the external world. These patients often showed excessive withdrawal or introversion and a general avoidance of human relationships. They, however, were not to be confused with schizophrenic patients; rather, they represented distortions, or pathological elaborations, of factors or tendencies to be found in all individuals.

Most recently, the schizoid personality has been described by DSM-III, the revised third edition of DSM (DSM-III-R), and DSM-IV as a relatively delimited syndrome that focuses on the clinical features of social indifference or social unease in interpersonal relationships. A full descriptive definition of the schizoid personality disorder would include all of these definitions, and yet all of them taken together would not do justice to the phenomenology of schizoid pathology.

Before proceeding further down this focused phenomenological path, one should note that the descriptive, presenting clinical picture can at best only be a red flag for the clinician, a signpost that may call the clinician's attention to a possible diagnosis. Masterson (Masterson & Klein, 1989) has stressed that most of the borderline patients he treats in the outpatient setting would not satisfy the DSM-III or DSM-III-R criteria for borderline personality disorder. Certainly the same could be said for the narcissistic personality disorder, where closet narcissists probably greatly outnumber those with exhibitionistic narcissistic disorders (1993). A similar state of clinical affairs is true for the schizoid disorder of the self. The schizoid disorder described in DSM-III and DSM-III-R identifies a type of severe, generally lower-level schizoid disorder that corresponds roughly to the stereotypes of the schizoid disorder held by both clinicians and the lay public.

DSM-III performed the important function of beginning to lay the groundwork for defining a schizoid spectrum or dimension by splitting the diagnosis of schizoid into three categories: schizoid, avoidant, and schizotypal. In actuality this was not a splitting of the concept schizoid, but an extension of the concept to include a range of pathology.

DSM-III-R reversed the trend toward making the schizoid diagnosis more inclusive and moved it once again in the direction of exclusivity by essentially eliminating the more severe forms of schizoid pathology, as well as the milder forms. How was this accomplished? By moving the schizotypal patient closer to the schizophrenic patient by the addition of criteria for odd, eccentric, or peculiar behavior, the diagnosis of severe schizoid pathology is made less likely. Indeed, these features are traditionally associated with a diagnosis of simple schizophrenia. The diagnosis of the avoidant personality also underwent change in DSM-III-R.

> The DSM-III concept of avoidant personality disorder was essentially social withdrawal due to hypersensitivity to interpersonal rejection. It was distinguished from schizoid personality disorder by the presence of a desire for affection and acceptance.

DSM-III-R was making note of the close association between avoidant and schizoid disorders and was making the distinction based primarily on the subjectively reported intensity of the desire for object relationships. However, DSM-III-R went on to conclude:

> The DSM-III-R concept of avoidant personality disorder differs markedly in that it now corresponds to the clinical concept of phobic character and is no longer mutually exclusive with schizoid personality disorder.

DSM-III-R made the diagnosis of a mild schizoid disorder almost impossible. Avoidant personality disorder was no longer mutually exclusive with schizoid disorder. Also, the description of the avoidant personality was blurred almost totally with the diagnosis of social phobia. Hence there was little place for a range of schizoid pathology.

DSM-IV makes some changes for the better and some for the worse. Perhaps what is most significant is that it once again makes changes for the diagnostic criteria for the avoidant personality disorder, although not for the schizoid or schizotypal disorders. Once again, the problem of solely using descriptive criteria is evident in the continual attempts to refine the definitions of these disorders along (what should be) a schizoid spectrum. DSM-IV removes the criteria associated with social phobia from the diagnosis of avoidant personality disorder and thus reverses the trend toward making social phobia and avoidant personality disorder synonymous. At the same time, avoidant personality is again seen as discontinuous with schizoid personality disorder and so is deprived of the treatment strategies that might follow.

Can descriptive psychiatry do better? With the publication of DSM-III we entered the age of criteria and, for better or for worse, the importance of criteria is greater than ever. Can we identify common criteria for a range of schizoid disorders from severe to mild? Perhaps it has already been done.

Harry Guntrip in 1969 described nine fundamental characteristics of the schizoid personality. As these nine characteristics combine both objective features and subjective impressions, they were unsuitable for DSM-III, DSM-III-R, and DSM-IV. They go much further than our current classification systems in presenting a comprehensive, descriptive overview of the schizoid personality and the range of schizoid psychopathology. Therefore, these nine characteristics can be used as a descriptive starting point for achieving an in-depth understanding of the intrapsychic world of the schizoid.

GUNTRIP'S CHARACTERISTICS

The nine characteristics that Guntrip (1969, pp. 41–44) identified were as follows:

1. Introversion
2. Withdrawnness
3. Narcissism
4. Self-sufficiency
5. A sense of superiority
6. Loss of affect
7. Loneliness

8. Depersonalization
9. Regression

In the following, those characteristics are discussed in greater detail, including the author's own elaboration of the phenomena from clinical experience.

Introversion

According to Guntrip, "By the very meaning of the term the schizoid is described as cut off from the world of outer reality in an emotional sense. All this libidinal desire and striving is directed inwards toward internal objects and he lives an intense inner life often revealed in an astonishing wealth and richness of fantasy and imaginative life whenever that becomes accessible to observation. Though mostly his varied fantasy life is carried on in secret, hidden away."

The schizoid person is cut off from outer reality to such a degree that he or she experiences outer reality as dangerous. It is a natural human response to turn away from sources of danger and toward sources of safety. The schizoid individual, therefore, is primarily concerned with avoiding danger and ensuring safety. This is why such persons will describe their experiences with external reality using such terms as wariness, caution, fear, and risk, as well as safety and danger. These aspects of experience are so much more a part of the world of the schizoid at every level of organization, from higher level to lower level, than those aspects most frequently associated with the schizoid—indifference, coldness, or uncaring. These more common descriptions of the schizoid experience apply generally only to those schizoid individuals who have never become patients.

The introversion that Guntrip describes focuses on the enormous, rich, and complicated fantasy life that is part of the person's inner world. The amount of time spent absorbed in fantasy can be extraordinary, ranging from minutes to hours each day. A schizoid young man described how he had spent much of his childhood in an empty refrigerator box in his home, fantasizing for hours at a time. This was his primary way of feeling comfortable and of escaping from the anxieties (dangers) associated with external reality. The box was his safe place, his nest, his haven.

Withdrawnness

According to Guntrip, withdrawnness means detachment from the outer world, the other side of introversion.

Guntrip's simple observation that the process of introversion will result in the appearance of detachment and withdrawnness cannot be dismissed. However, a fundamental distinction must be drawn here between sign and symptom, between objective observation and subjective reporting, and between external world and internal reality. While there are many schizoid individuals who will present with obvious withdrawnness (a clear and observable timidity, reluctance, or avoidance of the external world and interpersonal relationships), this defines only a portion of such individuals. There are many fundamentally schizoid people who present with an engaging, interactive personality style. These patients belong to the category I describe as *secret schizoids*.

How is the apparent contradiction resolved? One need only ask the secret schizoid what his or her subjective experience is in order to resolve the riddle. What the patient will describe is how he or she may be available, interested, engaged, and involved in interacting in the eyes of the observer, while, at the same time, he or she is apart, emotionally withdrawn, and sequestered in a safe place in his or her own internal world. While withdrawnness or detachment from the outer world is a characteristic feature of schizoid pathology, it is sometimes overt and sometimes covert. When it is overt it matches the usual description of the schizoid personality. Just as often, it is a covert, hidden internal state of the patient.

Several points are important to review at this time. First, what meets the objective eye may not be what is present in the subjective, internal world of the patient. Second, one should not mistake introversion for indifference. Third, one should not miss identifying the schizoid patient because one cannot see the forest of the patient's withdrawnness through the trees of the patient's defensive, compensatory, engaging interaction with external reality.

Narcissism

According to Guntrip: "Narcissism is a characteristic that arises out of the predominantly interior life the schizoid lives. His love objects are all inside him and moreover he is greatly identified with them so that his libidinal attachments appear to be in himself. . . . The question, however, is whether the intense inner life of the schizoid is due to a desire for hungry incorporation of external objects or to withdrawal from the outer to a presumed safer inner world."

The need for attachment as a primary motivational force is as strong in the schizoid person as in any other human being. Where, however, does the schizoid find the object of attachment? Will the schizoid look for the love object out there (external) or will he or she, defensively seek and settle for the love object being in here (internal)? The narcissism of the schizoid—that is, the fact that his or her love objects are inside the person—is a consequence of the fact that it is only by identifying those love objects as being inside that the schizoid will feel safe from the anxieties associated with connecting and attaching to objects in the real world.

The narcissism of the schizoid is also related to the fundamental capacity for self-containment. Self-containment is the ability to self-regulate one's internal affect states, especially to keep anxiety and depression within manageable limits. This capacity for self-regulation of dysphoric affect states is particularly striking and developed in the schizoid disorder of the self, in contrast to the underdeveloped capacity found in borderline and narcissistic self disorders. No one probably has a greater capacity to be alone with himself or herself than the schizoid individuals. The schizoid has had to learn how to self-regulate these core affects because he or she has had no other option.

Guntrip's question about whether the source of the intense inner life is to be found in the desire for hungry incorporation or withdrawal from the outer world can now be answered. The narcissism of the schizoid has nothing to do with envy or the desire to possess the valued object. It is not to be mistaken for the normal infantile, expansive narcissism of early life, or for the pathological narcissism exhibited by the grandiose self of the pathological narcissistic disorder. The narcissism of the schizoid reflects the withdrawal from the outer world to a presumed safer inner world.

Self-sufficiency

According to Guntrip, "This introverted narcissistic self-sufficiency, which does without real external relationships while all emotional relations are carried on in the internal world, is a safeguard against anxiety breaking out in dealing with actual people."

The more that schizoids can rely on themselves, the less they have to rely on other people and so expose themselves to the potential dangers and anxieties associated with that reliance or, even worse, dependence. The vast majority of schizoid individuals show an enormous capacity for self-sufficiency, for the ability to operate alone, independently and autonomously, in managing their worlds. The conscious awareness of this capacity for self-regulation, self-containment, and self-sufficiency is often highly developed early in the life of the schizoid. There is a kind of adultomorphism that goes on with the schizoid, unlike with many other disorders of the self. This premature taking on of adult capacities and responsibilities often dramatically distinguishes the schizoid from other self disorders. It may become manifest in early childhood. It has been given social recognition through such expressions as the latch-key child and the parentified child. These are often sad expressions of a child's capacity to mobilize internal resources prematurely because of an inability to rely on external resources that either are not there or are not perceived as being there.

Sense of Superiority

Guntrip states, "A sense of superiority naturally goes with self-sufficiency. One has no need of other people, they can be dispensed with. . . . There often goes with it a feeling of being different from other people."

The sense of superiority of the schizoid has nothing to do with the grandiose self of the narcissistic disorder. It does not find expression in the schizoid through the need to devalue or annihilate others who are perceived as offending, criticizing, shaming, or humiliating. The meaning and function of the sense of superiority were described by a young schizoid man in the following fashion: "If I am superior to others, if I am above others, then I do not need others. When I say that I am above others, it does not mean that I feel better than them, it means that I am at a distance from them, a safe distance. It is a feeling of being vertically displaced, rather than horizontally at a distance." By the last sentence the patient was conveying that whether he felt superior (vertically displaced) or withdrawn and introverted (horizontally at a distance), the fundamental issue was *maintaining a safe distance from others*.

Feelings of superiority, narcissism, and self-sufficiency must be understood in terms of their function in order to make a correct diagnosis. If the function of such feelings is to achieve narcissistic goals and to enhance the grandiose self, then one is probably dealing with a narcissistic disorder. If it is a way to protect the individual against unbearable danger and anxiety and to enable the patient to achieve and maintain safety, not grandiosity, then one is probably dealing with a schizoid disorder.

Loss of Affect

According to Guntrip, "Loss of affect in external situations is an inevitable part of the total picture." Because of the tremendous investment made in the self—in the need to be self-contained, self-sufficient, and self-reliant—there is inevitable interference in the desire and ability to feel another person's experience, to be empathic and sensitive. Often these things seem secondary, a luxury that has to await securing one's own defensive, safe position. The subjective experience is one of loss of affect. For some patients, the loss of affect is present to such a degree that the insensitivity becomes manifest in the extreme as cynicism, callousness, or even cruelty. The patient appears to have no awareness of how his or her comments or actions affect and hurt other people.

More frequently, the loss of affect is manifest within the patient as genuine confusion, a sense of something missing in his or her emotional life. Often the patient will complain, "I don't know what I am feeling," or "I don't know if I am feeling." All of these manifestations of loss of affect reflect the sacrifice made by the schizoid in the capacity to invest emotionally in others because of the need to invest so intensely in himself or herself, protectively and defensively.

It is necessary to distinguish the loss of affect that Guntrip described from the different process of emotional numbing that is expressed by many patients and is a dissociative phenomenon. The schizoid experience is not one of numbness, but one of uncertainty and confusion. Schizoids are not unable to feel. They are uncertain about what their feelings are, mean, and represent, and so often feel unable to put their experiences into words that can be shared with and understood by others. Emotional numbing, the experience that one is literally numb or unfeeling, is associated with posttraumatic states. Schizoid disorders and posttraumatic disorders are not mutually exclusive, and, in fact, their simultaneous appearance in the same individual may make for a difficult diagnostic problem.

Loneliness

According to Guntrip, "Loneliness is an inescapable result of schizoid introversion and abolition of external relationships. It reveals itself in the intense longing for friendship and love which repeatedly break through. Loneliness in the midst of a crowd is the experience of the schizoid cut off from affective rapport."

This is a central experience of the schizoid that is so often lost to the observer. Contrary to the familiar caricature of the schizoid as uncaring and cold, the vast majority of schizoid persons who become patients express at some point in their treatment their longing for friendship and love. This is not the schizoid patient as described in the DSMs. The longings for friendship and love repeatedly break through, and, in so doing, put a lie to the portrayal of the schizoid as indifferent. Such longing, however, may not break through except in the schizoid's fantasy life, to which the therapist may not be allowed access for quite a long period in treatment.

There is a very narrow range of schizoid individuals—the classic DSM-defined schizoid—for whom the hope of relationship is so minimal as to be almost extinct; therefore, the longing for closeness and attachment is almost unidentifiable to the persons themselves. These individuals will not become patients. The schizoid individual who becomes a patient does so often because of the twin motivations of loneliness and longing. The schizoid patient still believes that some kind of connection and attachment is possible and is well suited to psychotherapy. Yet the irony of the DSMs is that they lead the psychotherapist to approach the schizoid patient with a sense of therapeutic pessimism, if not nihilism, because the psychotherapist misreads the patient by believing that the patient's wariness is indifference and that caution is coldness.

The most common presenting issue for the schizoid patients I treat is the wish for connection and relatedness. Specifically, the wish is either to have a relationship or to have a family and children. It is very common for schizoid individuals to present for treatment in their 30s and 40s, at a time when the possibility of a relationship is growing more tenuous and that of companionship seems to be getting more and more distant. The wish and hope for intimacy and generativity seem to be approaching a last-chance period in the person's life.

Depersonalization

Guntrip describes depersonalization as a loss of a sense of identity and individuality.

Depersonalization is a dissociative defense. Depersonalization is often described by the schizoid patient as a tuning out or a turning off, or as the experience of a separation between the observing and the participating ego. It is experienced by the schizoid when anxieties seem overwhelming. It is a more extreme form of loss of affect than that described earlier. Whereas the loss of affect is a more chronic state in the schizoid, the experience of depersonalization is a more acute defense against more immediate experiences of overwhelming anxiety or danger.

A profoundly schizoid young woman, who often described herself as being on the outside looking in on life, would experience depersonalization when she was forced to participate in group situations as a condition of her employment. Depersonalization—experiencing herself as outside her body observing the group and herself participating in the group—was her way of dealing with the intolerable anxiety of too great a closeness in an inescapable situation.

Regression

Guntrip defined regression as "representing the fact that the schizoid person at bottom feels overwhelmed by their external world and is in flight from it both inwards and as it were backwards to the safety of the womb."

Such a process of regression encompasses two different mechanisms: inward and backwards. Regression *inward* speaks to the magnitude of the reliance on primitive forms of fantasy and self-containment, often of an autoerotic or even objectless nature. Specifically, these kinds of regressive phenomena involve preoccupation with body parts (fetishes and perversions), hypochondriacal preoccupations, and somatic concerns. Some examples are a middle-aged man's preoccupation with prostitutes, an older man's focus on the feet of his companions, a young woman's continual but vague somatic discomfort and numerous visits to doctors, an older woman's preoccupation with her breath. The presence of sadomasochistic fantasies, and their occasional enactment in reality, is another aspect of this regressive phenomenon. Examples of these can be found in many cases of erotomania and spousal abuse, as well as in delimited sadomasochistic sexual encounters/relationships.

Regression backwards to the safety of the womb is a unique schizoid phenomenon and represents the most intense form of schizoid defensive withdrawal in an effort to find safety and to avoid destruction by external reality. The fantasy of regression to the womb is the fantasy of regression to a place of ultimate safety. An example is the experience of a schizoid man who at a very young age had buried deep within himself, in an impenetrable shell, all that was good and true, sensitive and feeling. The self that he presented to the world was an empty shell, while his real self remained safely buried, protected from assault, appropriation, or annihilation, awaiting a time when it could be reborn into the actual world, rather than be kept hidden, secret, and safe from harm.

The description of the nine characteristics first articulated by Guntrip should bring more clearly into focus some of the major differences that exist between the traditional, descriptive (track 1, DSM) portrait of the schizoid disorder and the traditional, psychodynamically informed (track 2, object relations) view. All nine characteristics are internally consistent. Most, if not all, should be present in order to diagnose a schizoid disorder. However, several additional diagnostic variables must be considered.

One, already mentioned, is that patients who are identified through objective criteria would probably correspond to either the avoidant or the schizoid personality disorders of the DSMs. Patients who would be identified as schizoid only through the subjective reporting of the patient would be referred to as *secret schizoids*.

Furthermore, many patients will show some characteristics more prominently than others. Clinical experience indicates that these nine characteristics can be grouped into three clusters of characteristics in a fashion that is useful for differential diagnosis. The first cluster is the pure schizoid cluster. The specific features associated with this cluster are withdrawnness, introversion, and lack of affect. The pure schizoid cluster is essentially synonymous with the scarlet thread that runs through the history of the development of the concept. These three characteristics must be present in order to make the diagnosis of a schizoid disorder. This cluster is the most direct and clear expression of the schizoid patient's need to maintain a safe, stable interpersonal distance from others. The following are examples of two patients who show a prominent pure schizoid cluster. In the case of the first example the cluster is evident; in the second it is "secret."

MANIFEST PURE SCHIZOID CLUSTER DISORDER. Mr. I. had spent most of his life alone. He described himself as a loner and noted that those people with whom he most closely worked also described him in this fashion. His colleagues acknowledged and respected his wish, and apparent need, to be alone, and they kept their distance. He had never had particularly close relationships throughout his life. Now in his mid-40s, he had been working most of his adult life as a mathematician. He is extremely competent and capable at what he does. He keeps minimal contact with his family. They live a great distance from Mr. I., and when they do come to visit, he reports that he feels intolerably uncomfortable while they are in his home, particularly if they decide to stay overnight. This discomfort has become so obvious that they rarely do stay over.

Mr. I. takes great pleasure in his work, which absorbs him almost totally. When not at work, he spends most of his free time in a hobby related to the stock market. He methodically and obsessively attends to the details of this avocation, spending hours each day absorbed in detail. He shows little need to make contact with people.

Why was I seeing Mr. I.? The answer to this question addresses once again the very deep, hidden longing present in even the most profoundly schizoid individuals. Mr. I. had begun to experience feelings that his aloneness and isolation were less desirable and more disconcerting. He reflected more about the future, and he saw a life in which the opportunity for the pleasures associated with relatedness was slipping quickly away. He had had no sexual relationships and, although he expressed some interest in and mild curiosity about sex, he did not have any strong feelings of loss about the lack of sexual intimacy. He did have a vague feeling, however, of wanting something more in the way of connection and communication with others. The only reason for this vague feeling and for his seeking treatment at the time he did seemed to be his age and the awareness of life passing him by.

Mr. I.'s efforts at connecting to others during his treatment were poignant expressions of both the wish and the fear connected with relationships and of the kind of adaptations that the schizoid patient makes in order to try and balance these wishes and fears. A typical interaction with a male acquaintance would proceed as follows: Every week or so this friend would visit Mr. I. and they would agree either to watch a movie or to listen to music. The evening would pass with both sitting in the living room watching the movie or listening to the music. Neither would initiate a conversation with the other. After several hours, the evening would end. Both men would feel somewhat gratified (and neither would have made an interpersonal demand on the other).

It would be easy to see in this example only the distance that each party maintained interpersonally. What is less obvious, but just as important, is the connection maintained. In some ways, this behavior on Mr. I.'s part was reminiscent of the practicing child as described by Mahler, who can play safely and comfortably at the mother's feet or within a certain radius of the mother without having to interact, except occasionally turning to the mother for emotional refueling. There is no suggestion that Mr. I. was arrested at the practicing subphase of separation-individuation. The intention is to convey the quality of play of which Mr. I. would avail himself at times, when such play could be conducted safely and within carefully designed parameters. The schizoid patient who could always play so safely would perhaps play much more, but such conditions of carefully titrated interaction are not easily found or imposed.

Mr. I. also described an emerging heterosexual interest while in treatment. This took the form of a continuous, albeit infrequent, contact that Mr. I. maintained with a very distant cousin who lived approximately 1,000 miles away. Mr. I. kept up a correspondence with this woman after having briefly met her during a family social event. Mr. I.'s letters to this woman were romantic and intimate, as were her responses. There was an occasional, brief telephone call. Actual meetings were once a year. Mr. I. would extensively fantasize about a more intimate relationship with this woman, even about marriage, fantasies that he would very occasionally share with his therapist and even with the woman. However, during his six years in treatment, nothing more came of the relationship beyond the interaction already described. Any possibility of taking action on his fantasies was halted by his concern that such a relationship would be intolerably "intrusive on my space and time," and, "I have such a good thing going now, why should I do something that might ruin the relationship?" He never did.

SECRET PURE SCHIZOID CLUSTER DISORDER. Mr. R., a man in his 30s, presented with an affable, friendly, outgoing demeanor with just a hint of reserve and shyness. Well liked and in a job that required a fairly high degree of interpersonal interaction, he conducted his life in a generally engaging fashion.

After work he would participate in social events with his colleagues. He felt that it was part of his job requirement that he maintain these social connections. His free time was often spent playing various sports, and he was on several sports teams. He was very popular among his peers.

In his personal life, he had a long-standing relationship with a woman and they had lived together for several years before his beginning treatment. Although he reported some feelings of closeness with this woman, he said he always felt a barrier separating him from her and from all others. There was always, as he put it, "a limit to the closeness." He stated, "I can get only so close and then it feels like I get on a parallel track with the other person, like the rails on a railroad track, and I can get no closer. I don't know how to get closer, and I don't know if I want to get closer." His subjective emotional experience was that of anxiety, experienced when he felt that the woman knew too much about him because he had shared too much with her. These anxieties were evidenced by his unwillingness to consider marriage, despite the long relationship. The woman saw it as a difficulty with intimacy on his part and made the questionable distinction that the problem lay not in the capacity for closeness, but in making a commitment to marriage. This is how his friends saw it too, often teasing him about his reluctance to get married. What was essentially an extreme sense of anxiety and even danger around getting close was rationalized as a fear of responsibility and commitment.

Mr. R. had presented for treatment because subjectively he was experiencing increasing frustration, both at work and in his personal relationship. He was feeling a growing wish to have greater closeness. Yet he was equally aware of a growing dysphoria associated with his efforts to do so. By all outward appearances, no one would have identified Mr. R. as schizoid. Always with a smile on his face and a friendly word on his lips, Mr. R. would satisfy no one's objective criteria for schizoid disorder.

Mr. R., however, was profoundly schizoid. Examination of his subjective experience revealed the essential core of schizoidness. Withdrawnness, introversion, and lack of affect were no less a part of his life than they were of Mr. I's, but they were manifest pervasively in his internal world and little, if at all, in external reality. Mr. R. revealed over time his profound feelings of disconnectedness from others and the amount of his time spent in fantasy, often the preferred place to be. This sociable, friendly man spoke with great pain (and unconscious irony) about whether he could experience real feelings and whether he was fundamentally lacking in his affective life. He feared that he was a kind of android, going through life pretending to experience and feel, but not really doing so. He wondered whether his external persona was a mask worn over what was essentially a shell of a man, devoid of the capacity for genuine feeling.

The pain that he felt when recounting his anxieties about his affective life belied his interpretation of affective impairment. This is a striking example of the schizoid conflict about experiencing affect, and hence of the manifold defenses erected against the experience of that affect, even to the point that this patient effectively convinced himself that he was devoid of, or at least impaired in, this fundamental capacity.

Mr. R. was an excellent example of the secret schizoid. The real intrapsychic state of affairs only becomes apparent in discussion and interaction with this patient, because of his willingness gradually to expose his internal world. If the patient is willing to share internal experience, then the core cluster characteristics appear and make the diagnosis of schizoid disorder of the self possible.

These two presentations of the schizoid patient—the manifest and the secret pure schizoid cluster patient—represent two different points on the continuum of differential diagnosis. The manifest schizoid disorder is easily identified, but the secret schizoid disorder is much harder to diagnose. The other two clusters of characteristics that derive from Guntrip's nine characteristics represent two additional points of interest and diagnostic confusion along the differential diagnosis continuum. The second cluster is the *pseudonarcissistic cluster* and includes the features of narcissism, superiority, and self-reliance. The third cluster is the *pseudoborderline cluster*, which contains primarily the features of loneliness, regression, and depersonalization.

It is important to remember that all nine characteristics described by Guntrip can generally be found in all schizoid patients. However, the reason for making these distinctions among the manifest, secret, pseudonarcissistic, and pseudoborderline patients is that different relative proportions of these features may be present in different patients.

The pseudonarcissistic and the pseudoborderline presentations are relatively common. They are important to identify because, while they are essentially variations of the secret schizoid, they present distinct differential diagnostic problems.

The pseudonarcissistic cluster describes a group of patients whose presenting characteristics—narcissism, self-reliance, and superiority—focus on a need to maintain autonomy and independence in the face of conflicts around interpersonal distance. The patient will appear to have a narcissistic disorder. The narcissism of this schizoid patient, however, is unlike that of the person with narcissistic disorder of the self and does not have as its goal or function the enhancement of a grandiose self or the enactment of feelings of specialness or entitlement. For the schizoid patient, life goals are not related to the typical narcissistic ones of power, wealth, beauty, or even perfect misery or martyrdom. Rather, the narcissism of the schizoid patient is designed to help the patient maintain himself or herself at a comfortable distance from others. The schizoid patient's narcissism is intended to enable him or her to feel above others, not with the goal of being better than them, but, with the objective of being safe from having to rely on or depend on another person. This is an important diagnostic distinction, since many schizoid patients are first incorrectly diagnosed as having narcissistic disorders due to the misinterpretation of the meaning of the patient's presenting picture.

PSEUDONARCISSISTIC CLUSTER DISORDER. Mr. B. presented for treatment at the age of 35 with the chief complaint of not being appreciated at work and of quarreling with his immediate superiors over his failure to receive what he had anticipated would be a substantial bonus. His initial sessions consisted of a litany of complaints about being misunderstood by his bosses and by the women whom he met in his personal life. While his work history had been stable and he had held his current job for 10 years, his personal history was far more unstable. His relationships with women lasted for only brief periods before he found some reason to stop seeing them. His longest relationship, when he was 22 years old, had lasted for one year. It was the only relationship in which he had been sexually intimate. He explained that since then he had been able to satisfy his sexual needs for the most part through narcissistic masturbation, by which he meant masturbating in front of a mirror with anal stimulation.

In the initial sessions, he described with annoyance and bitterness his feeling that no one appreciated him. He stated that his talents were unrecognized and unacknowledged. He really was, he maintained, superior to those with whom he worked and to the women whom he dated. When others did not recognize his superiority, he felt strangely invisible. At times these feelings would escalate rapidly into brief episodes of terror, which he guessed to be "some sort of panic attack." He expressed his needs with a pervasive sense of entitlement, from the kind of office he felt he deserved at work to the responses from other people in every area of his life. It was my assumption (not stated by the patient) that he must feel that everyone in his life should feel as he felt, should think as he thought.

This initial presenting picture suggested the diagnosis of a narcissistic disorder of the self—in fact, a fairly typical exhibitionistic narcissistic disorder meeting all the criteria of grandiosity, entitlement, feelings of being special, and demand for one-mindedness (fusion or merger). Yet there were features to Mr. B., and a quality to many of his pronouncements, that led me to consider a primary paranoid state or a schizoid disorder.

While his work history was stable and he performed competently and capably, he worked best alone and was most receptive to praise in the form of bonuses. Verbal compliments or praise seemed not to matter nearly as much to him as did more tangible rewards. He said that he knew he worked well and that he did not need anybody to tell him that. The use to which he put his tangible rewards (salary and bonuses) were far from exhibitionistic. He decorated his own home to his precise tastes and needs with little need to show it off to others. The women he dated were rarely brought home because he feared that they would "mess up" or disturb his home in some ill-defined manner.

The more he described his interpersonal life, the more disturbed it sounded. There was a quality of object distancing associated with a lack of safety or a wariness. It became clear that he did not avoid people because he felt superior to them, but rather that he felt superior to people in order to avoid them, together with his fear of being manipulated and controlled by them. Mr. B.'s sense of superiority or narcissism was not utilized to pursue narcissistic goals. It was in pursuit of safety. To be above others was not desirable because of something inherent in that position (grandiosity or specialness), but was simply one way of being apart. Exploration of his life more generally revealed that he was equally likely to utilize withdrawal (feeling invisible), or even feeling below others ("I feel inhuman at times"), in order to maintain a safe distance.

The patient's narcissistic masturbation was a striking example of the capacity for self-containment. The mental image (fantasy) that accompanied the act was that of being watched by the woman with whom he had been most recently. The feeling tone associated with this fantasy was not one of being admired by the woman, but of feeling connected to her. In a similar fashion, he preferred talking to women on the telephone to being with them in person. Although he initially had requested medication for his panic attacks, it soon became apparent that these were not spontaneous, medication-responsive panic attacks. The precipitant was invariably his feeling of being invisible to others; this was the trigger to his feeling of cosmic aloneness, which he described as feeling like a living dead person, a zombie "like in a horror movie." Throughout the abbreviated period of treatment, he experienced no anxiety attacks because, as he reported, he felt "connected to this world because I am connected to you . . . not alone. . . ."

Rather than being narcissistic, this patient displayed the quintessential characteristics of the schizoid patient, and his was a relatively severe schizoid disorder. He operated in his internal world according to the unique object relations units of the schizoid, and his basic, operative dynamic paradigm was the schizoid dilemma.

The pseudoborderline cluster—loneliness, regression, and depersonalization—highlights a particular segment of schizoid patients who are in more active retreat and who feel more threatened by being disconnected from the world of object relationships. These features, which are typically described by many of those with borderline disorders, have a very different function for the schizoid patient. For the borderline patient, they serve the eventual function of maintaining closeness to the object, whether through the longing generated by loneliness, through the caretaking generated by helplessness and regression, or through the frantic need to make contact, generated by the disconnected (even though safe) feelings associated with depersonalization.

For persons with schizoid disorder of the self, these features reflect another way of being apart from (specifically, below) others. The schizoid patient understands the unwillingness to participate with others as due to his or her having no right to participate in their company because of self-imposed isolation (loneliness), dysfunction (regression), or alienation (depersonalization). The pseudoborderline schizoid patient has a self representation of feeling like a monster and a freak. Although this is a "bad" self representation, it is different from the borderline patient's experience of badness. Schizoid patients are bad because they are different, strange, set apart from others, and unable to experience love. Borderline patients are bad because they are guilty, inadequate, failures, evil or insignificant, and undeserving of love.

These descriptions may clinically blur, especially when trying to differentiate a schizoid disorder from a borderline disorder with distancing defenses. Several concepts help this differentiation. The bad self of the borderline patient is related to the experience of abandonment and rejection for efforts at real self-activation. The bad self of the schizoid patient is related to feeling different, associated with the fear and terror that accompanies the need to accommodate to social and interpersonal demands and expectations.

PSEUDOBORDERLINE SCHIZOID DISORDER.   Ms. S. was in her early 40s and was separated from her husband when she was referred because of increasingly severe anxiety, which had arisen in the past year, apparently in tandem with the growing estrangement from her husband. Her one child, a son, was approaching adolescence, and this too seemed to trigger additional separation anxiety. The patient dramatically described her enormous need for other people, her need to cling desperately to others, particularly when there was the slightest hint or anticipation of anxiety. She characterized herself as extremely dependent in this regard. She spoke of her need for constant reassurance and of an intolerance of being alone for fear of what might happen. She additionally described frank experiences of depersonalization, which frightened her and sent her running to her son or to call a friend in order to feel protected.

Her early history seemed to support the hypothesis that excessive abandonment fears were at the core of her disorder. She had had a severe, disturbed relationship with a very narcissistic (possibly psychotic) mother and a passive, withdrawn father. The mother had used constant threats of abandonment and expulsion from the home, alternating with praise for compliance, as her way of controlling the patient.

While the patient had been referred with the diagnosis of borderline disorder and demonstrated acute intolerance of being alone, a fear of feeling loneliness, much passive-dependent behavior, a clinging to protectors, and depersonalization, she nonetheless did not have a borderline disorder. First, and most significant, the patient did suffer from extreme panic disorder with agoraphobia. Many of the behaviors that led the referring therapist to the diagnosis of borderline disorder were intimately connected with her attempts to manage this overwhelming and misunderstood state. During nonsymptomatic periods, Ms. S. demonstrated a clear capacity for self-containment, self-management, and self-reliance, in stark contrast to her behavior during and around acute episodes. Despite her manifest symptomatology and its self-distorting capacity, Ms. S. was basically a survivor, confident of her own capacities to manage, except in those situations that she experienced as beyond her control (which they were). At times of acute panic, however, she would cling to anyone who was around.

Far from being prone to separation stress at her son's adolescence and her separation from the husband, Ms. S. actually experienced both with pleasure and a sense of freedom. Ironically, one of the greatest problems in the marriage had been the conflict generated by the husband's wish for closeness and Ms. S.'s need for distance.

CONCLUSION

In summary, this chapter has attempted to present a comprehensive, descriptive overview of the schizoid disorder of the self. Similar to the Masterson Approach to the narcissistic and borderline disorders, this overview has stressed that descriptive psychiatry can only be the starting point for effective diagnosis and treatment. A concept of schizoid that is broad enough to enhance differential diagnosis and clinical usefulness, without making the concept a diagnostic wastebasket, is the objective. With that in mind, the concept of schizoid introduced descriptively here has attempted to integrate what is most useful from the DSM and from the object relations theorists, especially Harry Guntrip.

A reasonable descriptive classification of the schizoid disorder has been proposed as a starting point, which rests on the following:

1. The schizoid disorder should be clinically subdivided into secret schizoid, avoidant schizoid, and classical schizoid disorders.
2. The classical schizoid diagnosis (DSM-IV) should subsume the diagnosis of schizotypal. A clear distinction should be made between the concept of schizoid as character pathology and of schizoid as schizophrenic-like for clinical purposes. The concept of schizotypal is a diagnostic hedge without sufficient justification and does more harm than good by blurring fundamental distinctions that are clin-

ically important. For practical, clinical purposes, patients who would be diagnosed as schizotypal should be given a clinical trial of treatment for schizoid disorders, albeit with severe schizoid pathology.

3. The diagnosis of avoidant schizoid disorder (DSM-IV criteria for avoidant disorder) should be used to describe the schizoid who demonstrates less withdrawnness, introversion, and loss of affect. Again, for practical, clinical purposes, the avoidant personality disorder of DSM would be treated as a milder form of schizoid pathology.

4. The term "secret schizoid" should be used to indicate all those patients who do not look schizoid or avoidant but who, upon questioning, subjectively report most, if not all, of Guntrip's nine characteristics of schizoid pathology. Three characteristics are essential: withdrawnness, introversion, and loss of affect.

5. The notion of a secret schizoid was foreshadowed in the Masterson Approach by the concept of the closet narcissistic disorder, that is, the diagnosis rests on structural characteristics, which are enduring, and not symptoms, which are state dependent.

6. Descriptive psychiatry can only point the way and alert the clinician to possibilities. Differential diagnosis is fundamentally a multidimensional process, one that begins with description but must be completed by the integration of descriptive phenomena with developmental considerations, with an understanding of intrapsychic structure, and with a clinical trial of response to different therapeutic interventions.

REFERENCES

Guntrip, H. (1969). *Schizoid phenomena, object relations and the self.* New York: International Universities Press.

Masterson, J. F. (1993). *The emerging self.* New York: Brunner/Mazel.

Masterson, J. F., & Klein, R. (Eds.) (1989). *Psychotherapy of the disorders of the self.* New York: Brunner/Mazel.

CHAPTER 3

Developmental Theory

Ralph Klein, M.D.

There are several questions that need to be addressed when considering the issue of developmental theory and its application to the understanding and treatment of the schizoid disorder of the self.

How much attention should be paid to developmental theory? How important is an understanding of developmental theory to the actual clinical treatment of a patient? Is developmental theory something argued over by individuals who have little need to address the more pressing issue of treatment?

Clinicians who primarily focus attention on what to do and when to do it often bypass the question that lies at the heart of both developmental theory and clinical practice. "Why do we do the things we do?" Developmental theory is the foundation for understanding the way people come into being—how they become and what they become. By defining the normal processes of becoming, developmental theory allows the clinician to determine more easily what is pathological. For example, a clinician may hear a patient express a fear of enslavement. What meaning can one give to this statement? Is it a normal, predictable part of human experience? Is it part of an engulfment fear that is inevitable as the infant emerges out of the state of infantile symbiosis? Is it an exaggeration of a normal process that reflects an understandable reaction to a hovering or overprotective parent or caretaker? Or is such a fear or anxiety a reaction that is perpendicular to the normal plane of human experience? If the developmental theory does not require a symbiotic period or an inevitable struggle over engulfment versus separation, then a fear of enslavement would represent a clear detour or deviation from the normal developmental pathway.

Without a firm foundation in developmental theory, much clinical prac-

33

tice would be adrift in a sea of uncertainty, and clinicians would operate on the principle of "flying by the seat of one's pants" or making interventions that seem to feel right at the moment.

For all these reasons, clinical psychiatry without developmental theory could never be psychodynamic psychiatry. From Freud to the present day, psychodynamic psychiatry has been a marriage of descriptive psychiatry and developmental theory. This was true of the psychoneuroses; it is true today of the disorders of the self. Without this felicitous marriage of observable phenomena and theoretical constructions, clinical psychiatry, and, in particular, the field of characterology, would consist of meaningless lists of criteria (as in the DSM) with no overarching, comprehensive way to organize the understanding of human nature and pathology—those stable, relatively inflexible, continuous ways of behaving, thinking, and feeling in relation to the world.

Developmental models of the mind are what distinguish descriptive psychiatry from psychodynamic psychiatry. Within the scope of psychodynamic psychiatry the choice of a therapeutic intervention is largely determined by the nature of the understanding the developmental model provides.

A note of caution before proceeding further. Developmental psychology—the study of the mind of the infant, the infant self, and the interpersonal world of the infant—has only established itself as a science in the past quarter of a century. The models of infant psychology that will be examined and from which clinical hypotheses will be drawn are in an embryonic state of flux, revision, and expansion. Such hypotheses must be viewed as tentative, and the therapeutic implications of such theory must continue to be tested in the clinical laboratory.

What are the unique developmental issues for the schizoid disorder of the self? To answer this question, one must first look at the two most current and prominent developmental theories that inform the clinician about the individual's process of coming into being. These two theories are generally referred to as *separation–individuation theory* and *the developing senses of self theory*. Their originators and major proponents were Margaret Mahler (Mahler, 1968; Mahler, Pine, & Bergman, 1975) and Daniel Stern (1985) respectively. Both theories are informative, clinically applicable, and, despite efforts to stress their dissimilarities, show much overlap and are fundamentally complementary.

It is important to understand the unique perspective of each theory as applied to the understanding of character more generally. Then one can focus more narrowly on understanding the developmental issues relevant for the schizoid disorder of the self within both theoretical frameworks.

Mahler's description of the psychological birth of the human infant and the phase of separation-individuation has been used extensively since the early 1960s in understanding and working with normal children and clinical populations. In the area of characterology separation–individuation theory has been most successfully applied to elucidating the genesis of the borderline personality disorder (Masterson & Rinsley, 1975). In the Masterson Approach, extending separation–individuation theory to include the narcissistic disorder of the self focused on the developmental arrest as occurring in the period before the rapprochement crisis, leaving infantile grandiosity largely intact and unmodified. The match of theory to clinical observation has never been as comfortable or as good a fit for the narcissistic disorder as for the borderline disorder of the self (Masterson, 1981).

Where does this leave the schizoid disorder of the self? Must one find a place for the schizoid disorder within the subphases of separation-individuation? Undoubtedly one could; the question is whether one should. Perhaps, as with the narcissistic disorder of the self, this would raise as many questions as it would answer. Therefore, rather than trying to do so, it might be better to reexamine the fundamental concepts of separation–individuation in order to identify what would be clinically enhancing rather than restricting and that might, in the process, provide a crucial area of overlap and similarity with developing senses of self theory.

Separation–individuation theory makes one central, fundamental assumption about the developmental process that should be highlighted. It states that there comes a time in development (the timing of which is largely irrelevant, or at least is secondary to the fact of the process itself) when the child begins to move beyond symbiosis as an operational principle of mental functioning and toward a capacity in mental life to distinguish internal world from external reality, and, most important, to distinguish internal self representation and internal object representation.

It is important to keep in mind that throughout Mahler's writings the concept of symbiosis refers to two different mental operations. First, it applies to the concept of the dedifferentiation between internal world and external reality. This concept of symbiosis has to do with failures in stabilizing ego boundaries and is associated with subsequent pathological states—specifically, childhood symbiotic psychosis. More generally, the failure consistently to distinguish internal world from external reality leads to persistent failures in reality testing and a fundamentally psychotic organization of mental functioning.

The second mental operation that Mahler uses the term "symbiosis" to describe refers to a purely intrapsychic state of affairs. Its relation to external reality is a secondary issue. This mental operation involves the dedifferentiation between self representation and object representation. It deals only with the representational world of the infant. This purely internal symbiosis, or dedifferentiation between self and object representations, does not primarily deal with the infant's perception of external reality, but rather addresses the infant's thoughts, ideas, and feelings about himself or herself and others, what he or she is like and contains as a human being, and what the object is like and contains. The emphasis here is on subjective experience, not on external reality. The operative words are *memories, feelings, fantasies,* and *ideas* about oneself, the self representation, and about the other, the object representation.

Internal symbiosis, this second principle of mental functioning, thus describes the infant or young child's inability to differentiate correctly (separate) his or her experiences of himself or herself and ideas about himself or herself as distinct from (operating from a different center of initiative than) the child's fantasies, feelings, and experiences of what the other, the object, is like, is feeling, and is experiencing.

Internal symbiosis is unrelated to the issues of reality testing and of differentiating internal world from external reality. It is related totally to the capacity to distinguish self and object representations. Clinically, this means that while *external* symbiosis (the first definition) applies to psychotic states, *internal* symbiosis applies to the domain of characterology and the disorders of the self. This lack of clarity of usage on the part of Mahler in her writings has unnecessarily impeded the understanding of the notion of symbiosis (albeit internal symbiosis) as it applies to the disorders of the self. Moreover, it has been a basic reason for the appearance of marked incongruity between the developmental theories of Mahler and Stern.

The first meaning of symbiosis (external symbiosis and the function of reality testing) is relevant to understanding the disorders of the self only insofar as it helps to understand the tendency of many lower-level disorders of the self to exhibit regressively delimited micropsychotic and pseudopsychotic episodes. Here one can clearly see the application of the concept of external symbiosis as a process of mental life that violates the boundary between internal world and external reality.

Far more applicable to the disorders of the self is the notion of internal symbiosis and the change in this aspect of mental functioning that is at the heart of the rapprochement subphase of separation–individuation. Mahler's concept of the dedifferentiation of self and object representations states that for the infant and small child there is a significant developmental period during which the child is unable to differentiate two independent centers of initiative. This means operationally that the child is unable to separate clearly the memories, feelings, and experiences of the self from the imagined memories, feelings, and experiences contained in the other. Mahler's concept of internal symbiosis, therefore, seems to refer clearly to a specific process (age-appropriate distortion) in mental functioning that allows the child to believe that other people think and feel the way the child does.

With these two definitions of symbiosis in mind, the subphases of separation–individuation can be reconsidered. Differentiation and practice subphases seem to describe well the mental experiments that the child conducts in order to achieve the twin goals of clear separation of internal world and external reality and of the separation of internalized self and object representations.

The rapprochement subphase begins with the process of differentiation of self and object representations largely achieved. The child is well on the way to consolidating this new aspect of mental functioning. The essence of the rapprochement subphase (which its name implies) is that a time in development has been reached when the child is aware that the other does not automatically think and feel as the child does. The person in external reality is no longer assumed to mirror the internal object that the child has long recognized as feeling and thinking as he or she does. Now the object in external reality mirrors an internal object representation that has its own unique thoughts and feelings. The child has entered a newly defined interpersonal world that reflects that child's newly achieved mental status, and the child must approach the object at a different level of understanding and with the new operation of mental functioning.

Much of the essential aspect of rapprochement has been described as the child's acute awareness of his or her separation from the object. The emphasis too often has been on separation from the object in external reality. The crucial focus should be on the child's separation from the internal object representation and the assumption of like-mindedness and like feelings.

The reason why separation–individuation theory and the borderline disorders have fit together so well is that the description of mental functioning characteristic of rapprochement fits all the disorders of the self as a central organizing principle. This distinguishes the more severe, psychotic level of organization from the level of organization characteristic of the disorders of the self.

By the very nature of the term "rapprochement," separation–individuation theory implies that there must now be an active negotiating process that will take place between the child and the other, both the other defined as the representative of external reality and the other defined as the representative of the internal world (internalized object representation). The consequence will be new interpersonal relationships and new internalized object relations. When Masterson (Masterson & Rinsley, 1975) first elucidated the genesis of the borderline disorder, he pointed to the crucial failure of maternal emotional availability during this newly emerging period in the child's intrapsychic reorganization. The mother's emotional unavailability in providing the conditions for creating a healthy deal or contract was the first of two crucial developmental failures. The second failure related to the unhealthy, unrealistic, distorted conditions of relatedness that the parent did present to the child. In the case of the future borderline disorder, these conditions are described in the classic paradigm: reward for regression, withdrawal in the face of separation–individuation or self-activation.

As described earlier, when Masterson extended separation–individuation theory to include the narcissistic disorder, problems arose in matching clinical observations to theory. While a developmental arrest could easily be postulated at the pre-rapprochement crisis period, with the preservation of a fundamental state of like-mindedness or internal symbiosis, problems in matching levels of ego functioning with levels of developmental arrest arose. Masterson proposed several possible solutions, but concluded that no explanation seemed totally adequate. An additional explanation suggested by separation-individuation theory is that the child, in actively negotiating with developmental capacities that have been achieved, elects to mobilize those conditions of relatedness that had served so well previously. Such an explanation requires only the theoretical shift away from a primary adherence to the concept of developmental arrest, and toward the substitution of a theory of reactivation or remobilization of modes of mental functioning previously available, but relegated to a secondary position in terms of primacy of mental functioning.

Having considered the concepts of separation–individuation theory, symbiosis, and rapprochement, the two questions posed previously can be answered. Is separation–individuation theory compatible with the theory of the developing senses of self? And what useful developmental theory can inform the clinician's understanding and treatment of the schizoid disorder of the self? The discussion of separation–individuation theory has already suggested answers to these questions.

In answer to the first question, the work of Mahler and Stern shows considerable overlap. Stern went far in supporting Mahler's fundamental assumptions by operationally defining and subjecting to rigorous examination the concepts that Mahler had described. The result is that Stern articulates a position that is almost identical to that described by Mahler. What are the similarities?

Stern initially described four developmental senses of self: emergent, core, subjective, and verbal self experiences or organizations. To these he later added the narrative self. Most important for purposes of comparison with separation–individuation theory are the core and subjective self organizations. The core sense of self established the child's sense of personal self-identity as a physically separate, cohesive whole. It integrated the capacities of self-agency, self-coherence, self-affectivity, and self-continuity into an organized center of initiative. The principle of mental functioning associated with this organization of self experience was described by Stern as the principle of one-mindedness. Operationally defined, this meant that the child experienced the self and the other (as external object and internal representation/evoked companion) as sharing the same focus of attention, intentionality, and affective state. This is an operational definition of internal symbiosis, of the similar mental content and affect state shared by the self and object representations.

Stern further described the principle of mental functioning associated with the subjective self as that of separate but interfaceable minds. This closely resembles Mahler's description of mental functioning during the rapprochement subphase of separation-individuation. Separate minds means the capacity to differentiate the content and affect states belonging to the object (representation) from that belonging to the self (representation). Interfaceable means the capacity to negotiate meaning and understanding between these now separate centers of initiative. The mental functioning described by Stern as associated with the subjective self emerges as identical to the mental functioning associated with the rapprochement child. The task of negotiating the conditions of relatedness, attachment, and shared mutual meaning, of interfacing, are no different during the rapprochement subphase than during the domain of intersubjective relatedness.

Several additional points should be noted when comparing and contrasting the theories of Mahler and Stern.

It is intriguing to note that if one were to apply the theory of the developing senses of self to clinical psychopathology, one could easily correlate the mental mechanism of one-mindedness associated with the core self with those clinical manifestations of mental functioning found in the narcissistic disorder of the self and generally referred to metaphorically as merger and fusion. One-mindedness seems an appropriate operational definition of merger/fusion metaphors. The grandiose self can now be operationally defined to mean an individual's conviction that others think and feel as the self does, a state of affairs in which the self has a very hard time conceptualizing the possibility that others could think or feel differently. One could again postulate that the narcissistic disorder demonstrates an early form of mental functioning, as Masterson has already postulated. However, the same criticisms that one encounters in the application of separation-individuation theory would be present in applying senses of self theory.

In addition, Stern has emphasized that the progression from emergent self organization to subjective self organization is largely a biological/ maturational achievement that can only be detoured by massive insult (such as severe mental retardation or childhood schizophrenia).

There are two other points where the theories of Mahler and Stern clearly diverge. Both seem to be issues of secondary importance. The first has to do with the concept of normal autism, a Mahlerian notion that developmental psychology has successfully refuted. The second has to do with the timing of developmental events. Although the descriptions of the mental processes are remarkably identical in the two theories, the timing of these events is remarkably dissimilar. For Mahler, the period of rapprochement is noted to be between 15 and 22 months, while for Stern, the domain of intersubjective relatedness and the primacy of the subjective self organization is identified as between 7 and 15 months. There seems to be no way to explain this discrepancy between observational and experimental data.

One can now proceed to attempt to apply developmental observations to the schizoid disorder of the self.

1. The schizoid patient is clearly capable of distinguishing internal world and external reality. The patient is not psychotic. The introversion and use of fantasy in no way reflect a malignant, autistic transformation of personality. Therefore, the schizoid pathology is in no way a *forme fruste* of schizophrenia or a point on the schizophrenic spectrum. A schizoid patient is no more prone to psychotic regressions or episodes than is the patient with any other disorder of the self.

2. The schizoid patient has achieved the capacity to differentiate internal self representation from object representation. The schizoid patient does not operate with the theory of one mind. The mental processes that govern the person's internal and interpersonal life are those best described by Mahler's characterization of rap-

prochement or by Stern's characterization of separate but inter-faceable minds (the subjective self).

3. At this stage in the evolving understanding of schizoid pathology, it is more useful to explore the conditions of attachment and the nature of the interpersonal negotiation that may play a decisive role in the genesis of the schizoid disorder than to be concerned with the specific timing of developmental events. What is important is that the genesis is early and is mediated (at least) by the parent–child interaction.

4. If one puts aside issues of developmental timing and does not become trapped by specific phase issues, one can easily note that the narcissistic and borderline disorders of the self reflect different patterns of negotiated relationships between the self and the other at a time when the self is psychologically capable of making these new kinds of deals or contracts. Similarly, one must attempt to define for the schizoid patient the specific conditions of attachment, the nature of the deal or contract that the schizoid patient enters into in order to experience the acknowledgment and affirmation that come with attachment, while avoiding the anxiety, conflict, and trauma that come with nonattachment. A comprehensive description of the representational world of the schizoid patient, developmentally informed, is the goal. No clinical objective is served by fitting the schizoid patient into a developmental straitjacket. Specifically, there is little clinical use for, or need to define, a developmental spectrum for the three currently described dimensions of psychopathology: narcissistic, borderline, and schizoid.

5. In placing rigid developmental phases in the background and in moving principles of mental functioning and the precise nature of the working models of attachment into the foreground, what becomes of the notion of a spectrum disorder? The idea of a spectrum or range of severity within a defined dimension of psychopathology has often been coordinated with developmental levels. The best, and most clinically useful example of this practice has been the description of higher-level borderline patients as being farther along in the rapprochement period, while lower-level borderline patients have been assumed to demonstrate developmental arrest during early rapprochement. The advantages of this schema are many. It explains a range of functioning, because the later the arrest (it is argued), the more intrapsychic is that structure that has been laid down and is available for use. Further, ar-

rest later in rapprochement could explain the predominance of abandonment fears in higher-level borderline patients, as opposed to the prevalence of engulfment fears in lower-level borderline patients. Masterson (1978) has fully articulated this point of view. It works well. But perhaps it works so well not because these are principles applicable in a narrow sense to the borderline disorder, but because they are principles of human maturation and development more generally.

The question remains: Is the concept of developmental levels a prerequisite to the concept of a spectrum or range of pathology? The answer is *No.* An equally suitable explanation is one that utilizes a multifactorial contribution to the clinical manifestation of any particular dimension of psychopathology, whether narcissistic, borderline, or schizoid. Masterson has summarized this multifactorial contribution with the notion of nature, nurture, and fate (1988). All three factors must invariably play a role in the final clinical manifestation of self structure and organization. What unique constitutional or temperamental factors contribute to the genesis of the schizoid disorder of the self? It is unclear. There can be no simple one-to-one correlation; for example, between the "slow-to-warm-up" infant and child and the later manifestations of schizoid pathology. But equally clearly, temperamental and constitutional factors *do* play a role. What these are remains to be discovered.

Fate plays its inexorable role in the final organization of self-identity; such factors as illness, loss, injury, coincidence, and luck play powerful parts in defining one's personal and interpersonal worlds.

Nurture is most compelling to the psychodynamically oriented clinician. The nature of the attachment, the conditions of relatedness, are surely also properties of the parent–child relationship. But a specific working model of attachment is not a homogeneous phenomenon. Any working model, or interpersonal contract, has an endless number of variations. A working model of attachment is not a contract chiseled in stone, rigidly defined and unalterable. Whether one has more or less intrapsychic structure laid down may be less important than the qualitative aspects of those structures. Are they totally rigid and unbending or flexible and malleable? Are they reinforced structures or temporary havens? Have they been used repeatedly and habitually or are they episodically and sporadically mobilized? The answers to these questions (along with the factors of nature and fate) may have as much explanatory value for the variety and range of clinical manifestations within a dimension of pathology as does the concept of developmental arrest.

Chapter 4 deals specifically with the representational world of the schizoid disorder. It looks at the specific nature of the conditions of attachment that are presented to the schizoid patient, and of the deal made between the schizoid patient and the significant others in his or her world. The nature of the schizoid patient's internal, representational world—the essential nature of schizoidness—is a consequence of the deal that is negotiated.

REFERENCES

Mahler, M. (1968). *On human symbiosis and the vicissitudes of individuation.* New York: International Universities Press.

Mahler, M., Pine, F., & Bergman, A. (1975). *The psychological birth of the human infant: Symbiosis and individuation.* New York: Basic Books.

Masterson, J. F. (1981). *The narcissistic and borderline disorders.* New York: Brunner/Mazel.

Masterson, J. F. (1978). *Psychotherapy and the borderline adult.* New York: Brunner/Mazel.

Masterson, J. F. (1988). *The search for the real self.* New York: Free Press.

Masterson, J. F., & Rinsley, D. B. (1975). The borderline syndrome: The role of the mother in the genesis and psychic structure of the borderline personality. *International Journal of Psychoanalysis, 56,* 163–177.

Stern, D. (1985). *The interpersonal world of the infant.* New York: Basic Books.

CHAPTER 4

Intrapsychic Structures

Ralph Klein, M.D.

To examine the intrapsychic structure of the schizoid patient is to explore the heart, the essential nature, of schizoidness.

What is the specific schizoid paradigm? In other words, what conditions does the schizoid experience that must be converted into a working model of attachment? What kind of deal does the schizoid negotiate in order to gain the benefits of attachment while avoiding the anxieties and dangers of nonattachment?

The answers to these questions come from listening to patients. The scientific loopholes are many and obvious. The greater the number of patients that one can listen to, however, the more accurate and applicable the answers become.

Masterson has clearly defined the nature of the borderline and narcissistic paradigms. For the borderline disorder, the fundamental paradigm is reward for regression, withdrawal in the face of self-activation (Masterson, 1978). For the narcissistic disorder, the fundamental paradigm is, "I am perfect, but I need you to affirm it," or, "You are perfect, and I can bask in the glow of your perfection" (Masterson, 1981, 1993).

For the schizoid individual, the process of negotiation, of deal making, is unlike that for any other self disorder. The nature of the schizoid problem is unique. Unlike persons with borderline and narcissistic disorders, the task, or fact, of negotiating itself seems insurmountable to the schizoid patient. The schizoid patient asks: Is any negotiation possible? For the schizoid patient, the existence of a communication network is in doubt. This can be put in developmental terms. The principle of mental functioning during rapprochement asserts the separation of self and object representations, so that like-mindedness is no longer assumed. Daniel Stern (1985) described this newly achieved mental state as a theory of separate but interfaceable minds. Both theories imply the need to approach, or interface with, the object in a new fashion, one that must develop new understandings and meanings. In order to connect, interface, and share, a communication system must be in place.

In order to negotiate a deal, one must have two parties willing to come to the negotiating table. In order to complete a telephone call, one must have two people, two telephones, and a wire over which information can flow. Borderline and narcissistic patients have a basic belief in the possibility of communicating and negotiating. Continuing the metaphors, persons with these two self disorders believe that negotiation is possible, that there are usually two parties able (if not always willing) to come to the negotiating table, and that there is a working telephone line. If the call is placed, someone will pick up. For those with borderline and narcissistic disorders, the main problem is in the nature of the negotiation, not in the act of negotiating itself. In these disorders, problems arise because each party comes to the negotiation with a clear agenda that he or she tries to impose. True connecting, interfacing, and sharing are replaced by impingements and reactions to impingements. The results of the so-called negotiating process for borderline and narcissistic patients are the paradigms described earlier. Essentially, it is a proposition to "take it or leave it," but a proposition nonetheless.

For the schizoid patient, the initial problems are quite different. There is no conviction, no basic assumption, that a communication network is in place or is even possible without grave risk and danger. The primitive agony or unthinkable anxiety (Winnicott, 1965) is complete isolation because there is no means of communication. The intensity of the affective experience for the schizoid patient is no less intense than that accompanying any other disorder of the self. The potential agony or anxiety for the schizoid patient carries with it the most profound potential experience of despair.

There is a refrain in a song from the Broadway show "1776" that goes: "Is anybody there? Does anybody care? Does anybody see what I see?" These questions elucidate problems at the heart of the schizoid conflict, in contrast to the narcissistic and borderline patients. A narcissistic patient is constantly asking, or demanding, that everybody else see what he or she sees (one-mindedness, merger, fusion). The borderline patient is constantly asking, "Does anybody care?" and will adjust his or her life in whatever fashion it is necessary to guarantee that there is somebody who cares. The schizoid patient is first and foremost asking the question, "Is anybody there?"

For those with borderline and narcissistic disorders, there is someone at the other end of the communication network. The task is to discover those specific conditions of communication or interfacing that will allow the patient to experience a sense of acknowledgment, affirmation, and approval. Narcissistic and borderline individuals go through life attempting an unending series of maneuvers, machinations, and schemes in order to secure for themselves that acknowledgment, affirmation, and approval.

For those with borderline and narcissistic disorders, the problem is finding the key that will unlock the supplies and gratification they need and want. For the schizoid patient, the very existence of the key is in doubt. There is a far more desperate interpersonal state of affairs for the schizoid patient than for the borderline or narcissistic patient.

How did this desperate state of affairs come about? What is it in the nature of the early parent–child interaction that leads an individual to a sense of near hopelessness about the possibility of relatedness? The subjective experience of many, if not most, schizoid patients is that their efforts at relatedness were of no avail and encountered either indifference or neglect. At their worst, the experiences of the schizoid patient were, and continue to be, fraught with danger and the possibility of being manipulated, coerced, or appropriated.

The schizoid patient's subjective experience is not that of being a vital cog in the family system, be it healthy or pathological; rather, the experience is of being a dehumanized, depersonified function that can be called on to serve a purpose, any purpose, and then can be consigned again to the back shelf until another service or function is required. As a child, the schizoid patient experienced a response from the parent—a look, a cue— that was confusing, and so the patient was unable to interpret it and use it for affective orientation. Or the schizoid patient experienced a response, a look, of almost scornful derision because the child had even turned to the parent for that kind of affective response or affective information. In either case, there was the experience of nothing being communicated back.

A child in this situation is left to his or her own devices. The crucial problem for the future schizoid patient is that the other person is not available to provide the kind of cues or responses that the child needs at those critical moments in life when decisions cannot be made by the child alone; rather, the child requires active input from another. The experience of the schizoid patient was not one of a consistent pattern of negotiation that informs the child about what must be done in order to get acknowledgment, affirmation, and approval. The consistent pattern is that one can be called on to perform particular functions at particular times with no particular rhyme or reason. Acknowledgment comes about through the person's availability to perform whatever he or she is called on to do. One patient described this as being a "human dust buster" for her family. She said that she "hung in the closet quietly. I was neither seen nor heard. But when I was needed to do something—different things at different times—I was called out, taken out of the closet, used, and then returned." It was, in her words, a "back-shelf existence."

This schizoid patient performed her functions well, and in so doing experienced a sense of self-value. This is true for many, perhaps most, schizoid patients. However, the notion of function in this context is one that is devoid of affect. The schizoid patient's experience of self-value is one that is devoid of interpersonal affective affirmation.

The experience of schizoid patients is that they were not living, dynamic parts of the family systems in which they grew up. They experienced themselves as being treated as objects without unique feelings, used and manipulated for whatever shifting purposes they were called on to serve. Schizoid patients, in describing such experiences, use certain metaphors over and over, such as feeling like a puppet or an android or, most frequently, feeling like a slave. In childhood, the future schizoid patient begins to rely more and more on internal feedback than on external feedback. If a person cannot confidently expect some sort of acknowledgment, let alone affirmation and approval, of his or her actions by another person, then the person is forced to turn to cues and feedback from other sources in order to guarantee some sort of affirmation. Otherwise, the person would experience life as an endless series of episodes in which his or her words or feelings were cast into a pit in which they would never hit bottom, creating no response, or even an echo, from the environment. This is an inherently terrifying experience similar to the primal agony of falling forever (Winnicott, 1965, p. 76).

A phenomenon, which is part of the history of many schizoid patients, dramatically conveys, and confirms, the kind of subjective experiences that have been described. Schizoid patients will frequently report that around the age of latency—generally between the ages of seven and nine—they became aware of the fact that no matter what they did, they could not expect, or rely on, their parents or caretakers for the acknowledgment, affirmation, and approval they wanted and needed. This was a conscious awareness at the time and not a retrospective awareness reported as part of a historical reconstruction. Patients report the conscious feeling at that time that their parents did not love them and that there was absolutely nothing that they could do to get their parents' love. That experience is uniquely schizoid. Narcissistic and borderline disorders are characterized by the endless efforts to uncover the treasure chest of interpersonal supplies that lies tantalizingly just beyond reach. These efforts have no end point. For the schizoid patient, such efforts must take into account and circumvent the reality of the experience of parental unavailability.

EXAMPLES

The following brief vignettes describe the kinds of histories that are often heard from schizoid patients. They are not incompatible with other kinds of psychopathology. There is no pathognomonic schizoid history. But there are prototypical experiences that one might expect and that point to the possibility of a schizoid disorder.

The Case of Ms. J.

Ms. J. was born into a family characterized by chronic unpredictability and instability. Her father was a minister who was repeatedly hired and fired by various congregations, necessitating multiple family moves. Her mother was a very disorganized woman who had "multiple nervous breakdowns." Ms. J. felt that neither of her parents had ever really heard her or understood her. At around three years of age, she had surgery for a bowel obstruction, and she recalled being told by her parents in the hospital that if she cried, she could not come home. Ms. J. also reported that the mother had the last of her severe breakdowns when the patient was eight and that her father deserted the family shortly thereafter. She stated that at that point she finally gave up hope that she would ever receive any sort of consistent stability or, more important, love from her family.

The Case of Mr. J.

Mr. J. reported that he had been born strangling—the umbilical cord had been wound around his neck. This served as a metaphor for his entire childhood, and perhaps for his entire life. His father was described as a passive man who suffered silently and was "afraid to act like a man around my mother." His mother was erratic and angry most of the time. Mr. J. remembered how hard he had tried to figure out what set her off in order to prevent her outbursts of rage. He never was able to, and so could never avoid her verbal, and occasionally physical, abuse. Mr. J. said that at around the age of seven he decided "not to love my parents anymore," and subsequently he remained true to that decision.

The Case of Ms. M.

Ms. M. had a memory from early childhood of her mother turning her back and walking out of the room as Ms. M. was standing in her crib crying. This memory pervaded the patient's entire history. There was evidence that her parents would leave her unattended for long periods during the day when the patient was between two and five years of age. Both parents were very religious, and Ms. M. was not permitted to associate with anyone outside of the family's own religious group. She felt alienated from her family, frightened by her father and uncomforted by her mother. She described herself as afraid, shy, and unable to make friends throughout childhood.

As is evident from these examples, the schizoid patient usually has a family history of severe chronic misattunement between child and parents during the early, formative years. Is anybody there? Does anybody care? Does anybody see what I see? Throughout the life of the schizoid patient, the answer to all three questions has usually been *No*. Given the historical and developmental state of affairs as described, what will be the nature of the resulting intrapsychic structure of the schizoid patient?

INTRAPSYCHIC STRUCTURES

The schizoid patient's internal world consists of split object relations units. Whether splitting is a normal, developmental mode of mental functioning or a defensive operation called on to organize conflict and chaos is not relevant here. What is important is that splitting is a ubiquitous clinical phenomenon. It is a useful way of organizing the great variety of experiences encountered. Human infants tend to dichotomize experience, or at least it is clinically useful to conceptualize the human patient as doing so. The organization of internalized object relationships makes good use of this concept. One can view the organization of the representational world as divided into two fundamental patterns. One pattern is that of successful relatedness or attachment, which could be termed the attachment unit. This unit describes those behaviors, feelings, and actions (all part of interpersonal negotiation) that are part of the person's experience of being connected to others, of garnering or winning other people's acknowledgment, at least, and affirmation and approval, at best.

There also exists another pattern of experiences of intrapsychic and interpersonal life. These experiences crystallize around the failures to achieve successful attachment or around interruptions in the state of attachment. The pattern is that of fundamental nonattachment, and the associated object relations unit might be called the nonattachment unit. In other words, in intrapsychic and interpersonal life there is the state of feeling connected to others, no matter how conditionally, and then there is the state of feeling unconnected to others when acknowledgment, approval, or affirmation is not forthcoming.

This simple dichotomy (split) holds for all relationships, including all the disorders of the self. In most healthy relationships or in those relatively successful disorders of the self, the state of attachment (the relative continuous activation of the attachment unit) is the norm. Interruptions in connectedness and attachment are infrequent, transient, and easily repaired. In most self disorders the attachment unit is tenuous and interruptions in attachment are frequent, prolonged, and not easily repaired.

In the borderline disorder of the self (Masterson, 1978), the attachment unit is the *rewarding object relations unit (RORU)* and the nonattachment unit is the *withdrawing object relations unit (WORU)*. In the narcissistic disorder of the self (Masterson, 1981), the attachment unit is the *omnipotent object/grandiose self unit* and the nonattachment unit is the *aggressive object/empty self unit*. It should be noted that both units are still relational units. The nonattachment unit brings with it anxiety and dysphoria; it is not the same as detachment.

What is the nature of the split object relations units for the schizoid disorder of the self? There is a basic attachment unit and a basic nonattachment unit, as in the borderline and narcissistic disorders of the self. This statement may seem surprising in view of what has been emphasized regarding the difficulties and dangers of object relatedness and connectedness for the schizoid patient. However, no description of those difficulties and dangers contradicts the principle of the motivational primacy of object relationships for all human beings. The schizoid patient has an inherent need to achieve the gratifications associated with object relatedness. The striving for object relationships—the wish to reach out to and hold onto others—has as much motivational power for the schizoid patient as it does for anyone else.

The basic attachment unit of the schizoid patient is the master/slave unit, while the basic nonattachment unit is the sadistic object/self-in-exile unit.

The relational unit that primarily defines the schizoid patient is the sadistic object/self-in-exile unit. Thus there is a striking difference between the schizoid patient and patients with narcissistic or borderline disorders in this regard.

"Home" for the schizoid patient is the nonattachment unit. Such patients usually "live" within the sadistic object/self-in-exile unit. As the poet Robert Frost said, "Home is where if you have to go there, they have to take you in." For schizoid patients, the self-in-exile is the place where they have to go and that will always take them in safely. Whereas patients with other disorders of the self are constantly struggling to live within their attachment experiences (the RORU or the omnipotent object/grandiose self unit), the schizoid patient's first and primary concern is to stabilize and secure his or her existence within the sadistic object/self-in-exile unit.

The sadistic object of this relational unit clearly evolves from the schizoid patient's experiences with others who are depriving, devaluing, and destructive. The sadism of the object is proportional to the degree to which the schizoid patient felt dehumanized and depersonified into a function. Many schizoid patients' histories contain examples of chronic neglect, abandonment, and physical and sexual abuse. The severity and pervasiveness of the sadism (malignant misattunement) are two of the clearest contributing factors to the concept of a continuum of pathological expression within the schizoid dimension of pathology. Experiences that have rendered the schizoid patient less flexible and more rigidly defended will result in the appearance of a lower-level disorder. In other words, the greater the misattunement/sadism, the higher will be the ratio of unattached unit to attachment unit and the lower will be the level of adaptive social functioning.

The perceived malevolence of the sadistic object discourages efforts at attachment. The quality of the malevolence differs from that found in the withdrawing object of the borderline patient and the aggressive object of the narcissistic disorder. It is unmodified by any specific gratification that the schizoid patient seems to offer the object. While the borderline patient may help the object to regulate affect states (especially the object's own depression or separation anxiety), and while the narcissistic patient may help the object to regulate its self-worth and self-esteem, the schizoid patient performs nonspecific functions, which lends a dehumanizing quality to the interaction.

Whereas the object representation of the nonattachment unit is sadistic, the self representation associated with that object is the self-in-exile. As stated previously, this is home for many schizoid patients—and, for those schizoids who never become patients, it is all too often a permanent residence. For schizoid patients, it is a bunker and, when necessary, an impenetrable fortress. A hospitalized schizoid woman who had made a serious suicide attempt described how she felt that she lived most of the time "in an icy fortress similar to the one that Superman has somewhere at the North Pole." At the extreme, therefore, the experience of the self-in-exile is that of the self as impenetrable to the intrusions or infringements of others.

Most schizoid patients are a select population from the larger pool of schizoid persons, and schizoid patients who present for treatment demonstrate a different quality in their experience of the self-in-exile. The schizoid patient has more conscious expectations and hopes about the possibility of successful attachments. The nature of the self-in-exile has a less intensely inaccessible quality than that described by the patient above. The most accurate characterization of the self-in-exile for most schizoid patients is that of a safe haven, rather than of an impenetrable fortress. The schizoid patient attempts to live in a safely defined and defended world.

Safety is a key word for the schizoid patient. It is defined as being far enough away from others so as not to be exposed to sadism, intrusion, and appropriation, but yet not so far away as to be exposed to the threat of total isolation and alienation. The self-in-exile makes safety possible. The self-in-exile self representation enables the schizoid patient to achieve a comfortable, relatively anxiety-free distance, intrapsychically and interpersonally, rather than being dangerously close to or dangerously far from others.

The self-in-exile as safe haven is typical for the schizoid patient. Mr. R., for example, described how he spent hours during his childhood in a huge, empty refrigerator box that his family kept in the basement. It was his safe home away from home where he could fantasize freely. It was a place of safety and security, away from intrusion and fear. The time spent in the box and his fantasies while there represented his quintessential safe place.

Ms. G., a middle-aged schizoid woman, easily described her ability to be with others, while never leaving her safe place behind. Her experience of safety and of a stable self-in-exile was achieved through the simple process of withdrawing affect. She could be in the presence of others, even at large gatherings, and yet, essentially she would still be alone. She stated, "I could be with others and feel absolutely nothing." This kind of depersonalization or emotional numbing reflected her capacity to withdraw the affect from a situation, leaving her in that place of safety in the larger perceived place of unsafety in her interpersonal world.

Both broad definitions of the experience of the self-in-exile, as a safe haven or as an impenetrable fortress, emphasize the importance of safety associated with the nonattachment unit. Many descriptions of schizoid phenomena begin and end at this place. These two characterizations might easily be identified with the DSM-IV descriptions of the avoidant personality and schizoid personality disorders. The avoidant personality seeks a safe haven, whereas the schizoid personality strives to establish an impenetrable fortress. Even the nine characteristics presented by Guntrip represent views of the safe place and the impenetrable fortress. To stop at this point in understanding the schizoid patient would be to understand only half of the internal world of the schizoid, for nothing has yet been said about the dangers associated with the self-in-exile or the attachment unit and the associated conditions of attachment. To complete the picture of the internal world of the schizoid patient, both of these phenomena must be understood.

How can a place of safety be unsafe? What possible dangers could be associated with the self-in-exile? To understand the nature of this danger, one must first understand that some schizoid persons go too far in their efforts to achieve a safe place. The most intensely schizoid patient, while preserving some potential or hope for attachment or relatedness, may so strive to create an impenetrable fortress that the potential will be buried so deep as not to be visible to the observer, or even to the patient. This type of schizoid patient usually maintains a hold on the experience of hope or potential for relatedness only through the realm of fantasy, divorced from any real interaction with the world. The existence of a fantasy life reveals the deeply hidden wish for attachment. Consciously, however, such patients may express their experience of exile in terms of having gone beyond the point of no return. It is as if, as schizoid patients move to the periphery in their efforts to find a safe place, there comes a time when they may feel that they have lost the capacity to reverse the process and have gone beyond the gravitational pull of human relationships. The experience beyond the safe place is then described as an endless space, a bottomless pit, and cosmic aloneness. One schizoid patient used the metaphor of an astronaut at the end of a space-walk tether or cable. To have that tether cut off is to be cast into endless, empty space. It is an experience of total isolation and aloneness, being cut loose from the forces that bind that person to others.

It is at this point in the potential experience of a schizoid person that suicide becomes a real possibility. When every possible thread of connection has been severed, when the flame that lights the potential way to human attachment flickers and goes out, when any possibility of utilizing even fantasy as a way of maintaining relatedness is lost, then the schizoid person loses the sense of being held in the world of object relationships. The terror associated with that state may be the precipitant for a serious suicide attempt. Schizoid patients, however, will not be serious suicide risks—no matter how hopeless and depressed they may sound—as long as they are able to maintain some relationship, or even the hope of some relationship. For some schizoid patients, the lifesaving relationship may be with the therapist. The therapeutic relationship is often the lifeline that ties the schizoid patient to the world of object relations and keeps the patient from the despair and agony associated with total isolation. Only if the therapeutic relationship, along with every other relationship, comes under stress and is experienced as fatally ruptured will the schizoid patient, while in active treatment, become an acute suicide risk. Often such risk is heralded by the patient's use of the word "despair" to describe his or her emotional state.

Most schizoid patients do not attempt suicide. But the discussion of the phenomenon is not important because it is the termination point for a few persons, but because it is part of the internal world and is a potential danger for all schizoid individuals. For some schizoid patients, its presence is like a faint, barely discernible background noise, and rarely reaches a level that breaks into consciousness. For others, it is an ominous presence, an emotional sword of Damocles. In any case, it is an underlying dread that they all experience. More significant, it is a primary force operating in the internal world of the schizoid patient—the anticipation of the experience as a possible outcome of distancing (exile) defenses—that alerts the schizoid patient to the possibility of going too far. It is a warning signal that tells the schizoid patient: "Beware!"

Therefore, in addition to the fundamental motivation toward object relations and attachment possessed by all human beings, the schizoid patient is held in the world of object relations by the awareness—vague at times and clear at other times—of the terror that awaits if one loses or relinquishes the capacity to communicate with others. This potential primal agony or unthinkable anxiety works as a counterforce against all the schizoid patient's defensive efforts to withdraw, retreat, and find safety from the sadistic-object world.

Several characterizations of the self-in-exile experience have been described: the safe place or haven, the impenetrable fortress, and the point of no return. But other capacities associated with the self-in-exile experience, and which Guntrip emphasized, allow many schizoid patients to occupy a much closer place in relationship to others. The nature of this kind of home, this experience of the self-in-exile, is one that can best be characterized by the terms "self-sufficiency" and "self-reliance." The feeling of safety still comes about through distance; however, this distance is built on positive qualities of self-containment and self-regulation, as opposed to the more negative quality of pure distance creation by withdrawing from others. While the schizoid patient is able, in this place, to feel a safe distance from others, it is a safety that comes through greater self-confidence, and the patient is willing to accept the challenges associated with the need for attachment.

Such schizoid patients are far more able to risk closeness, or the appearance of closeness, than are those patients occupying the positions previously described. They are more likely to maintain personal, or at least occupation-based, relationships. They may marry and have children. They may be involved in professions that involve interactions with others and are capable of maintaining some aspects of social relatedness, although often delimited, with a number of people. For these schizoid persons, life's affective experiences are not shrouded in obtuseness, mystery, or confusion. Feelings can be identified and utilized interpersonally, although in a limited and circumscribed fashion.

Prototypic of this kind of adjustment is the schizoid couple, whose relationship often has the appearance of early-childhood parallel play. The partners share in many activities—living together, raising children together, and enjoying each other's companionship as a protection against isolation and alienation. But affective experiences are not really shared. Feelings are rarely discussed. Often both parties take pride in their independence and independent functioning. This is a classic example, as Masterson (1972) has called it, of making a virtue out of necessity.

Another schizoid man described his life with his nonschizoid wife in the following fashion. While, for the most part, they lived happily together, he said that when he felt that the interpersonal demand to share feelings was too great (as, for example, when there were significant sad or happy life events), he would go "blank face," by which he meant that his face would become devoid of all expression. The subjective counterpart was the feeling of mild anxiety or emotional safety. His wife was aware of its happening, and accepted it with varying degrees of distress. His children also recognized this occurrence and would joke, "Dad is tuning us out again." This example is important not because it demonstrates the patient's ability to withdraw affect, but because it emphasizes his ability to interact in the world while confident of the capacity to self-contain and self-regulate his affect states. In the course of his treatment, these capacities, while always available, became increasingly ego dystonic. In fact, his awareness of his dissatisfaction with this response was the beginning of his experience of a "whole new level of experiencing the world."

With this final characterization of the self-in-exile, one can see that the range of homes for the schizoid patient may be quite varied. At one extreme can be found the person, seemingly well functioning socially, who at times displays an aloofness and a pride in the ability to be independent and self-reliant. At the other extreme is the person who explicitly conveys the message to others to keep away, and who is willing to settle for a self-contained world that admits to no interpersonal need for other people.

Several additional examples convey the varying living arrangements the schizoid patient may make.

Ms. A. described her sense of being at a distance from others as "the feeling of having one's nose pressed against the window of life. You are outside in the cold and inside everyone is happy and warm. You stand there watching the activity going on inside, but [are] afraid, or unwilling, or unable to act. I don't know what it is like to go inside and join in the activities." Ms. A. was describing her awareness of the fundamental desire, even longing, for connection, and yet the experience, self-imposed, was that of being set apart from the world. She was an observer, not a participant. She was outside in the cold, and she noted that everyone inside seemed to be having a better time. This portrayal is typical of those offered by schizoid patients. Ms. A.'s statement of fear, of an unwillingness or inability to go inside, reflects the schizoid patient's genuine difficulties and dilemma. Ms. A. was asked how she was attired in the fantasy. She responded that while she was "out in the cold," it was not that she was actually cold because, in fact, she felt wrapped in many layers of protective clothing. This was a metaphoric description of her capacity for self-reliance and self-sufficiency. She did not feel threatened by being out in the cold, and could take care of herself quite well. The conflict was present because she did not want to remain outside all the time, no matter how safe that was. The price of total safety is total exile.

Mr. A., in describing his feeling of distance from others, stated, "It is a feeling of being alienated, marooned, isolated . . . it is like you are a stranger in a strange land. An alien. Totally losing contact and being cast into a bottomless void. I feel like a real-life man without a country." Schizoid patients frequently describe an impairment in the capacity to pick up on the social cues that are necessary in negotiating one's interactions with others. Mr. A. strongly felt that he did not have a clue as to how he was expected to act or as to how he should expect others to behave. It is comparable to the experience of awakening in a foreign land, a totally different world, where one is unaware of the customs, laws, and traditions, and, in addition, does not understand the language that is spoken. In other words, there is no vehicle for communication. The characterization of alien is quite typical for schizoid patients because it conveys the sense of being dropped into the middle of a strange world.

The sadistic object/self-in-exile unit that has been described is the object relations unit by which most schizoid patients are known. It is the experience of the schizoid patient to which descriptive and clinical psychiatry has been almost solely addressed. The final feature of this unit is the affect that links the object representation and self representation. The affective tone that suffuses the nonattachment unit of any of the self disorders has been given the generic term "abandonment depression" by Masterson (1972). It is an umbrella term that includes all the particular dysphoric affect states associated with the experience of nonattachment or of interruptions in attachment.

The general affective coloration of the abandonment depression of the schizoid patient can be described as the feeling of being free, but isolated. The patient is free from the anxieties and dangers associated with attachment, but is isolated from the gratifications and joys associated with relatedness. The price of freedom is the feeling of life lived somewhere along the continuum of emotional exile. The affects associated with exile and nonattachment are predominantly depression and rage, emptiness and void, isolation and alienation.

Depression results from the experience of having to forego one's real self and, rather than living spontaneously, having to live reactively, responding to the needs, expectations, and impingements of others. To live falsely is to live with a profound sense of depression and melancholy.

Anger and rage result from the feeling of having no choice, of being presented with no options. The price of freedom is exile. Take it or leave it. Additional sources of rage include (1) self-hatred and criticism associated with the self-blame used as an explanation for why bad things happen, (2) identification with the aggressor (sadistic object) associated with reenactment and mastery, and (3) talionic impulses, associated with the wish for revenge at any cost (Masterson, 1981).

Emptiness and void emerge with depression as the experience of the impaired real self, the result of the growing awareness of identity diffusion that underlies the defensive false-self experience.

Alienation and isolation, actual or anticipated, are the affects that give a unique character to the schizoid patient's experience of the abandonment depression. This is the unique experience of loneliness, dread of cosmic aloneness, and terror associated with living with the possibility of the loss of the ability to communicate with another human being.

So far, only half of the story of the schizoid patient has been told, and so only half of the intrapsychic structure has been described. If the description were to conclude at this point, one would have to be content with the characterizations of schizoid pathology that have been passed on from previous generations.

The other half of the internal world of the schizoid patient is the attachment unit of the split object relations units. The need for human attachment and for object relatedness exists as a fundamental motivational force for the schizoid person, as it does for all human beings. In the internal world of the schizoid patient, this need, the attachment unit, is denoted by the metaphor of the master/slave unit. The master/slave unit is the primary attachment unit. There is enormous variation in the degree to which this unit is activated in the schizoid patient's internal world and external reality. At one extreme, it may be activated not at all in reality or in fantasy. When this unit fails, the schizoid patient has no choice but to retreat into an impenetrable fortress and live in exile. At the other extreme are those schizoid patients who are willing to take considerable risks and accept the challenges that come with activating their attachment units, but who only do so when they are confident in their ability to mobilize self-contained, self-affect-regulating defenses whenever intolerable affective involvement is demanded.

For all schizoid patients, however, regardless of the level of activation of the master/slave unit, the characteristics of the unit remain remarkably similar. The master/slave unit is a specific object relations unit that involves a unique perception of the object representation, the self representation, and the linking affect.

What is meant to be conveyed by the designation of the object representation as the master? A schizoid patient who makes an effort at relatedness (in the internal world or external reality) is likely to experience the object as being manipulating, coercive, and appropriating. The object is enslaving and imprisoning. The conditions of attachment, therefore, are fraught with danger and fear. Attachment is perceived as hazardous to the schizoid patient's health. The quality of attachment can only marginally be characterized as emotionally gratifying and sustaining; it seems to fulfill only the most basic needs associated with relatedness. At times, it may only function to exert the gravitational force necessary to keep the schizoid patient from hurtling beyond the point of no return. Based on previous developmental and historical considerations, the schizoid patient's experience of the object as master should be easy to construct.

Object as Appropriator

Appropriation implies that schizoid patients feel that everything and anything that they have that is of value will eventually be laid claim to by the object. Ideas, fantasies, abilities, possessions—all will be used by the object for the object's own purposes and own needs, with a total disregard of ownership as it rightfully resides in the patient. All will be used whenever the object wishes to use them, and for whatever function the object wishes to use them. The experiences of appropriation can be annihilating—a form of terror for schizoid patients. One schizoid man, in attempting to describe his sense of horror when growing up, compared his experiences of appropriation to the terror of the humans in the movie *The Invasion of the Body Snatchers*. In this classic movie, the humans were drained of the essence of their humanity, their minds and souls, by the alien invaders. They looked the same, but everything of value about them had been appropriated.

Another experience of appropriation is the feeling that one is not allowed any private world, any experience of a private self. One schizoid patient described her childhood as one in which she was recruited to be the caretaker for the succession of siblings who followed. Others are caretakers for their parents. None of this is done with the sense of pleasure or of satisfaction that comes when persons work, live, and share together toward the accomplishment of a goal. The appropriator calls on the patient to serve a particular function without regard for the patient's feelings. The appropriator believes that children (or the schizoid patient) should be seen (only when needed), but never heard. The appropriator neither rewards regression nor expects perfect mirroring. Appropriation is a form of depersonification, converting the patient into a function.

Appropriation can take many forms. At times, the appropriation may be blatant; at other times, it may be subtle. Mr. W. described his experience of appropriation, which seemed to start with his parents' refusal ever to have doors locked, or even shut, in his home. This almost psychotic intrusiveness and hypervigilance on the part of his parents left Mr. W. with the feeling that nothing he had could be kept private. For him, the open door became a symbol of the feeling that everything he was and had was there to be used by his parents, and that he was nothing and had nothing to which he could lay claim or of which he could feel ownership. Privacy was impossible, including the right to his own body. For example, his parents would always check on him at night to make sure that his hands were outside the covers, and he could never lock the door when he used the bathroom. He was discouraged from identifying himself as a sexual being. Mr. W., an extremely schizoid man, grew up with very explicit feelings of being asexual.

Mr. H. described his experience of appropriation in the following way. Whenever he would have an idea about what he wanted to do with his future and mentioned it to his mother, he felt that the idea would be lost to him forever because his mother would take it and use it to fuel her own fantasies and needs. She would alter or shape it to her specifications so that it no longer belonged to him. The idea or goal had been appropriated to provide emotional gratification for his mother, as opposed to any acknowledgment from his mother that the goal involved the patient's wishes, needs, or feelings. For example, the patient could never introduce a girlfriend to his mother without the prospect of a long lecture on how that girl met (or, more likely, failed to meet) the mother's specifications for a girlfriend. No sport played, interest pursued, or career considered was evaluated or even thought of in terms of the patient's feelings; rather, all were considered in terms of how they made the mother feel about herself, what she could tell her friends, and how they furthered the mother's success in shaping her son to gratify her needs. The patient described how he could never fight his mother on these issues, since he felt that all power eventually flowed from her to him. Her control was absolute. If she laid claim to something, it was hers. There was no sense in fighting. Surrender was inevitable.

Manipulation and *coercion* are closely allied experiences of the master. Both terms suggest that the schizoid patient's own experiences and feelings are disregarded or ignored by the object, the other. The experience of the schizoid patient is that of being used by others for the purpose of gaining the other's own ends without regard for herself or himself. Manipulation and coercion imply exerting control over another person rather than necessarily appropriating the other person. This quality of experience was best recounted by Mr. H., who described the nature of his relationship to others, especially his mother, as that of being a puppet sitting on his mother's lap. It was the feeling that every body part, every action, and every emotion was subject to the control of the object. It feels, as Mr. H. said, "like having one's strings constantly being pulled." The quality of manipulation and coercion is also often depicted by the metaphor of being a robot or an android, programmed to perform whatever function the object wishes.

The object as appropriator, manipulator, and coercer is all implied in the term "master." The self representation linked to the experience of the object as the master is that of a slave. The nature of the attachment of the schizoid patient to the object—in the internal world and external reality— is like the relationship of a slave to the master. The essence of enslavement is that one possesses nothing that can be called one's own. In a master/slave relationship, there is no private ownership. One exists to serve the master. Anything of value may be taken away: one's spouse, children, even life. The master/slave relationship suggests a fundamental disregard for the humanness of the other person. For all those reasons, the feeling of enslavement or imprisonment is common among many schizoid patients. The object is the master; the self is the slave. The object is the imprisoner; the self is the prisoner. Following are some characterizations of the master/slave unit as described by patients.

Ms. R. expressed her view of the fundamental experience of attachment as being a loss of control. Her description of her family relationships was that of an endless battle of wills. And in the end, she felt, she would surely lose. She felt that if she ever tried to be close to her parents in any way, she would have had to give up her self totally and become their live-in slave. Ironically, Ms. R. had presented for treatment at a point when her elderly, sick father was threatening to move in, so that the patient could be his full-time nurse. The expectation was that the patient would give up her job and devote her life to assisting him. No one in the family had asked the patient how she felt about this assigned role. The inability to acknowledge the patient's own feelings and wishes was as strong now, when the patient was 39 years old, as when she was a young child. Although Ms. R. had lived her entire adult life away from her family, there was no acknowledgment of her having any life apart from that to which she was assigned by the family.

Mr. H. expressed similar fears when he described how his mother's words or actions, or even facial expressions, would "drain all the energy from me." Although he was now 24 years old, he reported that the only picture of him in the family home, where he was still living, showed him at the age of five or six sitting on his mother's knee, like "a puppet on a ventriloquist's knee . . . I was trapped . . . unable to move or act except as she commanded me to do. I had a mind of my own, but it made no difference. No one cared and no one asked. I simply mouthed the words that she wanted and expected to hear. And if I didn't submit, I felt I would be discarded. Put aside. I would be away from her control, but I would be alone, exiled. To stay connected, I had to be her slave."

For the schizoid patient, the price of attachment is enslavement. A condition of relatedness is imprisonment. To be connected is to be in jail. If this is the experience of schizoid patients when they try to connect, why do they still try? They do so, first, because of the essential, fundamental human need to experience oneself in a relationship with another human being. Moreover, the master/slave relationship is the conditional aspect of how the schizoid person views relationships. This is what is possible—but it also is *only* what is possible. This is what relationships are like. Schizoid patients believe that any interpersonal relationship has to be a mirror or reflection of the internal, intrapsychic state of affairs, that the master/slave relationship is the only way in which people relate. If one wants to be connected, if one wants to be attached, if one wants to have an interpersonal relationship, it has to abide by the conditions imposed by the master/slave relationship.

What is the alternative? To be free is to be in emotional exile. Thus the choice is to be enslaved or to be in exile, to be attached or not to be attached. This is truly a Hobson's choice for the schizoid patient, the essence of the schizoid dilemma. Neither the state of exile nor that of enslavement is a felicitous state. Either is experienced as dysphoric, or as containing the seeds of dysphoria. Just as the schizoid patient experiences anxiety and danger around being too far because of the threat of going beyond the point of no return, so does the patient experience anxiety and danger around being too close, with its potential for total appropriation.

Perhaps most schizoid persons choose the state of exile as their primary residence. Certainly most choose, or tolerate, some form of enslavement as the price of living attached. But perhaps most characteristically, one sees in most schizoid individuals the continual alternation between these two fundamental states of being: attached and nonattached, enslavement and exile. Ms. B. described her life in this fashion: "I have difficulty relating to people. I'm limited because it has always been hard to share myself with people. If I depend on you, that implies being controlled [master/slave unit activated]. So, when I try to relate to people, to you, I have to keep a gap between what I'm saying and what I'm feeling [sadistic object/self-in-exile unit activated]." Mr. C. described, "Trying to relate to someone, to share feelings, is like traveling down a road. First it is smooth, then it becomes gravel, then sand. Then it is a cattle path with rocks and ditches. It becomes dangerous [efforts to relate become more anxiety ridden and threatening]." He continued: "You realize you are hopelessly off course. Help from the other person is not going to be there. The further you get in, you just cannot rely on other people. You will be left right where you started with your own devices and your own problems. You just have to take care of yourself [activation of the sadistic object/self-in-exile unit experience of self-reliance and self-sufficiency]."

For Ms. A. and Mr. B., the choice is never total enslavement or exile. Rather, life is a constant alternation between these two choices and a striving to find a suitable compromise. The quintessential example of schizoid compromise is fantasy.

Fantasy

In the life of the schizoid patient, fantasy is extraordinarily important and has a variety of functions. Most often, fantasy is viewed as a component of a person's withdrawal from the world, a turning inward and away from others. Viewed in this fashion, fantasy would be a core component of the self-in-exile. But it is far more complicated than that. *Fantasy is relationship by proxy.* It is a substitute relationship, but it is a relationship nonetheless. It is, for the schizoid patient, an ideal, defensive, compensatory relationship. It is an expression of the self-in-exile because it is self-contained and free from the dangers and anxieties associated with appropriation. It is also an expression of the self struggling to connect to objects, albeit internal objects. Fantasy permits schizoid patients to feel connected, and yet still free from the imprisonment of the master/slave unit. In short, in fantasy one can be attached (to internal objects) and still be free.

While, for the schizoid patient, fantasy seems to be an answer to the problem posed by the schizoid dilemma, it brings with it its own problems. This is also true for the therapist working with the schizoid patient. Fantasy has the capacity to stabilize and strengthen the self-in-exile structure. It enables the schizoid patient to achieve a greater degree of self-containment and self-reliance. Fantasy does not need objects in external reality to gratify the fundamental need of relatedness. Thus it can enhance the schizoid patient's ability to live in exile without feeling isolated. Fantasy allows the schizoid patient to live in a relationship but without danger, neither too close nor too far. It is a prime example of a schizoid compromise.

Fantasy plays such a pervasive role in the life of most schizoid persons that it probably comes closer than any other single characteristic to being a sine qua non of the schizoid state. Of course, most people make use of fantasy; it is a part of their internal worlds. As another expression of the creative, spontaneous self, it *enhances* experience. For the schizoid patient, it *substitutes* for experience. This is a critical difference and the critical problem with fantasy as compromise.

Schizoid patients will vary in the degree to which they use fantasy as relationship by proxy and as a stabilizing force for the self-in-exile. Those who are not able to utilize fantasy will be that minority of schizoid patients who are prone to substance abuse. For the schizoid patient, drugs or alcohol take over the function of fantasy as a substitute relationship; that is, the substance becomes a dehumanized object. The illusion of a relationship is often fostered, an illusion promoted by the mind-altering action of the substance itself.

More typically, the fantasy life of the schizoid patient is broad, deep, and rich, and yet, at the same time, covert, unexpressed, and intensely private. Schizoid patients may mobilize fantasy for hours every day. It can become a primary preoccupation of the person's waking life. Or fantasy may be resorted to in a more circumscribed, delimited fashion during periods of unusual anxiety or danger. While any theme is possible, particular themes tend to run through most schizoid fantasies. The fantasies of the schizoid patient are most often interpersonal fantasies that focus on relational themes of an intense nature. Romantic fantasies that sound like romance novels, caricatures of real relationships, are common. Fantasies that sound like sagas or thrillers and are associated with strong feelings are frequent. All of those fantasies are marked by an aliveness and a presence of affect that are frequently absent from real-life interactions. That is the point and the purpose: relationship by proxy. The fantasies of schizoid persons are far less given to themes of narcissistic grandeur, success, impersonal adulation, or escape.

Following are some typical fantasies reported by schizoid patients. One patient recalled that as a young girl four or five years of age, she most enjoyed playing alone with her many dolls, with which she would construct elaborate and extensive fantasies of family life. These fantasies could go on for the entire day if she were uninterrupted, which was frequently the case. By that age, she also could read very well, and she began a lifetime habit of creating very small and safe places for herself, such as in a closet or under a desk, where she would curl up and read for hours. She would supplement her reading with fantasy. One fantasy was that of being Superwoman, a powerful woman whom no one could harm. Rather than focusing on themes of power or perfection, her focus was on the endless romances she would have with Superman. Together they would fight the world of cruel injustices, their true identities known only to each other.

A middle-aged schizoid man described his fantasy as "an ideal haven from the danger of being with people." He stated that his favorite fantasy was "being the leader of the first moon colony. I am there with my family and about two dozen other people. I can escape from this painful world, yet I am still involved with people. People who look up to me and who need me." This patient's need to be the leader and to be looked up to did not reflect narcissistic needs, goals, or ambitions, but rather his need to be in control, self-reliant, and dependent on no one.

The young schizoid woman described as always feeling on the outside with her nose pressed up against the glass separating her from real life reported her fantasies of gala dances and parties, in which she would play the role of such characters as Cinderella and Eliza Doolittle. In reality, she rarely left her home.

Of additional note is the sadomasochistic plot of the relational fantasies of some schizoid patients. It is not difficult to understand the origin of these particular fantasies, as they represent an infusion of master/slave relationships into the attachment themes of the fantasies in a manner that poses no threat because the patient is in complete control of the fantasy. The patient owns it. It cannot be appropriated unless it is revealed, and it need not be revealed unless the patient wishes it to be. The role played by the patient may be that of either sadist or masochist, of either master or slave, because of the complete control that fantasies allow. One schizoid woman gradually revealed elaborate fantasies that were a part of almost every waking hour, and were of a sadomasochistic nature, involving an extraordinary array of objects, people, animals, acts, and outcomes. An intensely schizoid young man reported working his way through graduate school by writing pornographic novels. His editor had congratulated him on his "limitless imagination."

Even though the fantasy life of a schizoid patient is so important, it often is unrecognized by the clinician. This is so because, as stated previously, the fantasy life of the schizoid patient is hidden. Many schizoid patients will either deny the presence of fantasies if questioned directly about them early in treatment, or will hint that they are a part of their lives, but they will minimize them and will rarely share more than the vaguest outline of what the fantasy life is about. Fantasy is the one aspect of the internal world that the patient has been able to safeguard throughout life. It could be private and retained as such, beyond the grasp of the object, which could not know of its existence. While everything else might be lost or appropriated, the fantasy life would remain safe. Most schizoid patients are, therefore, reluctant to reveal their fantasy lives. Fantasies are not easily shared, and the more important the fantasy, the harder it is to share. Fantasy is the safe place of last resort in the world of object relations, of attachment.

Ultimately, however, no matter how safe, understandable, and useful the role of fantasy is, it is a defense that must be revealed and relinquished to a great extent. First and foremost, for the schizoid patient, fantasy is relationship by proxy, a substitute relationship. Keeping this in mind, the therapist will realize that while communicating his or her thoughts and feelings is the first great risk for the schizoid patient in therapy, the last and greatest risk will be revealing and relinquishing the primary, defensive function of fantasy. If the therapist further remembers that the fantasy life of the schizoid patient is personal and private for good reason, then the therapist can show appropriate respect for this aspect of intrapsychic functioning, and not rush to intrude on it prematurely. The measure of the success of treatment will often be the extent to which interpersonal dialogue can replace internal dialogue, the extent to which real-life experience can replace fantasy.

Three years into treatment, a schizoid man went through the following sequence in a session. He expressed, for the first time, that he recognized his need for other people. This was immediately followed by the statement that he recognized that he could never love another person. Later, in the same session, he revealed, also for the first time, that he had extensive sadomasochistic fantasies that began when he was a very young boy. He continued to reflect that he had remembered the origin of these fantasies only in the past few days, after having seen a movie in which a young child was murdered. He had, to his surprise, suddenly felt happy and had begun to laugh aloud, to the astonishment of those sitting near him. While telling the story, the patient was scanning me to observe my reactions.

This session took place at a time in the treatment when he was feeling particularly disturbed about our relationship and had begun to feel angry toward me. In reconstructing the meaning of the comments in that session over the ensuing period of treatment, several important themes emerged. The expression of his need for people was followed by his statement about his inability to love. He took a risk and took a step closer (to relationship), and then he became frightened and took half a step back. To acknowledge need was one thing, and he could do so relatively safely. But to acknowledge love was far more complicated, and far more demanding, risky, and dangerous. He was not ready to do that yet. The function of remembering and reporting his sadomasochistic fantasies at that time was manifold. The existence of the fantasies themselves was confirmation of what we had already surmised in the treatment about the nature of his relationship with his parents, essentially alternating activations of the master/slave and sadistic object/self-in-exile units. In sharing these fantasies with me for the first time, he was communicating his ability to feel safe enough with me to take that chance. Remembering the early origin of these fantasies was his way of confirming the validity of the work he had done in the treatment in reconstructing his past.

His experience of laughter in the theater, and his subsequent sharing of that episode with me, had a similar purpose. He wanted to show himself that he was so "perverted and strange" (his words) that he did not deserve (even if he had the ability) to love anyone. It kept him at a safe distance from his own desires and longings. But he also wished to portray himself to me as strange and perverted, so that I would impose a distance between us, further ensuring his safety by preventing him from getting closer. His understanding of the defensive, compromise, and safety functions of his sadomasochistic fantasies was pivotal in the progress of his treatment.

The description of the intrapsychic structure of the schizoid patient is the understanding necessary to successfully diagnose the schizoid disorder of the self. Armed with this understanding, one can begin to explore avenues of intervention that one hopes will result in successful treatment. Regardless of the myriad variations in presenting problems and therapeutic problems encountered in the course of therapy, the nature of the intrapsychic structure can be a map to guide the therapist through what at times will seem like complicated, or even incomprehensible, emotional terrain.

REFERENCES

Masterson, J. F. (1978). *Psychotherapy of the borderline adult*. New York: Brunner/Mazel.

Masterson, J. F. (1993). *The emerging self*. New York: Brunner/Mazel.

Masterson, J. F. (1981). *The narcissistic and borderline disorders*. New York: Brunner/Mazel.

Masterson, J. F. (1972). *Treatment of the borderline adolescent*. New York: Wiley.

Stern, D. (1985). *The interpersonal world of the infant*. New York: Basic Books.

Winnicott, D. W. (1965). Ego integration in child development (1962). In *The maturational processes and the facilitating environment*. New York: International Universities Press.

CHAPTER 5

Establishing a Therapeutic Alliance

Ralph Klein, M.D.

The psychotherapy of the schizoid disorder of the self rests on the foundation of treatment principles that were established by Masterson (Masterson, 1972, 1976, 1981, 1983; Masterson & Rinsley, 1975) for the successful psychotherapy of the disorders of the self. The concepts Masterson describes are fundamental organizers of the psychotherapeutic process, and apply as much to the treatment of the schizoid disorders as they do to the borderline and narcissistic disorders. They are therapeutic neutrality, the therapeutic frame and stance, the concept of transference acting out and how this must be converted to therapeutic alliance, and countertransference and countertransference acting out. Masterson has made a unique contribution to understanding these principles and implementing the techniques.

All of the concepts play an important role in the psychotherapy of the schizoid disorder, and each will be addressed briefly, first by reviewing basic definitions of the concepts, and then by considering the specific application of these concepts to the treatment of the schizoid patient.

THERAPEUTIC NEUTRALITY

Therapeutic neutrality is at the core of the Masterson Approach to psychotherapy. It is the foundation. Therapeutic neutrality is operationally defined as the therapist's ability to stay apart from actively intervening in a patient's life. The therapist who practices therapeutic neutrality avoids those interventions that are directive, involve advice giving, or make the therapist an equal partner in problem solving. Therapeutic neutrality allows exploration, questioning, confrontation, and interpretation. The notion of therapeutic neutrality is, most important, based on the conviction that it is absolutely necessary for a patient to assume responsibility for understanding, managing, and working on conflicts, anxieties, and maladaptive defenses. Therapeutic neutrality holds that the *process* of psychotherapy is the responsibility of the therapist, while the *work* of psychotherapy is the responsibility of the patient. The therapist is the organizer and guardian of the conditions that allow the work to unfold.

Therapeutic neutrality evolves from the therapist's certainty that becoming emotionally involved with the patient will sabotage the therapeutic process. It does not require that the therapist be a robot, a mirror, or a blank screen. The therapist is a full participant in the process through his or her interest in, curiosity about, and concern for the patient's impaired real self. There is a critical difference between concern for the patient's impaired real self and caring for or about a patient. The former is always the therapist's responsibility; the latter is always the therapist's failure. Caring for or about a patient is the proper attitude of a friend, lover, spouse, parent, spiritual advisor, and many others. However, it is not the job of the psychotherapist.

Therapeutic neutrality is not a dispassionate position. Those therapists who believe in its importance do so passionately. There are no modifications in the application of this concept in working with a schizoid patient. The anxieties and dangers that are part of the schizoid patient's internal and external world may evoke intense pathos from the therapist, and result in the introduction of parameters that the therapist hopes will make the schizoid patient feel safer or more connected. In fact, the opposite is true. The only real source of safety for the schizoid patient in the initial phase of treatment is the absolute confidence in the therapist's predictability, stability, and nonintrusiveness. The schizoid patient has to know where the therapist stands, and the only place where a therapist can stand that feels safe to the patient before a therapeutic alliance is established is at a safe distance, one that is predictable, stable, and nonintrusive.

THERAPEUTIC STANCE AND THERAPEUTIC FRAME

The definition of the therapeutic stance in the Masterson Approach is rooted in the concept of therapeutic neutrality. It begins with the therapist's expectation that a patient will be able to assume appropriate responsibility for his or her thoughts, behaviors, and actions. A patient for whom this assumption cannot be made, such as an actively psychotic individual, is not suitable for a psychodynamic psychotherapeutic approach. The therapeutic stance includes the conviction that all patients have to adjust to the demands of reality, to the conditions imposed by society and community, while at the same time maintaining a healthy real self that is creative and spontaneous.

This may seem obvious, but it is not. The therapeutic stance is one of positive expectations about the individual's responsibility to the self and to others. It addresses the patient's potential. To borrow a term from Vygotsky (1962), the therapeutic stance is in the zone of proximal development. The therapist places himself or herself at the outer boundary of the patient's potential. The patient is implicitly encouraged to fulfill those obligations and responsibilities to self and to others that have become blurred or distorted, but that the therapist anchors for the patient in reality and with clarity. In this way, the therapist is, as Masterson has stated, "the guardian of the real self." The stance of optimal, positive expectation cannot be unrealistic and beyond the reach of the patient, nor can it be the therapist's agenda, or a way of living, imposed on the patient.

The therapeutic frame is the operational arm of the therapeutic stance. It refers to all those conditions that one establishes as part of the therapeutic milieu. It is a set of conditions, obligations, and responsibilities that supports the therapeutic process. It sets forth a baseline of expectation that the therapist can use to point out, clarify, confront, or interpret a patient's attempts to disregard or distort those conditions of adaptation and responsibility to self, to others, and to the appropriate demands of reality.

There is no one ideal therapeutic frame. The operational conditions of the therapeutic frame can vary. One therapist's definition of what constitutes a therapeutic frame may be different from another's. The issue is not primarily the specific details or conditions of the frame, although the Masterson Approach does argue that certain conditions are essential. Sometimes the conditions will be so clear as to leave little room for argument. Such conditions would include prohibitions against the threat or use of violence or against the patient's presenting in the session in an intoxicated state. Any definition of responsibility for one's thoughts, feelings, or behaviors would obviously have to include not altering one's consciousness and not acting in a destructive way toward oneself or toward the therapist.

Other aspects of the therapeutic frame are more controversial. In the Masterson Approach, those aspects include the use of surnames when addressing patients, clear guidelines regarding payment and vacation policies (payments must be timely, debts must not be incurred, and vacation time must be defined), and the patient's financial responsibility for missed appointments. Other frame issues would involve the therapist's refusing to distort reality by being a librarian (lending patients books) or a secretary (lending patients a pen to write checks).

The point is not that all therapists should or must use the same definition of what constitutes an appropriate frame, but that there should be a frame in place, a set of expectations about the patient's responsibility to manage sessions and his or her life.

The therapeutic frame is as essential for working with the schizoid patient and establishing a therapeutic alliance as it is in work with persons with any disorder of the self. The reason should be evident. In addition to defining the patient's responsibilities clearly, the frame permits the schizoid patient to know securely where the therapist stands. Stability and predictability are enhanced. Further, the consistency provided by the frame minimizes distortions around manipulation and coercion. Treatment policies are not arbitrarily selected or imposed; there is a clear reason for all policies, which is established at the beginning of treatment. The schizoid patient may not like a particular policy, but the patient will not feel threatened by that policy.

The issue of frequency of sessions is one that some clinicians would include as a frame issue. Here an exception should be made for the schizoid patient. Whereas most psychodynamic psychotherapy must be conducted on a weekly basis in order for the treatment to have consistent meaning and impact, the initial (and perhaps prolonged) period of treatment of the schizoid patient can often best be carried out on an every-other-week basis. This schedule not infrequently is suggested by the schizoid patient, and it is a way for the patient to manage initial fears of imprisonment and enslavement. Until such time in treatment as it is clear to the patient that the therapist has no wish to enslave and entrap, every-other-week treatment may be optimal.

TRANSFERENCE ACTING OUT

No concept in the psychotherapy of the disorders of the self is more central than that of transference acting out. The patient with a disorder of the self comes into treatment seeing the world through the selective filter of his or her intrapsychic structure. The representational world includes very specific and inflexible ideas about the nature of what other people are like and what they contain, as well as the nature of what the self is like and what it contains. The internal world of the disorder of the self is constructed from these narrowly defined, frozen, internalized object relations.

The internal world of the schizoid patient consists of the two split object relations units described previously: the master/slave unit and the sadistic object/self-in-exile unit. These two basic units represent the fundamental ways in which the schizoid patient sees and experiences the self, others, and the relationship between the two. Transference acting out operationally means that the schizoid patient can only see the external world as a mirror reflection of the internal world. The intrapsychic filter removes all that does not fit the pattern of attachment that has been laid down historically in the internalized object relation. Practically, this means that the schizoid patient who presents for treatment can only experience the therapist as actively participating in either the master/slave unit or the sadistic object/self-in-exile unit.

In the initial stage of treatment, every patient with a disorder of the self sees the therapist only through the distorted projections of his or her internalized object relations units. The attachment units for the borderline and narcissistic disorders, while highly conditional, are also potentially more gratifying. For the borderline patient, the promise of a better state of affairs is in the form of the rewarding object, whereas for the patient with narcissistic disorder, it is in the form of the omnipotent object. For the schizoid patient, the initial treatment period is much more tenuous and fragile, since both internal units have strong anxieties and dangers associated with them.

The schizoid patient comes into treatment motivated by the inexorable push of the need for attachment. At the same time, the patient is convinced that the therapist, like most significant people in the patient's past, will attempt to reenact the conditions found in the master/slave unit or in the sadistic object/self-in-exile unit.

When the master/slave unit is activated (which must happen when the patient enters treatment), the schizoid patient believes that the therapist's primary intent, regardless of what the therapist might say, is to impose the therapist's own agenda on the patient. Specifically, the schizoid patient fears that the therapist, as well as all significant others, will attempt to manipulate, coerce, appropriate, imprison, and enslave the patient. The concept of transference acting out alerts the therapist immediately that the master/slave unit is operating for the schizoid patient from the moment he or she steps into the therapist's office. It is not just a state of affairs that operates in the patient's relationship with others. The concept of transference acting out further tells the therapist that the schizoid patient is not free to view the therapist as other than another master.

Is it any wonder that the schizoid patient approaches therapy in such a cautious, wary, uneasy, uncomfortable manner? The therapist is another potential master to the patient's slave. The therapist, no less than anyone else in the patient's life, will, it is feared, lay claim to anything of value that the patient possesses. The schizoid individual who comes into treatment is accepting or settling for the role of slave as the price to be paid for relatedness in order to accomplish the relational goals.

If the schizoid patient is not projecting the object representation of the master on the therapist, then the patient may be projecting the object representation of the therapist as the sadistic object. A sadistic object is one that is dangerous, devaluing, and depriving. To protect himself or herself, the schizoid patient must maintain a cautious, safe distance from the sadistic object.

The schizoid patient, in treatment or in life, will often accept some degree of master/slave relatedness as a condition of achieving some actual experience of connection with the therapist and with the world. However, when the experience is too appropriating, too manipulative, or too coercive, the fragile thread of connection may be broken because the price of attachment has become too high. The projection of the sadistic object takes over. This propels the patient into withdrawal and exile, but also into freedom. And once again the schizoid patient finds that the price of safety and freedom is exile and alienation. The schizoid patient who is willing to settle for connection at any price will expose himself or herself to the dangers associated with the master/slave unit. But once a certain critical line has been crossed and the projection of the sadistic object is experienced, the self has no choice but to retreat.

The two other major representational components of the intrapsychic structure are the slave and the self-in-exile. Through the process of projective identification (Masterson & Klein, 1989), both representations may be called into operation as part of the schizoid patient's experience of the therapist. In the process of projective identification, the patient projects aspects of the self representation—either the slave or the self-in-exile—onto the therapist, while simultaneously identifying with aspects of the object representations of the respective units. For example, when the schizoid individual is projecting those aspects of the enslaved self onto the therapist, the patient is attempting to introduce feelings of imprisonment, enslavement, and manipulation to the therapist while assuming the position of the controlling master. In the process of projection, the therapist learns what the patient's experience of the historical object was like. The past is being reenacted by the process of projection, and the patient experiences history repeating itself. In the process of projective identification, the therapist learns what the patient's self experience was like from the perspective of the feeling state of the patient. For the patient, history is again repeating itself, but from the safety and power of the object's position. Projective identification of the master/slave unit leads, therefore, to situations in which the patient tries to control, manipulate, and appropriate that which is good from the therapist.

Since it would seem better to be in the position of master rather than slave, why is this mechanism of defense not used more often? For projective identification to really work, the therapist must resonate with the projection. In other words, the therapist must accept the projection of the slave, in this example, and allow himself or herself to be manipulated, coerced, or appropriated. In simple projection, the therapist, as master, is under no pressure to act. In fact, if the projection is not identified, it will go on endlessly. In projective identification, the therapist is far more likely to experience dysphoria, and will be more apt to react by identifying the process in operation and acting to intervene to bring this uncomfortable state of affairs to an end.

Projective identification mechanisms may also involve the sadistic object/self-in-exile unit. In this operation, the aspect of the self, the self-in-exile, is projected onto the therapist. The therapist is experienced as distant, unrelated, uninterested, cold, and indifferent. The patient who has succeeded in sending a therapist into exile experiences a sense of control and power and the sadistic satisfaction that accompanies talionic revenge. Once again, the therapist must resonate with (accept) this projection, or its power is vastly diminished.

In summary, the schizoid patient usually comes into treatment projecting either internal object representation: that of the master or that of the sadistic object. Alternatively, however, the schizoid patient may project aspects of the self representations, either the slave or the self-in-exile, but these projective techniques require a more active participation (countertransference acting out) on the part of the therapist in order to be of use to the patient. Keeping these mechanisms in mind, the therapist treating the schizoid patient is now prepared for the initial therapeutic encounter.

Case of Ms. J.

Ms. J. provided one of my first extensive experiences with an overtly schizoid patient. When Ms. J. first presented for treatment, she described her conflict over feeling as if "everyone wants to control me, like my parents tried to do." During the initial weeks of treatment, I went from feeling like an interested observer to someone trying to "pull teeth" with my questions. I began to feel more and more like a sadistic object. The patient had extreme difficulty responding to any of my questions or interventions with anything other than long silences. It soon became clear that what I regarded as innocuous questions or helpful interventions represented to the patient my efforts to intrude on her and to control her.

The tools that one uses with most patients to convey one's curiosity, interest, and concern (that is, thoughtful questions and interpretations) seemed useless and counterproductive. Her responses, when she did speak, were usually one-word sentences. I could see no particular rhyme or reason as to why she answered some questions and not others. When she spoke spontaneously, her speech had a staccato quality. She would start, stop, start again, and then conclude, often in the middle of a phrase. It was confusing and infuriating.

Because I did not know then what it meant to be schizoid, I did not know initially how to understand this patient or how to treat her. Since I had some idea of what to do with borderline and narcissistic patients, I would change my diagnosis frequently and try various interventions, such as confrontation, mirroring, and interpretation. Nothing seemed to work. Everything seemed to be experienced by the patient as an intrusion.

The initial understanding of this patient came from an unlikely source: a 16-year-old catatonic schizophrenic girl I was treating at the same time. Like Ms. J., this patient refused to respond to almost any of my questions. Typically, a session would begin with my asking her a question. I would wait 5, 10, 15, 20 minutes until, finally exasperated, I would ask her another question. Finally, after many weeks of going through this routine, the patient turned to me and said, "Why do you bother asking questions if you are not interested enough to wait for my answer?" That was all she said. But she taught me something valuable that I was able to use to understand Ms. J. By not waiting for answers to the questions I was asking, I was conveying the message that my agenda was more important to me than was her agenda. She felt that what I was doing was only going through the motions in asking my questions. If I were truly a concerned and interested participant in the process, I would wait as long as it took, or at least I would pursue what was going on between us that so that the patient chose not to answer.

With this valuable assistance by the schizophrenic patient, I turned my attention once again to Ms. J. and tried to understand what she was trying to communicate to me by her relative silence.

In retrospect, I can understand and organize her behavior according to the structures previously defined. At times I would feel like an overbearing master trying to pry experiences, feelings, or thoughts out of Ms. J. I am not sure that what I was going to do with the information once I had it was important to me at that point in the treatment. It was important just to get it. This is a unique quality of appropriation. It is the having or possessing that is as important as what is possessed or had. The feeling that treatment was like pulling teeth was an example of slipping into accepting the sadistic object projection. Thoughtful questions had become a modified form of torture.

At other times, I felt manipulated and controlled by her as if her actions were purposeful. I felt like putty in her hands: unseen, unlistened to, being used for some as-yet-undecipherable reason, a mixture of self-in-exile and slave projections. I felt pushed away from her to such a degree that I had no place to go in sessions but into myself. I would often spend periods during the long silences that pervaded the sessions lost in my own fantasies (complete self-in-exile when the fantasies had nothing to do with the patient, and a form of staying attached to her when they did).

At the time, however, I did not have these structures in mind. I had simply begun to understand that all of my questions were in some way being experienced as a form of manipulation or as an effort at control, an intrusion into Ms. J.'s world. I realized that she had already told me something central to her conflict, which was her feeling that everyone wanted to control her as her parents had tried to do. While I had not forgotten this central theme, I had been unable to imagine that she could experience me in such a pervasively similar fashion. After all, I had reasoned, she was not schizophrenic or psychotically depressed. She could test reality. Did she not know that I was not like her parents? In reality, she knew that I was not her mother or her father. Emotionally, there was no difference.

I now had the answer to why my questions and interpretations were not working: transference acting out of the fear of being manipulated and controlled. My interventions were experienced as moves in some sadistic game that I was playing with her. Her intrapsychic structure left her no alternative but to feel that I was masquerading as a therapist. Sooner or later, she eventually reported to me, she was certain that I would figuratively peel back my mask of being a concerned therapist and reveal the underlying face of her mother or her father.

Armed with this new path to understanding what was motivating her behavior, I was able to proceed differently. I could sit for much longer periods quietly and comfortably and wait for her to proceed at her own pace.

At the same time, I now interpreted her need to keep a wary distance from me as she gradually tested the waters of the therapeutic relationship.

As I understood more, I began to convey more of that understanding to the patient. My interpretations were not elaborate or genetically based; they were simply explanations, almost narratives, of what I imagined her experience of me to be. This was my introduction to the usefulness and importance of interpreting the schizoid dilemma, or at least that part of the dilemma that had to do with my awareness that, as she took the risk of answering my questions, of communicating and conveying to me any of her thoughts or feelings, she was running the risk of experiencing the anxiety and dread that accompanied the feelings of being manipulated, coerced, imprisoned, and enslaved. I would interpret to the patient at those times my understanding of how my questions might seem like intrusions to her— at best, a stepping on her toes; at worst, trying to take from her the thoughts and feelings that she most valued. I would not make these interpretations as declarative statements but would mold the observations into the form of a question or a hypothesis to be tested. For example, I might say, "It seems to me that . . ." or "Could it be that . . . ?" or "My understanding of what you are saying is . . .". The emphasis was on conveying to the patient that the therapist had no specific agenda, let alone interpretation, to impose or that the patient was expected to accept.

For the first time in the therapy, Ms. J. began to acknowledge that my comments reflected how she felt. More and more frequently, she stated that what I was observing was exactly right. Similarly, I felt that I was beginning to enter the world of the schizoid patient. I was being introduced into the patient's master/slave world not by reenacting it, but by understanding it. For most of the first year of treatment, either I would patiently wait for the patient to communicate or I would interpret that part of the schizoid dilemma I had come to understand. The primary goal of this initial period was to enable the patient to understand that I understood how she felt—that any effort to interface with me was fraught with anxiety and danger.

I realized that the first and most important step in treating the schizoid patient was to make her feel safe, so that she could bring her self into the treatment. The defining condition for building a therapeutic alliance with the schizoid patient is safety. Her words, thoughts, feelings, and behaviors could be brought into the room and become a part of her interpersonal experience, without her fearing that I would try to appropriate or subjugate them to my own needs. I understood that this patient was not cold and indifferent or unconcerned about social relationships or her relationship with me. It was clear why interventions that worked with borderline and narcissistic disorders did not work with her. Confrontations, which are so crucial to the treatment of the borderline patient, were experienced by her as insufferable intrusions, attempts to control and manipulate. The patient did not have a problem in taking responsibility for herself, so confrontations could not be seen as strengthening the therapeutic alliance through clarifying the therapist's commitment to the competence of the patient's embattled and impaired real self. For this schizoid patient, competence was not the issue; communication was.

On those occasions when the patient had initially answered my questions, she had done so begrudgingly, with no underlying wish or belief that I would take over the management of her treatment, as would be the motivation for the borderline patient. Quite the contrary. Ms. J. complied with my questions because of a motivation to accept any condition as the price of relatedness. Responding to some of my questions was the price she was willing to pay for maintaining some connection to me.

Mirroring interpretations of narcissistic vulnerability, so useful in making the narcissistic patient feel understood, seemed to drive Ms. J. further and further away. The more empathic the interpretation, the more she seemed to retreat. I now understood why. My effort to feel into her experience by defining it emotionally was for her a potentially traumatic intrusion. Specifically, to say to this patient something like, "It is so painful for you to focus upon yourself that you withdraw into silence as a way of protecting yourself," would be intolerable. Precisely what would be therapeutically engaging for the narcissistic patient is anathema for the schizoid patient. To define the schizoid patient's emotional experience for the patient ("It is so painful . . .") creates the conditions for appropriation and depletion, not for understanding.

What might one say? One might rephrase the intervention as, "It seems to me that talking about yourself might be extraordinarily anxiety creating because it might bring you closer to me than you are prepared to be at this moment. . . ." The difference here is that the interpretation is (1) not declarative; (2) not affect defining, except in the broadest terms of anxiety or danger; and (3) referential to one part of the schizoid dilemma—being too close for comfort. While the mirroring interpretation accurately notes the patient's withdrawal as a form of self-protection, even this aspect of the therapist's defense analysis is off the mark because it inaccurately emphasizes the patient's possible difficulties with self-focus (maintenance and organization), rather than the patient's actual difficulties in interpersonal communication.

The more that I was able to interpret Ms. J.'s need for safety and her anxiety about and dread of risking communication, the more she was able to do so. Gradually, she accepted the fact that I was not going to impose my thoughts, feelings, and needs while appropriating hers. Increasingly, the therapy itself began to be a safe place where she could take risks and experiment around her initial goals, which had been her wish to find more satisfaction in interpersonal relationships.

At this point in the treatment, we were able to communicate much better, yet it still proceeded at an agonizingly slow pace. About a year and a half into the treatment, another incident occurred that was critical to my understanding of the intrapsychic world of the schizoid patient. Ms. J. went on a vacation. There had seemed little reaction on her part to the fact that the therapy would be interrupted for approximately three weeks. The exact date of the patient's return was not clear, and it had been agreed that she would call when she returned. About three weeks after she left, I received a message on my answering machine that said, "My name is Ms. J. I don't know if you will remember me, but I am a patient of yours and would like to make another appointment with you."

This message had a profound impact on me. I could have assumed that this was a striking example of a failure in object constancy or even object permanency. Had I left it simply at that more cognitive level of understanding, I would have missed something much more relevant and revealing. Instead, I decided to pursue the message with Ms. J. Had I attempted to do this much earlier in the treatment, it would probably have fallen into that vast range of questions that were perceived as intrusive. By this time, however, I had begun to establish a safe therapeutic alliance, and Ms. J. was able to tolerate my questions and explain to me her experience of having distanced herself so far from me, both intrapsychically and physically during her vacation, that she felt that she had perhaps gone beyond a point of no return.

Specifically, she described feeling that she had gone so far away that she questioned whether she would be able to retrieve herself or to retrieve me, or whether I might not be able to retrieve her. All three parts of this statement were concepts that provided important levels of understanding. First, she feared that she could not retrieve herself, that she might have gone so far away emotionally as to put herself into a place from which she could no longer find her way back, a place of total isolation and alienation. Second, she also felt that she might not be able to retrieve me, that is, to reestablish a connection with me, because she had gone so far that connection would be impossible. Third, she was also concerned that I might not be able to retrieve her. This concept involved projective identification mechanisms. One was to turn me into a function (slave) as she had felt herself to be, a function that could not reach out and connect to the significant people in her life, but could only stand by helplessly, passively, waiting to be contacted (connected to). Another was to identify me with her self-in-exile and then perceive me as being so driven into exile by her actions that I would have no need or wish to reach out and make contact with her. In either case, I would no longer have the ability or the desire to maintain a relationship with her.

I was now able, with Ms. J., to put together both sides of the schizoid dilemma, to understand the nature of her split object relations units. To my interpretation of the anxiety and danger she experienced when she tried to interface with me, I could now add that she repeatedly, defensively, and self-protectively withdrew from those risks, dangers, challenges, and efforts. By withdrawing, she was trying to reestablish a safe distance, a safe place where she could be free of anxiety. However, rather than freeing her from anxiety, this exposed her to different, equally dangerous results. She would be in danger of moving too far away, beyond the safety of exile, and beyond the point of no return—into the despair of irreversible alienation. Ms. J. showed me that the schizoid experience of exile brought with it not only self-containment, self-sufficiency, and self-reliance (safety), but also the implicit, underlying dread of alienation, the place from which she could no longer retrieve herself or me, and a place where I could no longer reach her.

I could now see the full extent of the schizoid dilemma, the struggle between the dread of appropriation and the dread of total isolation. At this point, nearing the end of the second year of treatment, I could now interpret fully to Ms. J. my understanding of her dilemma and the terrible anxieties she experienced. The full understanding of the schizoid dilemma and its repeated interpretation to the patient provided the essential key that allowed me access to Ms. J.'s internal world. I could now step into that world without causing her undue dread because my interpretation allowed her to feel safely understood. My interpretation in no way threatened a reenactment of either her perceived experiences of manipulation and appropriation, or her perceived experiences of being pushed away and cast off, devalued, deprived, and endangered. The conditions for establishing and deepening the therapeutic alliance were now present.

For practically every movement that the patient made in treatment, I now had a way of understanding the meaning of the move, and an intervention that would lower the patient's anxiety, resistance, and defense, thus promoting communication.

To summarize, there were principles that I finally understood in the treatment of Ms. J. that apply to the initial stage of the treatment of all schizoid patients, and that help to convert transference acting out to therapeutic alliance. As the case of Ms. J. demonstrates, converting transference acting out to therapeutic alliance is not facilitated by either confrontations or mirroring interpretations of narcissistic vulnerability. Moreover, empathy that is not a part of dynamic empathic understanding is not empathy at all. It is emotional invasion to the schizoid patient. Entry to the schizoid patient's intrapsychic world comes through interpretation of the schizoid dilemma. This is the foundation on which the therapeutic alliance is built. The consequence of this understanding, and the interpretation that flows from it, is a deep feeling of safety for the schizoid patient. There is no experience of emotional violation that can be present as a result of confrontation or mirroring interpretations.

Case of Mr. J.

Mr. J. was briefly described earlier as the patient who felt like a puppet sitting on his mother's knee. Initially, Mr. J. also struggled for many months in treatment to reveal his true feelings, thoughts, and needs. His style was quite different from that of Ms. J. All his comments seemed lifeless; his manner lacked animation. Facts were communicated fairly easily, but without aliveness of affect and often with a strong suggestion of compliance. Unlike the initial situation with Ms. J., it seemed that there was no question I could ask that was beyond Mr. J.'s ability to answer extensively. He was able to activate himself, for the most part, and to take charge of the session, supplying me with interesting details about what was going on in his life. Still, throughout the initial year of treatment, there was a remarkably shallow, disengaged quality to his communications. My own feeling, in response to being equally disengaged, had grown increasingly uncomfortable. Subtle at first, this feeling had become pervasive, and I had begun to experience enormous boredom and disinterest.

This feeling finally became the focus of my attention. I realized that despite the wealth of information Mr. J. had given me, he was not actually present in the treatment. At the beginning of the second year of treatment, I was clear enough about my feelings to begin to share some of these thoughts with the patient. I told him that I was experiencing him as being only partly there, as if I were in the presence of his shadow and not his real self. I further commented that I was not certain where the problem lay, but that I felt it was important to share my experience of him. He responded that he had no idea what I meant or what my problem was. The issue was dropped for the rest of the session.

In the next session, I picked up on the same theme. I acknowledged his dismissal of my observations, but I stated further that I had begun to wonder if my experience of him as being only partly present reflected a need on his part to maintain a safe distance from me. I wondered if perhaps he was accomplishing this by sharing some important details of his life, but draining these facts of their emotional tone and meaning. This time he responded by asking me to explain further what I meant. I continued, wondering whether the meaning of this way of communicating with me was to allow him to be close, but not too close. If so, then perhaps he was connecting to me, but was not really communicating with me.

Mr. J. was quiet for several minutes. He seemed to be thinking about what I had said, and since I did not feel that he was withdrawing or distancing, I sat quietly and waited. He then asked why I thought he might be doing that. Since we had previously discussed aspects of the schizoid dilemma in his relationships outside the treatment, I suggested that what was happening with me was a mirror of what we had discussed in his other relationships. In other words, he also had concerns about being too close to me, and these concerns generated their own anxiety, discomfort, and unease, which he managed by keeping one foot in the treatment and the other foot out of it—or, in this case, by putting some thoughts into the treatment while keeping his feelings out.

Mr. J. slowly began to confirm these observations, and, to go well beyond them. He told me, over a number of sessions, that while he had related many facts about his life, he had rarely told me his true thoughts, let alone his feelings. Essentially, he had told me only what he thought I wanted him to say. What was the meaning of this patient's compliance? Exploration revealed that it was not in the service of a borderline need to comply with the object in order to be taken care of, and to have the object help regulate the affect state of the patient, nor was it in the service of trying to mirror me in order that he might bask in the glow of my treatment of him as special, and thus enhance his core, narcissistic grandiose self.

Rather, it became clear that he had been willing to settle, as he said, "for the semblance of a relationship since I knew that I could not have the real thing." He added, "Some relationship is better than no relationship." He was describing his essential way of experiencing the world of object relations, of having to settle for a master/slave relationship, being a puppet and mouthing my words. It took several more weeks for him to reveal his concern that really communicating with me was a dangerous undertaking, not unlike the feelings that he had described about the other people in his life, especially his mother. Seemingly, I had been excluded from that group of feared relationships, but in reality Mr. J. had managed his fears by first removing himself from our relationship, which was exactly what he had done with everyone else in his world.

Mr. J. showed another behavior in the initial stage of treatment that was essentially a concrete representation of his effort to establish a safe, therapeutic distance and alliance. He would constantly change his choice of a seat, never seeming to be totally comfortable or at ease. Many patients, of course, spend the first few minutes in treatment (or in relationships, more generally) deciding what feels like an appropriate distance between themselves and others in a real, physical sense. But this behavior, which is a part of most individuals' initial interpersonal (and intrapsychic) negotiation, becomes for the schizoid individual a prolonged quandary in the real, physical world, and an interminable quandary in the intrapsychic, emotional world. What for most individuals is a momentary focus of attention for the schizoid patient is a lifetime focus of interpersonal and intrapsychic concern.

This state of affairs is often enacted in the schizoid patient's positioning in the therapist's office. When I first saw Mr. J., he had jokingly (sic) wondered whether he might sit in the hallway outside of my office proper, with the treatment conducted at that distance. Other schizoid patients will act out their anxiety or fear about distance by trying to sit behind pillows or other physical barriers that they place between themselves and the therapist. I have had patients initially request that they be allowed to sit behind the chair or couch in my office, or cover themselves with a blanket that was brought from home, or have only telephone sessions, all of which are dramatic efforts to regulate distance in a literal sense. Such efforts must be dealt with interpretively as a form of compromise or settling, and no allowances of this kind need be, or should be, made.

COUNTERTRANSFERENCE ACTING OUT AND COUNTERTRANSFERENCE

The fourth and final major concept to be considered in establishing a therapeutic alliance is the role of the therapist's emotional life in the therapeutic relationship. In the course of treatment, a therapist may have strong emotional reactions. When a therapist responds to, or resonates with, the transference acting out of a patient, the therapeutic alliance will be seriously compromised. Such reactions are designed as countertransference acting out in order to distinguish them from countertransference in the narrow, classic sense.

In countertransference acting out, the therapist is responding to something the patient is doing. Moreover, it is a reaction that the patient is consciously or unconsciously attempting to provoke in the therapist. The therapist's reaction is not peculiar to the individual therapist, but is a reaction that one might expect from almost any therapist who is unaware of the meaning and the proper management of the patient's resistance, as well as of the therapist's own reactions.

Countertransference acting out is to be distinguished from countertransference proper. Countertransference in the classic sense is a reaction that originates primarily in the therapist, not in the patient. It is a reflection more of unresolved, early developmental and interpersonal conflicts in the therapist than of anything in the therapeutic setting. It is primarily between the therapist and the therapist's past, and only secondarily (if at all) between the therapist and patient.

Knowledge of the schizoid patient's intrapsychic structure helps the therapist to understand and anticipate the nature of the patient's transference acting out, and, therefore, to identify and control his or her own countertransference acting out. Most countertransference acting out by a therapist treating a schizoid patient results from resonating with, or accepting, the patient's projection of either the object or self representation of the specific object relations unit. Any projective technique utilized by the schizoid patient (whether simple projection or projective identification) acquires its greatest power if it can trap the therapist into resonating with the projection. Projective techniques will have limited success if they cannot provoke the therapist into resonating with the particular projection.

The therapist must be aware of the patient's need not only to see the world through the screen of his or her intrapsychic structure, but also to impose on the world that same intrapsychic structure. Mental life is an active, not a passive, process. Experiences are not just passive phenomena, but are actively created. When working with any disorder of the self, the therapist will experience powerful projections that attempt to draw him or her into the internal world of the patient and make the therapist a coconspirator, rather than a guardian of the patient's real self.

What does this mean clinically for the therapist treating the schizoid patient? The schizoid patient may project the master object representation, which the therapist either will identify as such or unknowingly respond to by feeling powerful, strong, and manipulative. These feelings on the part of the therapist are often evidenced by the therapist's giving advice, directing, and subtly molding the patient, and expecting the patient to comply with those interventions. Ironically, the therapist who responds, for example, to the schizoid patient's request for help, information, or advice will only be reinforcing the patient's belief that the therapist has an agenda to impose.

The patient may alternately project the object representation of the sadistic, dangerous, depriving, and devaluing object of the sadistic object/self-in-exile unit. Again, the therapist will either stand apart from that projection or resonate with it and feel sadistic, dangerous, depriving, and devaluing. This is made manifest clinically most commonly when the therapist feels that he or she is not giving the patient enough (a form of deprivation), that he or she is not expecting enough (a form of devaluation), or that he or she may be pushing the patient too quickly and with too much impatience (a form of threat or danger).

What are the remaining major pitfalls of countertransference acting out? One need only recall the intrapsychic structure of the schizoid to have the answer. As described by Klein (Masterson & Klein, 1989, chap. 17), the self representation of a split object relations unit may be projected, while the patient identifies with the object representation of the respective unit (projective identification). Thus for the schizoid patient there are two major projective identification operations corresponding to the two fundamental split object relations units.

The patient may project the self representation of the slave, while identifying with the master. Once again, the therapist may remain neutral and not resonate with this projection, or may respond to the projection by feeling enslaved, trapped, manipulated, and appropriated by the patient, who is now perceived as being in control. The patient does feel in control. Part of my reaction to both Ms. J. and Mr. J. had been affected by this projection, and had been manifest by feelings of powerlessness, and by feelings that whatever I had of value as a therapist was heard, used momentarily, and then stored for use by the patient without further acknowledgment or credit. Typically, the pattern will become manifest when the patient uses an intervention and almost immediately turns to the therapist with the complaint that the therapist is not helping or doing enough. Understanding the process of projective identification allows the therapist to understand that the patient does find the intervention useful; however, the schizoid patient is often left with the choice of consciously acknowledging that fact and feeling enslaved, rejecting help and feeling hopeless and disconnected, or appropriating the intervention as his or her own, and, by so doing, getting the benefits of the interventions without the feeling of enslavement (but also without the feeling of a mutually shared experience). Once more the patient settles for part of a relationship in place of the whole.

The patient may also project the self representation of the self-in-exile while identifying with the sadistic object. As is true of all the projective techniques, this one also enables the patient to rid himself or herself of the acute, painful aspects of experience—in this instance, that of feeling alienated, isolated, and in exile. The patient invites the therapist to resonate with this projection. The therapist who does so will feel a distance from the patient, illustrated by boredom and inattention; disconnection from the patient; or even flight into personal fantasies during the session, which removes the therapist completely. The therapist who resonates with this projection will feel that the patient is doing this to the therapist, when, in fact, it is the patient who is keeping the therapist at a distance and making himself or herself unavailable to the therapist, who then feels uncomfortable and pushed to the periphery. In this instance, the therapist feels that he or she is not able to understand the patient, that he or she is not in tune with the patient, and is not the right therapist for this patient. It is an intense feeling of not being able to connect meaningfully with another human being.

The therapist's countertransference acting out can be put to positive as well as negative use. When it is being actively enacted between the patient and the therapist, there are all types of negative consequences, as just described. In short, any therapeutic progress or change is sacrificed as the treatment dissolves into endless repetitions of past experiences, in which the roles of the characters may change. At times, the therapist may be the reincarnation of the earlier objects in the patient's life. Alternatively, the therapist may be experiencing the various roles that the patient occupied and performed at various stages in his or her development (via projective identification). When the therapist responds with countertransference acting out to the patient's transference acting out, all that happens in the treatment is an ongoing reenactment of the past, which usually is potentially traumatizing to the therapist and certainly is retraumatizing to the patient. Regardless of which role is being played by whom, therapeutic progress is sacrificed on the altar of the past.

There is, however, a beneficial aspect of countertransference acting out. Once it has been identified by the therapist, it can be an invaluable tool in understanding the patient. It becomes available to the therapist as a window through which to look into the past. It is like observing a videotape replay of something that happened in the history of the patient. It provides a unique opportunity for the therapist actually to see into the life of the patient, and to understand first hand, in a sense, what is must have been like for the patient.

Will the countertransference acting out be put to good use or bad use?

If the therapist is an active player in the patient's drama and assumes the role that has been assigned, then the consequences can only be bad. However, if the therapist can step out of the role, see it as a role, and experience himself or herself as an observer or member of the audience (therapeutic neutrality), then the countertransference acting out can be helpful. In the treatment of Mr. J. and Ms. J., the identification of the countertransference acting out allowed the therapist to make those interventions, which ultimately led to significant breakthroughs in establishing the therapeutic alliance.

How can the therapist judge the state of the therapeutic alliance? In one sense, this already has been described. The essence of the therapeutic alliance is that it is a new object relations unit for the schizoid patient, one that provides a new lens through which to view the world of intrapsychic and interpersonal relationships. The relationship between patient and therapist is that new object relations unit; therefore, the degree to which the patient can view the therapist in a healthy, realistic fashion, freed from the distortions of the master/slave or the sadistic object/self-in-exile object relations unit, is the key determinant of a successful therapeutic alliance.

Other measures of the strength of the therapeutic alliance are available, specifically in changes in the nature of schizoid compromise and in changes in the quantity and quality of schizoid fantasy. These provide valuable mechanisms to ensure that the therapist is correct in the assessment. They are somewhat more objective criteria that should complement the judgments made (often with strong subjective overtones) about the therapeutic relationship. These criteria are also useful as an ongoing measure of the success of ego-reparative treatment, the goal of which is to repair the defects in the self without effecting a fundamental transformation in the structure of the self. Masterson (1978) has clearly drawn these clinical distinctions.

SCHIZOID COMPROMISE

One of the key criteria the therapist can use to validate the conviction of a growing therapeutic alliance, and the accompanying greater sense of therapeutic safety, will be the schizoid patient's effort to experiment with and alter the nature of his or her compromises. If the schizoid patient is feeling the safety of the therapeutic alliance, this should be manifest in a willingness to effect different forms of compromise solutions to the dilemma, both within and outside the therapeutic milieu. Operationally, this means that the patient should demonstrate greater risk taking and a willingness to accept the challenge to connect, communicate, and share thoughts and feelings, or at least actions, with others. In sessions, this would involve efforts to communicate thoughts and affective experiences more freely to the therapist. Outside the treatment, it should be manifest by efforts at making real-life interpersonal contacts and connections. There should be a slow, but perceptible, shift from relatively isolated activities to those that involve one or more persons, or even groups. In the secret schizoid, whose interpersonal skills appear to be intact, there should be the subjective reporting of a slow but perceptible shift from affect withdrawal and containment to affect sharing.

Everyone makes compromises in life, specifically in interpersonal relationships. This is reflected in the concept of a normal social self, one's social veneer. It is not to be equated with the concept of a false self, since it is adaptive and promotes social, communal living. It is, for most healthy persons, an aspect of functioning that is the surface layer of the real self, an acknowledgment of the fact that others have their own emotional centers, separate from one's own. For the schizoid patient, the concept of compromise has a unique meaning, which is a basic decision to settle for the semblance of a relationship to others without the reality of it. It is settling for something that approximates a real relationship, but never succeeds in achieving it. The closest one gets is either through the master/slave relationship or through fantasy.

Compromise means always having one foot in and one foot out. There are many degrees of compromise. Some are better than others; some are closer than others. The secret schizoid leans toward, while the classic schizoid leans away. Some schizoid patients marry, but remain too much apart; others never marry, but may share more with friends from a safe distance. One person's compromise is to be alone in a crowd; another person's compromise may be to share closely with one person, while excluding all others.

At the very least, the concept of a therapeutic alliance means the possibility of a better compromise, the possibility of closer approximations to, and possibilities for true attachment and sharing, shorn of defensive armor and emotional distancing. If the fundamental schizoid compromise is not too close and not too far, then the better schizoid compromise is closer rather than farther.

This concept of better compromise is anchored by the therapeutic alliance. It is also the goal of ego-reparative psychotherapy. It is only by working through in intensive analytic therapy that the concept of schizoid compromise shifts from a focus on better compromise as a pervasive goal of everyday functioning to a focus on no compromise or, more accurately, on the retention of compromise only in its communal sense. In other words, the goal of working through is to remove compromise as a fundamental principle or organizer of experience. The schizoid patient who works through is able to forego compromise, achieve true intimacy and sharing, and experience all the joys and disappointments of neurotic conflict instead of the anxieties and agonies of schizoid compromise.

FANTASY

Fantasy has multiple forms and functions for the schizoid patient. These change throughout therapy, and the nature of the changes determines to a great extent the ultimate end point of treatment.

Clinically, the function of fantasy for the schizoid patient in treatment can be divided into generalized fantasies involving multiple themes and specific fantasies involving the patient's therapist. Both kinds of fantasies may function to keep the patient from establishing a firm therapeutic alliance. They are alternatives (relationships by proxy) to creating a new object relations unit with the therapist, and act as protection against the risks involved in connecting to, and sharing with, the therapist. In this fashion, they are part of the general defensive makeup of the patient. Both kinds of fantasies may help the patient avoid the painful process of working through abandonment depression. Here especially, the patient may hold onto settling for (compromising) the relationship with the therapist (which takes place more in fantasy than in reality, and is often intense and intimate in nature), rather than proceed with focusing on the pain of working through.

Changes in the generalized fantasy life provide evidence of a growing therapeutic alliance. These include active efforts on the part of the schizoid patient to interrupt flights into fantasy and to make efforts to introduce real alternatives and real interpersonal interactions in place of fantasy. Change in fantasy and better compromise are close companions.

The following case reflects the complexity of the function of specific fantasies about the therapist in the progress of treatment generally, and in the firm establishment of the therapeutic alliance more specifically.

Case of Ms. M.

With Ms. M., the initial period of transforming transference acting out to therapeutic alliance extended over several years. This period was characterized by persistent timidity, aloofness, and, at the same time, subtle flirtatiousness. She seemed markedly schizoid in her adaptation, structure, and approach to treatment. During this period, I introduced the concept of the schizoid dilemma, and repeated this interpretation whenever the clinical material required it. I thought that would be enough to keep the treatment moving toward a gradual consolidation of the therapeutic alliance. But despite the fact that she seemed responsive to my interpretations, I found the work with her to be extraordinarily slow, even by schizoid standards. I found myself subtly impatient with her progress, despite my usual ability to be quite patient in working with schizoid patients. While I knew that something was wrong, for a long time I could not discern what it was.

It was only because Ms. M. had responded so well to the interpretation of the schizoid dilemma that I eventually was able to understand what was becoming an increasingly obvious therapeutic stalemate. Well into the third year of treatment, I was struck by the inconsistency between her integration of the interpretations and her failure to be able to move effectively into a solid therapeutic alliance, reflected by increasing risk-taking behavior, both inside and outside the treatment.

Concerned about her lack of risk-taking behavior and its meaning for the health of the therapeutic alliance, I began to share with her my feeling that there was something not right about what was happening. I reflected that while she seemed increasingly aware of and able to talk about the anxieties that she experienced, in her desire to be close to me, as well as in her need to distance from me, she seemed consistently unwilling to take risks and to accept the challenges of making these same efforts in the world outside my office. She responded with anger, resurrecting a theme that I had not heard for some time, that I was trying to control her and impose on her my agenda as to how she should live her life. I responded that I experienced no sense in myself of wanting to impose anything on her. In fact, I added, I was bringing up something that related to her initially expressed wish in treatment—the capacity to have a more intimate, gratifying, real relationship in the world. I concluded that, while I understood her sensitivity to any feeling about being intruded on and controlled, and since I felt none of that coming from within me, I was surprised at her reaction.

Her response was one of silence, neither affirming nor disagreeing with what I had said. Her expression was one of surprise and consternation. She looked hurt and betrayed. I had not seen those emotions so clearly in her expression in the treatment up to that time. There was a hint of tears in her eyes. I told her what I was observing and pointed out that this reaction was different than usual. She offered no comment and was silent for the remainder of the session.

Ms. M. continued her silence throughout most of the next session. I waited. With about five minutes left in the session, she spoke up and reported the following dream, which she had had two days earlier. In the dream, she and I were naked and attached together like Siamese twins from the top of the sternum to the groin. She stated that it was an image that was both confusing and exciting. We talked about aspects of the dream and she revealed fantasies, which had existed since the beginning of treatment, of having an intense relationship with me.

This was not simply an eroticized fantasy. Rather, it was an elaborate fantasy of an idealized, intimate, shared relationship that included romantic images. It became clear to both of us that part of her reluctance to experiment outside the treatment was based on a feeling that she would be betraying our relationship, which she had maintained in fantasy. This also helped to explain her hurt reaction when I brought up my awareness of her failure to experiment, to take risks in her relationships outside the treatment. As she saw it, I was betraying her by encouraging her to have these adulterous relationships with others while she was totally committed to her relationship with me.

With the revelation of this fantasy through the vehicle of her dream, I expected there to be a gradual shift in the patient's behavior and a gradual movement finally toward more experimentation outside the treatment. To my surprise, six months after the initial discussion of the dream, she still had made no movements to expand her connections. For some time, I had made the assumption that there was a firm therapeutic alliance in place, and that her fantasy about our relationship had been primarily an obstacle to the process of working through. As it turned out, I had been premature and overly optimistic in my interpretation of the meaning of these events. I again returned to the theme on which I had first focused six months previously: the contradiction between the work that she was doing in the treatment, and the lack of similar risk-taking behavior and progress outside the treatment. It was also at this time that I realized there were parts of the dream we had both ignored.

I remembered especially how she had first mentioned a feeling of confusion. I had not pursued that particular feeling with any degree of persistence up to that point. I had focused almost exclusively on her feeling of excitement and on the more romanticized nature of the relationship. Now I wondered specifically about whether the confusion in the dream was a cover for more frightening and dangerous feelings that continued to operate as a major obstacle to therapeutic progress. The focus now shifted to another aspect of our connection as described in the dream. As I asked her to describe more precisely the image in the dream, she reported that as Siamese twins we shared all the vital organs. In other words, there was only one heart, one set of lungs, one stomach, and so forth. Part of the dream also included her knowledge (which she had not indicated in our prior discussions) that I was the one who really possessed the organs, while she had a kind of parasitic relationship to me. Therefore, this meant that, should we ever be separated, all the life-sustaining organs would stay within me, while she would be left eviscerated, totally appropriated.

What I had missed in my understanding of the dream and its interpretation the first time around was the extent to which I was still a dangerous, potentially sadistic and destructive object for her. That aspect of the relationship with me had been the other part of the tremendous barrier to therapeutic progress generally, and to the establishment of a firm, safe, therapeutic alliance specifically.

Once these issues were exposed in their full, life-threatening intensity, the patient was gradually able to understand the full extent of the danger she perceived in relationships. She could then work with me toward building a stable alliance. The correctness of this focus was confirmed by the fact that the patient was now able to begin slowly taking risks in sharing feelings and connecting interpersonally outside the treatment. Furthermore, the way was cleared for her to engage fully in the working-through process, to face her abandonment depression in all of its intensity.

Several aspects of the case of Ms. M. should be highlighted. One is the extraordinary degree of wariness with which some schizoid patients will approach treatment. Ms. M. was intensely schizoid and occupied a place on the extreme end of the continuum of schizoid pathology, where the dangers are enormous and the terror potentially overwhelming. It can take an enormous amount of time and effort to build a therapeutic alliance, since the fears associated with taking this step may be deep and difficult to uncover. It should be stressed that the only reason the dread that Ms. M. felt could overtly become a part of the treatment to be discussed and overcome, was that the prior focus on the schizoid dilemma had begun to lay the foundation for the therapeutic alliance and for the possibility of being understood. Therefore, when I pointed out the contradiction between her behavior inside and outside the treatment, she was able not only to have the dream, but to tell me about the dream, and to give me the opportunity to enter further into her internal world.

Finally, one might ask why it was that I was unaware of this meaning of Ms. M.'s dream for so long. The answer once again brings the issue of countertransference acting out to the forefront. More precisely, what was in operation was the therapist's intense defensive effort to ward off succumbing to the patient's projections with countertransference acting out. I had been the subject of two massive projections from Ms. M.—the projection of the master and the other was the projection of the idealized, intimate partner. I had been resistant in some measure to exploring both of these projections. My resistance to the projection of the ideal sharer was clearly less intense than my resistance to holding the patient's life in my hands as a sadistic, powerful master.

One last form of countertransference acting out deserves mention. In response to either of these projections, a therapist may resonate with the patient and consequently feel vastly important to, attracted to, or seduced by the patient. The therapist may feel totally necessary to the patient's "going-on-being." The therapist may be swept up in the intensity of the projection and cross that thin, critical line between fantasy and reality in his or her own mind, enacting with the patient in reality the content of the patient's fantasy. I believe that many instances of inappropriate sexual or physical contact between patients and therapists take place between those patients who are fundamentally schizoid and those therapists who resonate with the schizoid projections.

REFERENCES

Masterson, J. (1983). *Countertransference and psychotherapeutic technique*. New York: Brunner/Mazel.

Masterson, J. (1981). *Narcissistic and borderline disorders: An integrated developmental approach*. New York: Brunner/Mazel.

Masterson, J. (1976). *Psychotherapy of the borderline adult*. New York: Brunner/Mazel.

Masterson, J. (1978). Therapeutic alliance and transference. *American Journal of Psychiatry, 135*, 435–441.

Masterson, J. (1972). *Treatment of the borderline adolescent*. New York: Wiley.

Masterson, J., & Klein, R. (Eds.) (1989). *Psychotherapy of the disorders of the self*. New York: Brunner/Mazel.

Masterson, J., & Rinsley, D. B. (1975). The borderline syndrome: The role of the mother in the genesis and psychic structure of the borderline personality. *International Journal of Psychoanalysis, 56*, 163–177.

Vygotsky, L. S. (1962). *Thought and language*. Cambridge, Mass.: M.I.T. Press.

CHAPTER 6

Shorter-Term Treatment

Ralph Klein, M.D.

The application of shorter-term treatment to the disorders of the self has long been a subject of controversy, and, for the most part, personality disorders have been viewed as incompatible with such treatment. Contrary to this view, Masterson and Klein (1989) have described the shorter-term treatment of the narcissistic and borderline disorders of the self.

There are several reasons why it is useful and appropriate to begin a discussion of specific therapeutic interventions in treating the schizoid disorder of the self with a focus on shorter-term strategies. Shorter-term treatment forces the therapist to focus therapeutic interventions in a systematic (even obsessive) fashion. The patients described here are those who were either suitable for shorter-term treatment or for whom shorter-term treatment was a reality-determined necessity. In either case, the techniques particular to the treatment of the schizoid disorder have to be implemented quickly and rigorously. For that reason, the techniques become highlighted when applied under the pressure of a shorter-term treatment approach.

Further, for many clinicians, the whole concept of shorter-term treatment of schizoid disorders represents an oxymoron. Nonetheless, a number of schizoid patients are well suited to the treatment approach. In reviewing the cases of schizoid patients with whom this therapist has worked over the past decade, approximately one third were treated with a shorter-term approach. The kind of schizoid patients treated and the reason for using a shorter-term model are exemplified by the following five patients. The first two are secret schizoids, the third is an avoidant schizoid, the fourth is a classical schizoid, and the fifth is best viewed as schizotypal.

PATIENT NO. 1. Mr. R. presented with the chief complaint that he was planning to be married in six months, and was experiencing overwhelming anxiety and ambivalence about this decision. He was constantly questioning himself, feeling that he could not decide whether marriage was the right or the wrong choice. Mr. R. was first described in Chapter 2 as an example of a secret schizoid, one who appeared to all as sociable, outgoing, and friendly, and who displayed none of the objective signs of schizoidness. What at first appeared to be a problem of an unwillingness to give up his freedom and settle down in a committed relationship (as his friends and fiancée viewed it) revealed itself to be a profound schizoid conflict.

PATIENT NO. 2. Ms. B. was also described briefly in Chapter 2. She had recently separated from her husband. Despite repeated attempts by the couple to live together, Ms. B. had concluded that it was not possible. Immediately after the separation, she said that she began to have "feelings that I had never experienced before." They included feelings of dread about being alone, experienced at times as paralyzing and terrifying panic. Ms. B. described her conflict as one of seemingly being caught between a rock and a hard place; she was able neither to live with her husband nor to live apart from him. Other frightening experiences included pseudohallucinatory hypnogogic phenomena that made her feel as though she were losing her mind. Ms. B. was also a secret schizoid. On the surface she appeared to her friends, and even to her family, as sociable, calm, "a rock of consistency," never depressed. Her separation anxiety and symptoms were almost as startling to her friends as they were to her.

Both Mr. R. and Ms. B. were relatively stable, successful persons with schizoid disorders who were presenting in crisis. Mr. R. was struggling with the anxiety associated with an incipient, anticipated master/slave situation (from which there would be no easy escape), and Ms. B. was struggling with the symptoms of a full-blown anxiety disorder, associated with the severing of an important attachment bond and with the anticipation of potential, isolation (intensification of her self-in-exile experience).

PATIENT NO. 3. Mr. F. had recently moved to New York, far from his family of origin. He said he had always felt extremely involved with his family, and yet strangely apart. His sense of involvement primarily consisted of his feeling that he was on call for his alcoholic father and detached mother. He had always been called on to provide whatever service either parent needed. However, part of him had always remained detached, and he saw himself as basically having always been on the periphery of relationships, a loner who would connect superficially to others but who knew that "when push came to shove, I had to be able to rely upon myself." He was surprised that the loosening of these chains of attachment (as he called them) to his family had created feelings of depression, even to the point of contemplating suicide. It was these acute suicidal feelings that brought Mr. F. to treatment.

Mr. F. satisfied all the intrapsychic criteria for a schizoid disorder and appeared as an avoidant schizoid. The acute loss of Mr. F.'s stable source of feeling, connected through the master/slave unit (chains of attachment), had led to the emergence of intolerable feelings of self-in-exile and of futility. As he stated it, "Living in New York is like living in exile." There seemed to be a need for quick intervention focused on his acute suicidal feelings, as he had seriously begun to plan a suicide attempt.

PATIENT NO. 4. Mr. C. was sent for treatment by an employee assistance program (EAP). He had been threatened with dismissal from his job if his behavior did not change significantly within three months. The immediate precipitant had been a verbal altercation with another employee who had been smoking in an elevator with the patient. Mr. C. had threatened to strike the offender. He had a history of incidents with other employees during the decade that he had been at his current job. This incident had been the "last straw" for his supervisor, who had placed him on probation and referred him to the company EAP. Mr. C. descriptively and structurally had a schizoid disorder, classic type. He had lived largely in his sadistic object/self-in-exile unit. When the stability of that unit was disturbed by events outside his control, he experienced an intolerable intrusion (activation of master/slave unit), and reacted with rage and withdrawal to the feeling of being endangered and devalued. Mr. C. was now in crisis—a crisis that he saw as being imposed from without, rather than as emanating from within, but a crisis nonetheless.

PATIENT NO. 5. Ms. Q. came to treatment with a mixed picture of anxiety and depression associated with hallucinatory experiences that seemed to be in the nature of ruminative or obsessional thoughts. Ms. Q. experienced this as "losing my mind" and "falling apart." The specific precipitant for those feelings was that she had been informed by her family that her invalid father was planning to live with her. A loner most of her life, she was 40, single, a virgin, and successfully employed in a job that required much travel. In response to the family's plan to have the father move in with her, she had experienced terror that was manifest by the symptoms noted. Ms. Q. still hoped ultimately to have a relationship, a companion in her life. Descriptively and structurally, Ms. Q. was a schizoid-disordered woman whose sustaining fantasy of attachment had been dramatically interrupted by the anticipated imposition of a dreaded master/slave relationship from which she felt powerless to escape. Her symptoms were increasingly paralyzing her, and she seemed on the verge of a psychotic decompensation with loss of reality testing.

Of those five patients who presented for treatment, four did remarkably well in relatively shorter treatments, none of which lasted beyond six months. Only one failed. Were there indicators of therapeutic success or failure? The main criteria of suitability for a shorter-term treatment approach can be summarized by the concept of "in and out." This means that the schizoid individual who presents in treatment with both clear and present internal and external conflicts is a potentially suitable patient for a shorter-term model. The "in" of "in and out," therefore, refers to the schizoid patient's experience of a disruption in a previously stable, intrapsychic structure. More specifically, it refers to a disruption in a previously stable compromise solution to the pressures and anxieties associated with the master/slave unit on the one hand, and the sadistic object/self-in-exile unit on the other. The interruption of a previously successful schizoid compromise (successful meaning stable and predictable) creates tremendous intrapsychic motivation for change in order to effect a new, stable, better compromise.

Four of the five patients described were internally motivated to change. Mr. R., Mr. F., and Ms. Q. all wanted to push away from exile toward greater connection and attachment. Ms. B. realized that her previous connection (compromise) had been unsuccessful, and that she needed a new compromise because her current state allowed her no calm or stability. Only Mr. C was not internally motivated to change, and he explicitly expressed the wish that he could get back to the way things had been before. As will become apparent later, this was not as simple as it had at first seemed. During the treatment process, it became evident that Mr. C. still harbored deeply buried hopes about the possibility of relatedness. However, it is doubtful that he would have initiated any effort toward consideration of greater connection had the external events not conspired to force him to do so.

At some point, all but Mr. C. would have acted on their motivation to push toward change. However, actual external events pushed them all to consider it. Mr. R.'s impending marriage, Ms. Q.'s family crisis, Mr. F.'s separation and move, and Ms. B.'s separation from her husband all served as acute external ("out") factors that encouraged reexamination and action in the moment.

The positive response indicators for shorter-term treatment with schizoid disorders of the self are, therefore, no different than for any disorder of the self. The presence of "in and out" (internal and external) motivators simultaneously pushes the schizoid patient to new compromise. If only one of the factors is present ("in *or* out"), the likelihood of the schizoid patient's taking up the challenge of change is far less.

What does the treatment process look like with these patients? The treatment process is defined in part by the patient's intrapsychic structure (what has to change) and in part by the overall treatment goal (the direction and objective of change). The patient's intrapsychic structure has already been described extensively. What are the general goals in the shorter-term treatment of a schizoid disorder? What are the direction of change and its objective?

    1. Lessen interpersonal (schizoid) anxiety.

Intrapsychically, this means helping the schizoid patient to experience a connection, a communication with another person (generally, but not necessarily, the therapist) that will not immediately result in the activation of the master/slave unit.

    2. Interrupt withdrawal and retreat.

Withdrawal, behavioral and affective, must be interrupted in order for the patient to take the risk and face the challenges associated with connection and with the inevitable accompanying sense of danger. Schizoid patients are all too willing to lessen social anxiety by withdrawal and retreat, and the myriad methods that they employ to do so much be interrupted.

    3. Promote interpersonal (social) communication or connection.

The less energy the person devotes to controlling the anxieties associated with either closeness or distance, the greater is the opportunity for shared interpersonal experience and the willingness to attempt to interface with another person (not the therapist) in a relatively safe, potentially emotionally gratifying fashion.

All three goals have an overarching, connecting thread: the objective of helping the schizoid individual to contain and manage the anxieties and dangers associated with the schizoid dilemma. None of the goals speaks specifically, or ultimately, to the objective of *eliminating* schizoid anxieties and dangers, or of *working through* the developmental determinants and origins of the schizoid patient's false self organization, so that the patient might be free of the wary vigilance that he or she must bring to the ongoing task of containing and managing the conflicts of his or her interpersonal world.

THE THERAPEUTIC PROCESS

Beyond the general goals, the therapeutic process involves the following steps to achieve those goals.

Step 1. Consensus Matching

The term "consensus matching" means that the patient sees that the therapist understands the schizoid dilemma. If there is a consensus between therapist and patient as to the nature of the schizoid anxieties, and the patient is aware of the therapist's knowledge of those anxieties, then the patient will feel that the therapeutic setting is less dangerous and risky. The patient has greater reason to hope and believe that the therapist will be respectful of the patient's anxieties. The patient will also be more aware of the effect that the therapist's words and actions have on the patient. How is consensus matching achieved?

First, the therapist must interpret the schizoid dilemma as soon as possible and as frequently as possible. The generic interpretation is: "*It seems to me that as you try to connect* (share, get close, communicate, take a risk), *you feel unsafe* (anxious, in danger, imposed on, intruded on), *and then you withdraw* (retreat, shut down, turn off, go into exile) *in order to feel safe* (free, in control, self-possessed, self-contained). *However, this place of safety brings with it its own anxieties* (dangers, alienation, isolation, disconnection, despair). This interpretation, either in part or in whole, should begin as soon as possible, even in the first session if it is indicated. The therapist can only convey awareness and respect for the schizoid patient's dilemma by openly and interpretively articulating that dilemma to the patient. Therapeutic patience is not enough. Respecting the patient's need to titrate his or her own risk taking by silence and acceptance is not enough. Allowing the patient to proceed at the patient's own speed is not enough. Active interpretation must complement the therapeutic stance. The therapist who conveys an understanding of the patient caught on the horns of the schizoid dilemma is taking the first and most important step toward consensus matching.

Second, consensus matching is further achieved by maintaining therapeutic neutrality. This fact is not altered by the length of the treatment (shorter-term or long-term treatment), by the content of the treatment (crisis or no crisis), or by the goal (containment or working through). Maintaining therapeutic neutrality, even in the face of an acute external crisis that might easily lure the therapist into wishing or acting to intervene in a more directive fashion, conveys to the patient the therapist's commitment not to step into the master/slave unit and not to impose the therapist's own agenda on the treatment. When the therapist "steps in" in this fashion, the schizoid patient feels, despite and regardless of the intent of the therapist, that he or she is being manipulated, coerced, imprisoned, and enslaved. Maintaining therapeutic neutrality conveys powerfully, as does the interpretation of the schizoid dilemma, the therapist's understanding of the nature of the schizoid anxieties. Of course, as with any patient, the presence of an acute internal crisis (that is, suicidality, homicidal intent, or psychotic decompensation) requires the therapist to take any and all actions necessary to protect the patient and others from harm.

A third technique to promote consensus matching is for the therapist to clarify the "in and out" aspects of the schizoid dilemma. The therapist must interpret the schizoid dilemma and the patient's anxieties associated with it in situations that arise not only in the therapeutic setting, but also in the patient's life outside the treatment. Equal attention should be paid to both. In so doing, the therapist conveys to the patient the therapist's understanding of the pervasiveness of the patient's anxieties and how they apply equally both in and outside of the treatment situation. This is especially important since many schizoid patients may present initially with the focus of their anxiety directed either toward being in treatment or toward their external conflicts and fears. The therapist should not be lulled into thinking if one is present, its counterpart is not. For the schizoid patient, anxieties are always present both inside and outside the treatment, even while the focus of conflict may shift from one to the other at different points in the therapy.

Step 2. Containment

What is meant by containment and how is it linked to consensus matching? Consensus matching promotes the patient's ability to conceive of a new distance in interpersonal relationships. It interrupts the fantasy or the expectation of inevitable enslavement or exile. The patient experiences less anxiety over potential appropriation into the master/slave unit, and is thus encouraged to interrupt his or her retreat. Flight into withdrawal and retreat, either exile, self-containment, or fantasy, is then interrupted. The desire and motivation to escape are also interrupted or contained. How is containment further promoted, encouraged, and accomplished?

First, the therapist must maintain a consistent interpretive stance. This means that the therapist, for the most part, will avoid using either confrontations or mirroring interpretations in the treatment of the schizoid patient. Confrontation will usually be experienced by the schizoid patient as an effort to impose an agenda and to manipulate and coerce the patient. For example, a confrontation of a schizoid defense might be, "Why do you pull back or retreat every time you take a step forward?" The content of this statement is correct; nothing else is. The borderline patient would probably hear such a statement as, "I support your impaired real self as it struggles to activate itself in the face of anticipated abandonment." The schizoid patients hears, "You should not pull back when you take a step forward." Such a statement immediately puts the schizoid patient on the defensive and propels the patient into greater withdrawal or compliance (enslavement). An agenda is being imposed, while, at the same time, there is acknowledgment, but no understanding, of the schizoid's dilemma. The first principle of consensus matching is violated.

Mirroring interpretations share a similar fate. For the narcissistic patient, the mirroring interpretation of narcissistic vulnerability is the road to feeling understood. For the schizoid patient, the mirroring interpretation is an unwarranted entry into the patient's internal world. For example, a generic mirroring interpretation would be, "It is so painful for you to focus on yourself that you turn to me in order to soothe the pain." Masterson (1993) describes the reaction of a narcissistic patient to this interpretation as, "I don't know how you do this, but somehow you slip in the back door and the next thing I know I'm thinking about something that makes me uncomfortable, and that I really don't want to think about". This is not the reaction of a schizoid patient. Mirroring is experienced by the schizoid patient as appropriating, while mirroring interpretations are intrusive and manipulative. In treating the schizoid patient, the therapist must always come in through the front door, and then only after knocking to make his or her presence known.

Maintaining a consistent interpretive stance that focuses on the patient's schizoid dilemma helps the patient contain the wish to withdraw defensively by making retreat no longer necessary. If the therapist is committed not to resonate with the master or the sadistic object representation, then the patient will have little reason to escape to the self-in-exile and will be able to contain the urge to do so.

The second technique for assisting the patient to contain the urge to withdraw and distance is to identify and clarify for the patient those efforts or tendencies toward retreat, both inside and outside the session. The principle is simple and well known: clarifying that there is a defense helps to interrupt the operation of that defense. In other words, when the schizoid patient is observed in a state of retreat, inside or outside the treatment, the therapist should bring this to the patient's attention. An example would be, "I notice that whenever you talk about feelings, you shut your eyes. I wonder what that means." This is neither a confrontation nor an interpretation; it is one of the numerous clarifications that helps to bring a defense or resistance to a patient's awareness. The therapist is making no judgment about the retreat that is taking place. The therapist is not pointing out to the patient the cost that such a retreat extracts in the patient's world, nor is the therapist empathically identifying such a retreat as a protection against painful self-exploration.

Another technique that will assist the schizoid patient to contain flight is to offer the interpretation that the patient's efforts at distance, withdrawal, or flight represent a compromise position, a compromise solution—in other words, a schizoid compromise. The interpretation of schizoid compromise is a central therapeutic strategy. This interpretation follows the interpretation of the schizoid dilemma as an anchoring therapeutic intervention, whether in shorter-term or in long-term, intensive treatment. Just as the interpretation of the schizoid dilemma integrates and conveys the therapist's understanding of the various anxieties that the schizoid patient experiences, so the interpretation of schizoid compromise integrates and conveys the therapist's understanding of the various defensive maneuvers on the part of the schizoid patient. An example drawing on that clarification would be: "I notice that whenever you talk about feelings, you shut your eyes. I wonder if this might not be a form of compromise, meaning that you want to talk about the feelings, but to do so while looking at me would feel too close. So you shut your eyes as a compromise. You can stay here and talk to me without feeling unsafe or in danger." The focus of the interpretation is on the defensive maneuvering and not on the schizoid anxieties per se. If the therapeutic moment were different and the therapist felt that the patient was withdrawing rather than compromising, the interpretation (of the schizoid dilemma) would sound different: "I notice that often when you start to talk about feelings, you shut your eyes and then fall silent. I wonder if you experience some anxiety talking about feelings with me, and so you shut your eyes and stop talking as a way of feeling safe again." (Whether the therapist would interpret the other side of the dilemma, the anxiety about being too far away, would depend on the therapeutic moment and the therapeutic consensus to that point.)

Interpretation of the schizoid compromise is essentially an interpretation that a patient's feelings, thoughts, or behaviors represent a compromise between the anxieties associated with too great a closeness and those associated with too great a distance. Interpretation of the schizoid compromise is an acknowledgment on the part of the therapist that a particular thought, feeling, or behavior serves that function, accomplishes that goal, and is selected by the patient as the primary way of managing to find his or her way safely between the dangers represented by the master/slave unit and those dangers associated with the sadistic object/self-in-exile unit.

The schizoid patient's anxieties are best understood by the therapist through the concept of the schizoid dilemma, and the therapist best conveys understanding to the patient through interpretation of the dilemma. The schizoid patient's defenses in reaction to those anxieties are best understood by the therapist through the concept of the schizoid compromise, and the therapist best conveys understanding to the patient through interpretation of the compromise. These two interpretations are the foundation of the therapist's understanding of what is theoretically and technically necessary to treat the schizoid patient. They allow the schizoid patient to feel optimally understood. Working in tandem, these interpretations are the twin foundations upon which a firm therapeutic alliance is built.

The discussion of schizoid compromise leads to the third and final step in the shorter-term treatment process.

Step 3. Closer Compromise

The concept of closer compromise means that the patient is able to experience the possibility of alternative, intermediate positions between the extremes of unbearable anxieties about appropriation and permanent exile. The patient is able to take risks by creating less interpersonal distance, and can attempt greater connection, communication, interfacing, or even sharing of ideas, feelings, and actions (acting in concert with others). Such efforts carry with them the possibility for achieving a more fulfilling and adaptive interpersonal (and intrapsychic) distance. Closer compromise means that while the vulnerability to the anxieties of the schizoid patient is not overcome, it is modified and managed more adaptively. The techniques associated with the achievement of this objective implicitly and explicitly acknowledge that vulnerability.

First, the therapist must continuously convey to the patient the idea that anxiety is inevitable, yet manageable. There should be no illusion that the schizoid anxiety and the vulnerability to such anxiety can be permanently dispelled or dispensed with—far from it. Such anxiety must be acknowledged and dealt with as best as one can. The patient is encouraged to tolerate greater and greater degrees of risk and danger in order to effect closer and closer relationships. The limiting factor is the point at which the danger becomes overwhelming and the patient must again retreat. In this process, far more interfacing with others may be possible, even though intense anxiety still lurks as an ever-present potential experience.

The second technique associated with the goal of closer compromise is a direct extension of the therapeutic stance of accommodation (anxiety is inevitable and must be managed) and focuses on the need for action. The patient needs to accept challenge, to endure risk, and even danger, by making efforts at connection or communication. This must be directly stated as the patient's responsibility. "It seems to me that in order to accomplish your goals, it is necessary to put yourself at risk," or "It seems to me that your willingness to come here (to treatment) and struggle with your anxieties must be mirrored by your willingness to challenge yourself outside of here," or "It seems to me that your efforts to connect with me are only half the battle; the other half must take place in the more dangerous arena of your life outside this office." Notice that several features characterize these interventions as hypotheses and clarifications rather than as directions. The therapist is always conveying that these are the therapist's impressions. He or she is not reading the patient's mind or imposing an agenda, but is simply stating a position. Also, the therapist's position is an extension of the patient's position or therapeutic wish ("your goals," "your willingness," and "your efforts"). Finally, the therapist specifically directs attention to the need for action outside the therapeutic setting.

The emphasis on action leads to the principle that equal attention must be paid by the therapist to the patient's efforts to connect and take risks both inside and outside the treatment setting. The therapist must watch what the patient is doing in the office and also in the greater world outside the office, respecting equally the pervasive nature of the schizoid anxieties and the pervasive ways in which the schizoid patient is pulled to compromise or settle for safety in both settings. The bottom line is action, because the willingness to compromise or settle for limited emotional supplies, fantasized or real, is a resistance or defense that is utilized more by the schizoid patient than by any other patient. A schizoid person will be inclined to nestle down within the relative safety of the therapeutic relationship. He or she is then likely to make it not the anchor of his or her efforts at relatedness and connection, but of all of his or her efforts in this area. The therapist who remembers the principle of divided attention will find it a useful platform from which to observe, monitor, and focus on the patient's inevitable, repeated slippage into compromise.

A final factor that contributes to the achievement of compromise is the continuing availability of the therapist. While this availability is implicit in shorter-term work with all patients should further conflicts or crises arise, in the shorter-term treatment of the schizoid patient another factor is at work. The therapist remains a beacon of attachment for the patient long after the treatment ceases. The patient/therapist relationship continues to function as a new, stable, safe, closer relationship for the patient that will afford protection against reexperiencing the feelings of enslavement in response to efforts at relatedness or the despair and futility associated with total isolation and exile. This function should be made explicit by verbalizing to the patient the therapist's availability for sessions, at the patient's request and not only should further conflict or crisis arise.

It should be emphasized that the steps described here not only are steps toward accomplishing the goals of a shorter-term treatment, but also are steps toward achieving a therapeutic alliance. A stable, solid therapeutic alliance provides the basis for a more adaptive and functional management of the schizoid patient's life, which is the goal of shorter-term treatment specifically, and the first goal of long-term, intensive treatment.

CASE ILLUSTRATIONS

Case of Mr. R.

Mr. R., a 22-year-old man, was planning to marry in six months, and had begun to feel extreme anxiety. He appeared outgoing and friendly, but there was a sense of wariness about him, which I attributed both to the anxiety he felt generally and to the stress of beginning treatment. It was with some surprise, therefore, that I listened to him describe in the initial session how he had always preferred "being on the outside of any commitment," and how he had been struggling with the decision to marry his fiancée for the three years he had known her. In briefly reviewing his personal history in that session, he remarked that he had always valued his independence highly. He described how he and his two brothers had practically raised themselves. "We were latch-key children," he said with equanimity. He was the youngest by a number of years, and had not been close to either brother. He stated that each brother preferred to go his own way.

His parents had been "not terrible, just disinterested." They were middle-class, hard-working people, and "just had no time for us." They had not been abusive or mean, rather, "They had, for all intents and purposes, not been there for me emotionally." He had felt close to a grandmother, whom he saw frequently. She died when the patient was seven years old, and Mr. R. recalled a defining life event around the fact of her death. Shortly after her death, he recalled waking at night terrified. He described the feeling as "total aloneness, a blackness that was overwhelming. I ran out of my room to tell my mother, but I could only stand before her shaking, unable to tell her what I was feeling. I felt that even if I found the words, she could not, would not understand. After a while she just turned her back and walked away." This experience was repeated, with minor modifications, a number of times until the patient was 10 years old.

Adolescence was remembered as generally a good time. He felt competent, did average work in school, had several friends, and went on to college. He commented in the initial session that he enjoyed solitary activities, since they gave him a feeling of freedom. For example, as a teenager he liked to get on his bicycle and ride alone for hours. When he was old enough to drive, his favorite activity was to drive, again alone, for hours, with a sense of pleasure and freedom.

He remarked that he had never discussed his future or his plans with his mother (his father died when he was 14), because he felt that she was not interested, or because "I had a vague feeling that something was wrong about it. I didn't want her to know. It was like her knowing would ruin it. I didn't want to hear what she had to say." He had met his future fiancée in college, where they had dated for almost the entire four years. He had graduated the previous year and was now living with his fiancée. He was unhappy with his current job, which he had taken essentially to earn money for graduate school. His plans were to relocate and begin school after the wedding. The decision to get married seemed to be mutual. Yet, having made the decision, Mr. R. began to have intense symptoms of anxiety.

This information was reported with relative spontaneity in the first two sessions. The only other significant bit of information was that he specifically indicated that he did not want medication. He wanted to be able to manage his anxiety "on my own."

Since there was clearly a limited period in which to conduct the treatment (approximately seven months or 25 sessions), I saw the need to make a diagnosis as soon as possible. I felt that the first hypothesis to be tested was that of a schizoid disorder. In short, the developmental history suggested that significant others were emotionally unavailable and were experienced as disinterested, unreachable, and potentially appropriating ("It was like her knowing would ruin it"). Distance from others, at times physically and at times emotionally, seemed to be a repeatedly mobilized defense and a readily assumed position. His relationship with his fiancée seemed beset with schizoid anxieties about being too close (marriage) and being too far away (letting her go and reexperiencing the anxiety of unplanned, uncontrolled aloneness). The importance of independence (self-containment and self-reliance) seemed to run as a thread throughout his life, from his childhood ("I valued my independence") to the session (his wish to manage the anxiety "on my own"). I decided to approach his presenting problems from the perspective that he had a schizoid disorder, was struggling with his anxieties, and had made an unsatisfactory effort at compromise.

The patient was late for his third session. He said nothing about his lateness. When I pointed it out, he answered that the traffic had been bad. I responded, "I like to share my impressions, my understanding of what I feel patients are trying to tell me. This way you know what I'm hearing and where I stand. I may be right or I may be wrong. I hope that you will tell me if I am wrong so that I can understand better. Let me tell you what my thought is now. I wonder if your lateness had a meaning. I wonder if you had become anxious telling me so much about yourself these past two weeks and decided to step back and get some distance, and if your being late was your way of doing that." My interventions have several purposes. In general, I want the patient to know that his or her words and actions have an impact on me, and that I am interested in what is being communicated. I am also interested in communicating my understanding to the patient. I am there, and I am interested. We are two separate minds trying to figure out where and how to interface. I have no need, however, to impose my understanding. I offer it as my experience of the patient and await confirmation or correction. I am not committed to an agenda. I want the patient to know where I stand. I am predictable, interested, curious, and concerned (the definition of therapeutic neutrality in the Masterson approach). If the patient is initially trying to establish a safe distance from (and with) me, one that is close, but not too close, then that process is facilitated if the patient knows where I stand. He or she can then experiment with where he or she stands (what the patient communicates or shares) in relationship to me without worrying about where I stand. Once these conditions of relatedness are established, I can begin to interpret the schizoid dilemma, in this instance, a broad, generic interpretation about the anxieties associated with connections and the need to regulate anxiety through regulating distance (this time by withdrawal in action, at other times by withdrawal of feelings or thoughts).

Mr. R. responded to my intervention by stating that, he had been apprehensive about coming to the session that day. Actually, he added, he had felt anxious, almost fearful. He paused. I asked him what he normally did with such anxiety or apprehension. My intervention at this point was purposeful. The patient had acknowledged the first part of my intervention, the existence of (schizoid) anxieties, but had repeated the defensive withdrawal by becoming silent. I wanted to demonstrate to him the fact of that withdrawal and focus attention on it in order to interrupt its operation. He responded, "Usually I just sweep it under the rug and go on. And if that doesn't work, I just close down."

We were already beginning to establish a consensus. I said, "It seems to me that when you begin to get close and reveal more about yourself, you begin to experience anxiety, even apprehension, about how the other person will react to you. Here the other person is me, but out there the other person may be your girlfriend. You seem to deal with the anxiety by shutting off the feelings, which is what I assume you mean by sweeping them under the rug or closing down." He said that was just the way he was, always keeping that distance. In fact, he went on, it was surprising to him that it was not working and that he had been experiencing such anxiety. Sometime, he said, "I wish I could just drop the whole thing—you, my fiancée—and just move to Hawaii. But at the same time, I don't really want to." He again fell silent for several minutes. I intervened: "You seem to have quite mixed feelings. On the one hand, sweeping things under the rug probably feels safe; on the other hand, maybe being under the rug doesn't feel so good. Maybe it has its own down side, its own anxieties, like feeling isolated." He nodded (consensus matching), but quickly defended, "Permanence, any permanence, scares me. It's hard for me to stay in touch. It is easier to let the feeling drift away." For my part, I was introducing the other half of the interpretation of the schizoid dilemma: the potential anxiety associated with the self-in-exile (under the rug).

This fundamental theme of the schizoid dilemma was repeated over the next several sessions whenever the opportunity presented itself. By the sixth session, the patient was increasingly talking about some of his earlier life experiences, all of which seemed to be related to some aspect of the schizoid dilemma. That kind of response makes it more likely that the interpretation is correct and is being integrated. Mr. R. spoke about getting little emotionally from either his parents or his brothers. There had been "no one to turn to, no one to ask." He told me that often his thoughts seemed simply to drift away, or he would become confused (depersonalization), or time would become distorted (derealization), or he would have private conversations in his own head for long periods (fantasy). He said, "I guess those are my ways of staying disconnected, of staying on the outside. I feel so uncomfortable when I think of permanence" (which for him meant connection associated with inevitable entrapment and enslavement). I took this opportunity to raise the concept of compromise: "It strikes me that your private conversations are not just a way of staying disconnected. They seem more like a compromise. They enable you to feel connected and disconnected at the same time."

In the next session, the patient told me something that he had never mentioned to anyone. He described how in his latency and preteen years he would spend hours each day playing alone in a large, empty refrigerator box that was kept in the basement of his home. In this box, he would construct elaborate plays, as well as conversations, in his head. This was the antecedent to his later flights of fancy on his bicycle and in his car, and to the private conversations that continued throughout his life.

Over the next two sessions, the patient returned to his memory of overwhelming panic with no one to turn to, which had begun at around the age of seven. He felt that this incident, with its sense of a total inability to communicate his feelings, of no one being there to respond to or understand his needs, was linked to his retreat into the refrigerator box. He elaborated on the fears of death and of the end of the world that often accompanied the episodes of panic. It was between the ages of seven and ten, as symbolized by these specific traumatic memories, that he lost belief in the availability of his parents ever to be there for him, to understand him and to love him.

He went on to describe how, over the ensuing years, he had increasingly experienced periods of having no feelings. He stated that he had countless "exits out of getting in touch with my feelings." And, he added, he thought that he would rather be a person who had feelings than one who had none. He then paused, and remarked that at the moment, he was feeling totally overwhelmed with anxiety about his fiancée and the marriage. He stated, "I'll be trapped by the permanence of it, and it terrifies me again." I intervened, "I suspect that getting in touch with your feelings pushes you out of the hiding place in your head, and potentially into thoughts about your fiancée and being with her. But being with somebody while feeling such intense need has never been a safe place to be. Like when you ran to your mother and she could not help. Being that close and that needy feels unsafe, more like a prison than a refuge."

He acknowledged this interpretation and elaborated, "It's times like this that I feel I have to get away. So I go inside myself." He paused at that point, and wondered aloud what he should do. "Should I feel? Should I commit myself? And if so, how? I'm trying to stay in touch a little longer with these feelings." He paused, and suddenly remembered an incident that had happened when he was 12 years old. He had been trying to convince his parents to get him a telephone for his room. Although he did not have many friends or plan to use the phone extensively, he remembered wishing very much to have one as a connection between himself and the world beyond his home. With sadness he reported that when his birthday arrived, his parents had actually bought him a phone, but the cruel irony was that it was an antique decorative telephone that was only for display and did not work. It was, in other words, a phone that connected to no one and over which communication was impossible. The session was over.

Mr. R. came in the following week for session 10, and was silent. He seemed to be drifting further and further away. After about 15 minutes of silence, I interrupted the withdrawal, noting, "You have been struggling with the decision whether to reach out, to take more risks. From the story last week it would seem you anticipate that some kind of cruel joke is out there waiting to be played on you by your fiancée or by me." He looked at me for another 10 minutes, and finally commented that it was easier to discuss these things with me than it was to discuss them with his girlfriend. I responded, "I'm sure it is, because I am much less potentially dangerous to you. You know that I have no particular agenda in my relationship with you because I am not a part of your world outside the walls of this office." In a long-term treatment, I would have accepted this comment, allowing a deepening alliance with me or fantasy about me to grow. But because of the limited nature of the therapeutic contract, I wanted to keep the patient focused as much on his relationship with his fiancée as on that with me.

In the following session (session 11), he stated that it had been an active week of feelings for him. He was surprised that it had not been bad or overwhelming, and, in fact, he had enjoyed the brief moments of longing he had experienced. He then told me that he realized he had "checked out" of his home, and away from his parents, when he was seven or eight years old. That was when he had become "independent." But it was an independence, he realized, that was born out of necessity, not out of choice.

This was a remarkable description of the self-in-exile: an attitude of independence born out of necessity, not out of choice.

In session 12, he said he wondered whether he would ever know what it meant to feel "intimately." He questioned whether he was really capable of having any feelings. He wondered whether he would ever want to take the risk of reaching out again. Then, after a brief pause, he said that he was again feeling nothing, that he had gone blank. I responded with an interpretation of the schizoid dilemma: "The more you share your thoughts, even your questions, with me, the more you experience some sort of anxiety or apprehension that seems to lead you to want to retreat again to your safe place of feeling nothing, of being blank."

The next two sessions were characterized by alternating efforts at connecting and withdrawing, both inside and outside the treatment. I would respond whenever possible with interpretations of the schizoid dilemma and compromise. In a typical interchange, Mr. R. told me about a particularly upsetting incident with his fiancée. She had raised the issue of whether they would buy a house after they were married. He had refused to discuss this with her, without providing any explanation. She had then been cold toward him for several hours. He had "gotten scared" at her silence, and had finally agreed to discuss his feelings about a house with her. Without any basis in reality, he felt that he had to "crawl back to her and beg forgiveness." He explained that it was now clear from this episode that his fiancée would use him as his mother had, and then ignore him when it suited her purpose. He was going to tell her that the marriage was off, but wanted to discuss it with me first. I responded, "Let me see if I have this right. Your fiancée brings up buying a house, which is a challenge to you to get closer and even more committed. You get scared at being trapped, so you withdraw from her without explanation. She responds to your withdrawal by getting angry, and withdrawing herself for a brief time. You, however, experience her silence as a threat to your feeling connected, and you feel tossed into emotional exile. You then get scared at her silence, which I think is that part of you that fears and does not want exile. But when you try to connect again by discussing the house, the feelings of submitting, even subjugating yourself, arise and you decide that exile is better than enslavement. Do I have it right?

He laughed, stated that I had said a mouthful, and decided that he would not do anything about the wedding plans until he figured out what I had just said. I laughed and said I thought that was a good compromise.

In the next session, he stated that he had decided that he and his girlfriend should live together for another year or two before making a decision about marriage. I responded that if he was doing this as a way of "treading water" and avoiding dealing with his anxieties, I thought his solution was a bad compromise.

In session 15, he told me that he had called his mother for the first time in many weeks. He was surprised at how upset he felt about "not caring more about her." He looked sad. He paused for several minutes, then looked at me and reflected that he felt I was forcing him to express feelings and he did not like it. I responded, "It seems to me that reaching out with your feelings, as you have just been doing, continues to feel dangerous and risky, as though you are being controlled, coerced, and manipulated. This is probably why you are feeling as if I am trying to 'make you' express feelings, when, in fact, I feel quite confident within myself that this is not my intent." (Again I am clarifying my position to the patient.) I continued, "I wonder if the feelings that you once experienced with your mother, as you have told me, are now being anticipated as potential experiences with me and with your fiancée. This is usually the time when you go inside, go blank, or start conversations in your head in order to feel safe." He responded with a striking description of the split object relations units of the schizoid: "When I am outside, I have no will to feel, yet when I am in, the place is very crowded and dangerous." I noticed that, for the first time, he was describing his outside place as one associated with a sense of discomfort, a place where he had "no will to feel."

Over the next several sessions, he more fully described the nature of his anxieties. He stated that his anxiety was a "physical thing at times, a tangible feeling, even a visual experience. It's a claustrophobic place and I feel afraid, unwilling to be with anybody. At other times, the anxiety is like a barren landscape, like a desert." This description of his outside place as barren, a desert, was further evidence of increasing dysphoria as he began to experience his exile more as a place of alienation and isolation and less as a place of safety or refuge. He wondered at this point, somewhat sardonically, whether his decision to marry had been a decision to live "in the desert but with someone" (that is, a better compromise). He adamantly reiterated his conviction that "being out was preferable to being in," that "being claustrophobic was worse than feeling detached."

I responded, "Living in the desert with someone strikes me as a compromise between being claustrophobic and trapped, on the one hand, and safe but alone, on the other. It seems to me that the critical question for your life is where you finally want to settle, both literally and figuratively." Identifying the compromise temporarily served to interrupt it, and led him to reflect more about the nature of his anxiety. He began to wonder whether he had always had his anxieties and fears. Were they, he wondered, "hard wired" into his system or had they gotten there because of his experiences? Had this patient been in a long-term treatment, these questions would open the door to the past and to an understanding of why he became the kind of person he was. But this was not intensive, long-term treatment; this was session 18 of a probable 25. His marriage date was five weeks away, and he had still not decided whether he was actually going to go through with the wedding. Therefore, I responded that in either case (hard wired or experience driven), and regardless of what had come first, the real question was whether he would take the risk and accept the challenge that comes with the effort to make a strong connection and communicate fully with another human being.

He responded by staying with the past, and he reflected, "My parents never explained things right to me; they never explained what was really going on at all. Perhaps it was that they just didn't want to hear me, or maybe that they could not really understand me, or maybe it was that they were incapable of understanding me." Obviously, the patient at this point was inclined to pursue an understanding of his "coming into being." In shorter-term treatment, the therapist must listen quietly without encouraging or discouraging the patient's exploration. The therapist allows the exploration to run its course and then returns to the here-and-now issues at hand. In this case, the patient returned by himself. He looked quite troubled during several minutes of silence, and then reflected that he was scared that "perhaps this marriage thing is driving me back to being disconnected. Everything seems to be spinning in my head."

I felt that his retreat at this point was due to his apprehension that perhaps neither I nor his fiancée, like his parents, could understand him. I said I thought he had heard my comment about risk and challenge as a possible command to take action, and I assured him that it was not. It was simply a reflection about how the world worked as I understood it. In other words, nothing ventured, nothing gained. But I knew, as did he, that the choice about how to "be," like the choice about how and when to proceed, could only be his. He replied that he was glad that I had said that, because if I had made a clear suggestion about what to do or how to be, then he would have been forced to do neither because the decision "would no longer have been mine. Even if it had been the greatest idea in the world, I would have had to reject it because it would no longer have belonged to me."

In sessions 19 through 21, the patient primarily talked about his battle with the state of being disconnected: "It's so easy and safe to be out there. Permanence, on the other hand, means commitment, which means potentially being trapped. I am constantly having to move in and out, in and out, to assure myself that I will not be trapped forever." He reiterated that his anxiety was about "sticking and never being able to be free, and also about spinning off and never being able to connect again." I reflected that his conflict was all laid out before him. He understood the anxieties and benefits that closeness could bring him, and yet was increasingly aware of the anxieties associated with distance. I added, "It seems to me that somewhere between these two places there could be a place that could be close, but not too close, a place that could be far, but not too far, a place where perhaps you and most people can live comfortably, even contentedly."

In session 22, the patient told me that he had decided to go ahead with the marriage, which was now only two weeks away. He stated, "I feel increasingly the pressure to go ahead. It is a pressure from within, not from outside, not from you or my fiancée, but from deep within myself." He said that when his girlfriend stated her wish to be closer to him, it felt more like an invitation and less like an intrusion. He reflected, "Fantasy has kept me company too much and for too long. I never truly liked being alone. I still don't. I sat in that refrigerator box for hours upon hours, but never truly enjoyed it. I just accepted it as the way it was and had to be. I guess that's what I've done most of my life. It's just the way things are, I would tell myself. Relationships were always like railroad tracks, always parallel, never coming together. That's the way it always has been and still is. What's different now is that I don't want it to be that way."

Over the next two sessions, the patient spoke of his relief at having made a decision and of his sadness at having to end the treatment. He recalled more memories. He remembered being sad as a child. Specifically, he recalled having a friend who had died of leukemia when the patient was around seven or eight years old. He linked the death of this friend to the experience of terror, aloneness, and maternal unavailability that he had described at the beginning of treatment. He realized he had never really felt attached to anything or anyone after that time, and he wondered if the feelings of sadness and disconnection had really started those many years ago. He commented that, in the previous week, he had experienced both anxiety and sadness when thinking about the end of the treatment, and had not felt disconnected from either. It surprised him. I reflected that rather than taking his old escape route, he was staying "in there" and wanted to struggle with the feelings.

In the next to last session, following the wedding, he commented that while he felt 70 percent connected to his new wife, he felt 80 percent connected to me. I stated explicitly that while the treatment was ending and he was leaving, I was staying in the same place, and if he needed to contact me in the future, he knew where I was.

In the last session, the patient concluded with the following: "I have been excited by this process. All the fears around change and decision. But now it is easier to deal with it all, the whole emotional part. Will I ever be emotionally attached to anything, to anyone, and not experience this anxiety?" (He is aware of his continuing vulnerability to schizoid anxieties, and wonders whether he will ever be free of that vulnerability.) He went on, "I find myself at times trying to go too fast, to do too much, too soon. It feels like I am going full tilt at times. Now I'm able to stop, to pull back, not all the way back, just to take time, to take a deep breath. To become more relaxed and then I can go back to it more slowly this time, steady. I am really trying to figure out relationships. When I am too close, there is still not a whole lot of 'I.' You know what I mean? Not a capital 'I,' it's more like just a small 'i.' Like I have become smaller, expose less surface to danger. When I am outside, when I am still having those conversations at times in my head, then I can still be all of me. But I don't want to live on a desert or in a refrigerator box. That's my decision. So that I must make room for others in my world. The way I want my world to be—it cannot be *either* you or me. It has to be you *and* me."

Case of Mr. C.

Mr. C. was the patient referred by his company EAP because of his threat to hurt physically another employee who had been smoking in the elevator. He was on probation, and a decision about employment would be made in three months.

When I first met Mr. C., he described himself as basically a shy and apprehensive person. He said he had always been that way. He stated that in situations where one could either hold back or go forward, he was generally the kind of person who held back. He stated that he really had no friends. In the past, he said, he had wished that his condition could be otherwise, and in some ways, he still did, but he had become used to having no friends, in large part because he had always found it difficult to interact with other people. This difficulty led him to feel and act in an isolated fashion. One of a series of jobs he had held in his adult life, he had been at his current one the longest, for ten years. His previous employments had also been terminated because of difficulty in getting along with his co-workers. He lived alone in his own home, in which he took great pride. Although he was in his late 30s, he was still a virgin and had had only two brief relationships. He had tried a series of dating services, but had never dated a woman more than two or three times.

In the first several sessions, Mr. C. was quite expressive about his feelings of being isolated and alienated. It was as if he were desperate to share these feelings with someone who could not hurt or threaten him and who had no real power over him. I had made clear to him that in no way would I communicate with the people where he worked. Their decision about him would be based on his behavior, performance, and what he told them, not on any report or evaluation that I would make, or on any contact that I would have with them. Perhaps because I made this clear, he was able to share very quickly his opinion that the deterioration of his behavior at work was, in fact, a significant problem. However, he stated, "I am not sure whether it is my problem or everyone else's problem." At the same time, he added that his personal life seemed dark and hopeless. Connecting his problems at work and in his personal life, he remarked that he was increasingly talking to himself at work. He often did this quietly under his breath; at other times, he spoke out loud. He remarked that this behavior had been one of his supervisor's concerns.

When I questioned him about this behavior, his response was succinct and to the point: "Talking to myself is better than talking to no one. Any communication is better than no communication at all." However, such longings were felt only episodically. Much more often he felt that he lived in the middle of an "emotional minefield," partly of his own creation and partly the creation of others. This minefield, contrary to what one might think, was really a safety zone, in the middle of which he lived. Around him was a 100-yard space that separated him from everyone else. Within this 100-yard radius were innumerable bombs that kept him safe from intrusion, because anyone who ventured into the area would be blown apart. However, this minefield also kept him from venturing out and contributed to his feeling of being alone and isolated. He described it as his safe place, which was half jail and half paradise. Although Mr. C. used the minefield as a metaphor, his depiction of his fantasy was so intense as to make it feel real.

I reflected back to him that he seemed to live his life on the horns of a terrible dilemma: "On the one hand, there is a wish to live safely, free from the intrusions and hostility of others. Yet, while this is a place of safety, at other times, it is one of extraordinary isolation and alienation. But if you attempt to reach out and make contact, which obviously part of you still wishes to do, there is a fear that such an effort will lead to your destruction at worst, while at best it will be a path to the unknown or the dangerous." I asked him how he was able to balance the pressure from both sides of his dilemma.

He responded that fantasy was his protection and his escape from other people. He said that his fantasies calmed him, and gave him a feeling of being in control. He revealed briefly the major theme of many fantasies, which was to be the leader of an expedition to the Amazon or the Arctic, where he would live with a small group of carefully selected colleagues. I reflected that his fantasies seemed to be a compromise between his wish to remain connected with others and to ensure his safety against unwanted intrusion. Interpretation of the role of fantasy as compromise tended to interrupt the compromise for a moment, and seemed to encourage Mr. C. to look again briefly at what possibilities might lie in real connection in real relationships.

This brief glimpse was made manifest by his willingness to look at what he might do at work to save his job. Yet it seemed that as soon as he began to consider these options, the specter of the master/slave unit loomed before him. He spoke in sessions 4 through 6 of his intense anxiety about authority and the attempts by authority figures to control him. He stated that, at times, his anxiety became a deathly fear of people generally and of what they would try to do to him. He reported that he had had those fears since early childhood. He remembered that it started with his parents, but that it included everyone. He felt that others were in control and that he could not communicate at all or talk his way out of any situation. Other people became larger than life, and more dangerous, huge and monstrous. This sense activated his fight-or-flight response, as he called it, which appeared either as withdrawal into fantasy or as explosive anger. Both had gotten him into trouble at work and in his personal life.

Most often, however, he felt defeated, immature, and strange. He felt that no one wanted to have anything to do with him, and that he just had to keep his distance and feel satisfied to be in a safe place most of the time, protected, with no one around. Authority, he said, was capricious and dangerous. I was less astonished by his powerful description of schizoid anxieties than I was by his willingness to communicate those anxieties to me. I assumed that it most likely was due to the combination of the clear, limited nature of our contact, his intense (albeit frustrated) hidden longing, and the ability of the interpretation of the schizoid dilemma to promote safety in the therapeutic relationship.

Therefore, I continued to interpret his schizoid dilemma at every opportunity. For his part, he continued to elaborate more and more on the experience of his self-in-exile. By the eighth session, he had described himself as being invisible, like an animal, subhuman, strange, weird, and "never being able to see the stop sign until after the accident has occurred." I would try to translate each description of his self-in-exile into relational language, in an effort both to interrupt the seemingly entrenched quality of his place of exile and to encourage potential efforts at interpersonal involvement. For example, when he would refer to his "animalistic, subhuman" behavior, I would respond, "I understand these feelings to be self-judgments, which place you so below or different from other people that you leave yourself only the option of remaining apart from others. You are telling yourself that you do not belong in the company of humankind; therefore, you deprive yourself of and excuse yourself from making any effort to be with others." In response to this interpretation, he reported the following dream at the beginning of the next session, the 11th: "I was digging and digging through a pile of manure until I finally found what I was digging for, which was a deeply hidden piece of gold."

I asked him for any associations he had to the dream. He responded that it had to do with what I had said in the previous session. He felt that it was valid. But, he added, he really felt that "to feel is to experience self-hatred. Self-control is the only true measure of self-worth." He defined self-control as keeping a safe distance from others. To change this behavior would be to make himself feel subservient and afraid. I understood and interpreted this to mean that any efforts at connectedness potentially activated the subservient (slave) role of the master/slave (relational) unit. He responded that to change his behavior was almost impossible. *He* said there was a core feeling that he was just not deserving, that to change would mean he was breathing air that others should be breathing. *I* felt his master/slave relational unit was ubiquitous in defining his interpersonal world. It was sealed so tightly that he did not even feel entitled to the air other people breathed. If the master/slave unit were activated by any efforts at relationship, he would be taking the risk of having the very air he breathed ripped from his lungs. In essence, relationship meant death. *I* said that I understood the extraordinary nature of his anxiety associated with making connections, and why he should try to escape at those times to a safe place or a safe fantasy. But, I added, I knew of no other way to get to the piece of gold but to dig for it, as he himself had expressed in his dream.

At the beginning of the next session, he reported another dream. He had been looking for a house. The house looked somewhat like an apartment, perhaps even like the therapist's office. There was an older man in the apartment. The man looked nice. But then the patient started to notice problems with the apartment. All of the doors had locks, except the back door. He thought to himself, "There is danger here." I interpreted this dream. "It seems to me that you are now feeling your fundamental dilemma about me, just as you have felt it about others in the world. I think you experience me as inviting you in to look around a new apartment, or a new world, or a new way of relating, but you fear that my invitation is really a ruse to trap you, and that the only way out of that trap is through the back door; in other words, retreating through your old escapes, to your old existence, your safe place." He acknowledged my interpretation with a nod, but said nothing else.

In the next session, he came in reporting that he had felt on edge all week—bitchy, estranged, confused, afraid, exploited, and ripped off. I interpreted that the more he shared with me and the closer he felt, the more dangerous it had become, and he was seeking ways out through the back door, specifically to his feelings of exile, which were manifest by his feeling confused, afraid, and exploited, just as before he had felt like an animal, subhuman and bizarre. He paused for several minutes. Then he asked, "Why am I acting like this? Why am I setting myself up? Why do I feel so confused? I can't get past that in order to approach. Why do I put off any possibility of change? Why do I do that?" The hope that the asking of these questions seemed to revive quickly receded.

By the next session (session 15), Mr. C. reported "being afraid, being much more afraid, having deeper fears than I have ever experienced. It is like an endless reservoir of fears." Briefly he wondered why he was so afraid, but he responded to his own question by stating that his reservoir of fear had filled over all the years of his life. It had been, he said, not one specific event that did it; it had filled day after day after day. I commented at this point that it had been my observation in life that often other people can play a role in helping to bail out a sinking ship or to drain an overflowing reservoir. I wondered aloud if there were not perhaps a better place between the prison of enslavement by capricious authority and the loneliness of the minefield. His response came from deep within the self-in-exile: "I'm afraid of myself. I'm afraid of living, afraid of growing. My fears are primal. It is like I have a reptilian brain and other people are malignant to me, malicious, capricious."

The three months were drawing to a close. Realizing that work remained to be done, I hoped that Mr. C. would continue in treatment after his probation period. I told him that over the next two sessions, but despair seemed increasingly present, and my interpretations had little impact. In the last session, his final words were, "I can make no peace with the world. I cannot fit myself into the world." He called me several weeks later to tell me that the final decision had been made at work, and he had been fired. He was going on unemployment and would spend some time at home thinking about what he wanted to do next. He ignored my invitation to call me to set up an appointment whenever he wished, and I have not heard from him since.

The contrast between Mr. R. and Mr. C. seems particularly striking and important. Mr. R. had been able to use the therapist as a participant in a potential, new object relations unit, one that stood in a realistic, healthy place between the master/slave and the sadistic object/self-in-exile units. The therapy could be an anchor for a new compromise between the extremes. As the therapist occupied a new place between the master and the sadistic object, so Mr. R. occupied a new place between slave and self-in-exile. For Mr. R., a better compromise was achieved, one that was not free of the vulnerabilities associated with the schizoid conflict, but was functionally able to transcend it. Mr. C., however, could not use the therapist or the therapy in this fashion. For a moment, I was that nice man who could potentially occupy a position between master and sadistic object. And for an equally brief period, he could occupy a position between slave and self-in-exile by reaching deeply within himself and experiencing the possibility of finding gold. Nonetheless, the therapy could not provide more than a momentary anchor for the hope of change. Why? For one thing, Mr. C.'s reservoir was filled to overflowing. Second, the time was too brief for the kind of work that Mr. C. needed to effect a better compromise. Third, the internal motivation for change had not been strong. Initially, it had been almost nonexistent, as Mr. C. had been responding only to his supervisor's referral. Still, the therapy had stirred some of the latent hope that lived deep within Mr. C., although it was too little and too late.

Cases of Ms. Q., Mr. F., and Ms. B.

Ms. Q. was the woman who feared that her father would move into her home, and that she would have to become his live-in nurse/slave and take care of him for the rest of his life. Over a nine-month course of treatment (36 sessions), she was able to accept her healthy entitlement to live in a position other than as a slave or self-in-exile. She said *No* to enslavement by refusing to take her father in. Instead, she offered to participate in finding alternatives, and when this was rejected, she reinforced her No by getting an unlisted telephone number. Equally important, she began to say *No* to exile, and began dating for the first time in her adult life. Content with the degree of freedom (compromise) she had achieved, Ms. Q. stopped treatment when her father entered a nursing home. Her psychotic features evaporated, as did her fears of having a nervous breakdown.

Mr. F. had recently moved to New York, was unemployed, and found it difficult to establish a new and better compromise apart from the ties to his dysfunctional family of origin. The severing of his family ties had led to near despair and suicidal preoccupation. Mr. F. responded dramatically to interpretation of the schizoid dilemma, and used the interpretation to propel himself into action. In the course of the 20-session treatment to which he had agreed, he set in place the conditions to effect the compromise he sought. He forced himself to seek work, which he found. He forced himself to seek social contacts. He joined a synagogue where he found a small group of single friends, and he stated that the new connections had dispelled his suicidal thoughts. With his schizoid anxieties intact, but armed with new understanding and a blueprint for action, he concluded treatment because he felt grounded, and stating, "I know where I stand in New York."

Ms. B., who had reacted with extreme anxiety following the separation from her husband, was also able to deal with her conflicts by effecting a better compromise, one that she felt consciously acknowledged both her wish for connection and her anxiety about being too close or too far. Armed with interpretation and understanding of the schizoid dilemma, she managed her compromise by agreeing with her husband that they would not proceed to divorce, but would make arrangements whereby they would live apart during the week and be together on weekends. This seemed an ideal arrangement for her and her equally schizoid husband. Ms. B. ended treatment after the arranged 24 sessions, content with her decision and free of the symptoms of anxiety. A year later, she called to ask for a referral to couples therapy, since she and her husband had decided that they wished to try slowly again to develop a closer relationship.

REFERENCES

Masterson, J. (1993). *The emerging self*. New York: Brunner/Mazel.
Masterson, J. F., & Klein, R. (eds.). (1989). *Psychotherapy of the disorders of the self*. New York: Brunner/Mazel.

CHAPTER 7

Intensive, Long-Term Psychotherapy

Ralph Klein, M.D.

A strong therapeutic alliance lays the foundation for therapeutic progress. The success of treatment, whatever the goals are, is directly related to the strength, stability, and capacity of the therapeutic alliance to anchor the therapeutic process. First and foremost, schizoid patients require a safe, non-threatening therapeutic alliance, one in which they do not feel that they have to battle for control. Rather, such patients require a therapeutic alliance in which they are truly free to establish their own distance and regulate the pace of their feelings, thinking, and acting.

The key word for schizoid patients is "safety." They must be certain that the therapist will not behave either as a master or as a sadistic object. The patients must be convinced that their transference acting-out distortions of the therapist as manipulative, controlling, dangerous, and devaluing are false. Much of the description of the treatment of the schizoid patient to this point has been devoted to helping the therapist address the patient's fears and distortions.

The therapist's interpretation of the schizoid dilemma allows the patient to feel understood and, therefore, safe. Interpretation of the schizoid dilemma is to the treatment of the schizoid patient what confrontation is to the treatment of the borderline patient and what mirroring interpretation of narcissistic vulnerability is to the treatment of the narcissistic disorder. It is the fundamental therapeutic intervention that converts transference acting out to therapeutic alliance and transference. The therapeutic alliance is a new object relations unit, a newly negotiated and implemented intrapsychic and interpersonal relational contract, that stands between transference acting out and transference, providing a clear view of both.

The therapeutic alliance is the most critical intrapsychic and interpersonal condition necessary for working through to take place. Once the alliance is forged, the process of working through is remarkably similar from one disorder of the self to another. The fundamental role of the therapist as facilitator of the process is the same in many ways whether the patient is borderline, narcissistic, or schizoid. It is during the working-through phase of intensive therapy with any disorder of the self that the concept of the therapist as a guardian of the process is seen most clearly. As the patient continues a process that has been set in motion by the creation of the therapeutic alliance, the therapist's main task is not to start the patient off or keep him or her going, but to keep the patient from swerving off course and becoming detoured or bogged down.

Working through is a concept that has been used extensively in the practice of dynamic psychiatry. Its meaning, in the Masterson Approach to the psychotherapy of the disorders of the self, is intimately tied to the concepts of the real and false selves and the abandonment depression. Drawing in part on the terminology provided by Winnicott, Masterson has defined the *real self* as the most spontaneous and creative aspects of self organization and as the experience of the self with others. In a disorder of the self, the real self is forced off the normal, healthy developmental pathway to actualization because of the overwhelming need to construct an alternative pathway, the false, defensive self. This *false self*, no longer spontaneous and creative, is primarily reactive. It is a self organization and an intrapsychic and interpersonal experience of the self with others, which must first attend and respond to the pervasive, ubiquitous impingements and needs of the object, not the self.

The false self should be contrasted with the *impaired real self*. The impaired real self is the term used operationally to refer to all of the deficits in real self organization that result from the developmental detour. This concept, together with the associated abandonment depression, lies at the core of all the disorders of the self.

The abandonment depression is an overarching, umbrella term devised by Masterson to describe a number of different affect states, all linked by the patient's experience of having to give up his or her spontaneous, creative self and then having to live according to the conditions imposed by the false, defensive self facade. Abandonment depression is a generic concept for describing the experience of a person who goes through life primarily reacting to the needs and impingements of others. However, it is far more complex than the notion of simple reactivity, encompassing also the concepts of dysphoria, distress, and despair.

In attempting to reflect the intensity of the affect states generated by a person's need to live so conditionally, Masterson (1972) long ago described the affects associated with the abandonment depression as the "psychiatric horsemen of the apocalypse." This powerful expression attempts to convey the affective experience of a person who lives under the conditions and proscriptions imposed by the false self. The range and quality of affects associated with the abandonment depression may vary somewhat from one disorder of the self to another, depending on whether the patient is narcissistic, borderline, or schizoid. Nonetheless, there is a great deal of overlap. Dysphoria, distress, and despair are all held in common. More specifically, suicidal depression and homicidal rage lie at the center of all of the abandonment depressions. Depression results from having to live incompletely and falsely, and rage follows from always having lived with imposed conditions, which leave the patient with no alternative but to conform. In working through the abandonment depression, both depression and rage inevitably appear as the patient remembers, feels, and understands the conditions of his or her coming into being and of the creation of the false self, and recognizes the need to dismantle the false self.

Other affective components of the abandonment depression also may vary. For example, in working through the abandonment depression of the borderline patient, it is evident that there is a vast reservoir of such feelings as helplessness, panic, fear, and guilt. The therapist should remember that these feelings are not just defensive operations of the false self, but also are descriptions of what the borderline patient feels he or she is like and what he or she contains; in other words, they reflect an experience of the patient's self-identity. For the narcissistic patient, shame, humiliation, envy, and emptiness coexist with depression and narcissistic rage to give the abandonment depression a unique quality, different from that of the borderline patient. Finally, the abandonment depression of the schizoid patient has its own "emphasized" affective components alongside the fundamental depression and rage. These components are intolerable anxiety, alienation, isolation, longing, devaluation, deprivation, and danger.

In the process of psychotherapy, one sees a two-tier effect. At the first level or tier, the patient is operating according to the false self. The false self displays the compensatory, conditional operations that the patient has used to ensure that he or she receives acknowledgment, affirmation, and approval from the intrapsychic and interpersonal other. As the defensive and compensatory operation of the false self becomes identified and clarified in treatment, the patient becomes increasingly aware of the mal-adaptive aspects of the false self. The patient then goes about attempting to find better ways of negotiating his or her relationship with the external world, ways that are more realistic and adaptive. The focus of therapeutic activity at this first level is on new and better negotiations with the exter-nal world. The impaired real self still exists. New ways of behaving are em-ployed to deal with old ways of feeling and thinking. Such a focus may re-sult in enormous gain for the patient in terms of successful functioning. It leaves fundamentally unchanged the old ways of feeling and thinking (the impaired real self), as well as the affects associated with those feelings and thoughts (the abandonment depression).

Working through is the second tier of psychotherapeutic work. Its goals are to change fundamentally the old ways of feeling and thinking, and to rid oneself of the vulnerability to experiencing those affects associated with old feelings and thoughts. A new therapeutic operation is called for: re-membering with feeling. What exactly needs to be remembered? One must remember with feeling the coming into being of one's false self. This means that one must remember with feeling the conditions and proscriptions that were imposed on the patient's ability and freedom to experience the self and the self with others. Ultimately, remembering with feeling leads the patient to the understanding that he or she had no choice in the process of becoming. The patient did not have the opportunity to choose from a selection of possible ways of experiencing the self and of relating to others. Rather, the patient had few options, if any. The false self that emerged was simply the best, and often the only, way in which the patient could experi-ence repetitive predictable acknowledgment, affirmation, and/or approval (the emotional supplies necessary for emotional survival), while warding off the affects associated with the abandonment depression.

If the goal of first-tier therapy is for patients to understand that they *are not* the way they appear to be and can act differently, then the goal of second-tier therapy, working through, is for patients to understand who and what they are as human beings, what they truly are like and what they truly contain. The goal of working through is not achieved by the patient's dis-covering some hidden, fully formed emotional homunculus, talented and creative, living inside. Working through is the process of slowly freeing one-self from the shackles of the abandonment depression in order to have the opportunity to uncover a potential. It is a process of experimentation with and experience of the spontaneous, nonreactive self and the self in rela-tionship with others.

The working through of an abandonment depression is a complicated, lengthy, and conflicted process. It is an enormously painful experience, in terms of both what must be remembered and what must be felt. It involves a mourning, a grieving, for the loss of the illusion that the patient had support for the emergence of the real self. The reality is far different. Ironically, it is also a mourning for the loss of an identity (the false self), which the patient constructed and with which he or she negotiated much of his or her life. The dismantling of the false self means letting go or relinquishing a way of being that has been, in a sense, all that the patient has ever known of himself or herself. Just as a bad relationship may be preferable to no relationship, so, too, a bad experience of the self is often better than no stable, organized experience of the self, no matter how false, defensive, or destructive that experience (or identity) may be. This dismantling of the false self in terms of its historical roots, as well as its reenactment in the present, is another fundamental component of working through. Dismantling the false self leaves the impaired real self with the opportunity to convert its potential and its possibilities into actualities.

It bears repeating that for the schizoid disorder, as for all the disorders of the self, treatment on the level of the first tier (reparative work) is not just patchwork. The patients described in the previous chapter were able to effect important changes in their relationships with others and to structure their worlds in ways that would allow them to be happier and far more successful.

The process of working through, however, brings with it its own unique rewards. Perhaps the most important element in the new self-awareness of schizoid patients as they work through the abandonment depression is the growing realization that they have a fundamental, internal need for relatedness, which they may express in a variety of ways: "I really understand that I want to be with other people," or "I really know that I want to be cared for," or "I want to be in relationship, to be connected." It is only through the working-through process that schizoid patients will understand with a certainty that this desire is at the core of their natures.

This feeling should be contrasted with the outcome of tier 1, or reparative work. Many schizoid patients will understand as part of the reparative work that a preferred solution (compromise) to the schizoid dilemma is being in relationships. Only schizoid patients who have worked through the abandonment depression, however, ultimately will believe that the capacity for relatedness and the wish for relatedness are woven into the structure of their beings, that they are truly part of who the patients are and what they contain as human beings. It is this sense that finally allows the schizoid patient to feel the most intimate sense of being connected with humanity more generally, and with another person more personally. For the schizoid patient, this degree of certainty is the most gratifying revelation, and a profound new organizer of the self experience.

Case of Mr. X.

Mr. X., age 40, presented for treatment at the conclusion of a somewhat stormy, ungratifying relationship over the prior 10 years. Despite the on-and-off nature of the relationship, he was quite distressed about its final demise. He stated that while he felt that his partner had always been controlling and manipulative, he had permitted it because "it was better to have this relationship than not to have any relationship at all." "Besides, he added, "compared with what else is out there, it didn't seem so bad. At least I felt alive and excited at times." At this point, however, he was able to say that he felt quite conclusively that he could no longer tolerate his lover's seeming need for total control or his own feeling of being invisible and unimportant in the relationship. "It is one thing to let her call all the shots; it's another to have to totally disregard my own feelings all the time, to feel like her servant, like a dog waiting for her to throw me some crumbs from the table." He continued, "I know it is better without her, but I worry that there is no one else out there. I'm not sure that I care if there is. Most of the time, I don't care. But when I do care, when I feel anything, it is loneliness. Maybe a little sadness."

Mr. X. had had a turbulent childhood. His parents separated when he was four years old. In retrospect, the patient wondered whether his mother had ever really wanted to have him. It was not, he said, so much that he felt that she had actively disliked him as a child. Rather, it was more that he felt like an intrusion with which she was not prepared to deal or tolerate. Early memories were sparse, but two stood out. One was of simply lying in his crib, playing with a toy horse. He knew there was no point in reaching out between the bars of the crib because no one would be there. In the memory, he did not care. He was content to play with the horse. The second memory was of repeated scenes of battling with his mother over his refusal to eat. He remembered that at times he would submit, while at other times he would clench his teeth and refuse. In either case, he felt "attacked," "under siege," and "like I was fighting for my life."

Following the separation of his parents, the patient lived with a series of relatives. This seemed to reinforce for him the idea that he was just a bother, too much for either his mother or father to handle. No home became permanent. He remembered moving frequently, often after only a year or two.

Although he lived at the homes of relatives, he always felt like a stranger. He kept to himself a great deal, attracting little attention or concern. He remembered feeling lost and unhappy, when he felt anything at all. There was nothing abusive about the homes where he lived, and his mother or father would visit regularly. Still, "I was always the fifth wheel, always on the outside looking in, never truly invited by any of my relatives to be a member of the family. Even if I had been, I'm not sure what I would have done. At times, I felt angry and ashamed, and in the early years, wanted to be back home, but more of the time I just didn't care."

He recalled that around the age of seven or eight, while living with a distant relative, he decided that he could find little solace in the presence or comfort of others. He retreated at that point into a rather extensive personal world of creative fantasy. He would play with the few possessions that he took from home to home, but more than that, he absorbed himself in drawing. He would occupy himself for hours with this interest, drawing pictures of superheroes to accompany the stories he wrote. The combination of his creative play, drawing, and writing created a safe haven, a resting place from the disappointments and feelings of unimportance and alienation that pervaded his real world.

The impact of the many moves throughout childhood and adolescence was profound. Their effect was demonstrated most dramatically and poignantly in one recollection from a time in late childhood, probably around the age of nine or ten, when he had moved to a new relative in a new neighborhood. He was dropped off at school the next day, but after school, he realized he had no idea of how to get to his new home. He wandered the streets for hours, feeling totally lost, confused, and despairing, "like an alien dropped into an unfamiliar, unfriendly, and unresponsive land." After many hours, as night approached, he went to the door of a house and tried to explain his situation to the woman who answered. He found he could say nothing. He just stood there; he could find no words. Through the intervention of the police and the school, his home was located and Mr. X. was able to return there.

Throughout these years, Mr. X. remembered never quite feeling a part of anything. He developed a few friendships, but always with the anxious anticipation that the attachments would end if he had to move again. He remembered some of these friends and how much he enjoyed the brief times he shared with them. Increasingly, however, even these feelings faded as he retreated more and more into his own private world. During this time he was usually viewed by others (family, friends, teachers) as a cooperative and friendly, if somewhat quiet, young boy.

At the age of 14, he returned home finally, to spend some time with his mother. By then, he had not heard from his father for several years, and he seemed not to care. In general, he reported feeling little about anything, including being back home with his mother. There were episodes of arguing with his mother, but for the most part, the relationship was distant. He always managed to do well in school, and he was able to graduate and go onto college.

The college years were recalled as a painful time. He felt as if they were one more displacement. He was isolated from those around him and became increasingly uncomfortable in the presence of others. He put his drawing aside and began to drink heavily over the next decade, from the age of 20 to the age of 30. He said that the drinking helped him to get through college. It also helped him to lose the first several jobs he held after college as an architectural artist and designer, a profession that allowed him to work on his own for the most part.

During and after college, he had some relationships with women, mostly of a sexual nature. He did not feel close to anyone. His relationship by proxy during that period was with alcohol. Until the age of 30, he largely lived (existed) in exile. He mobilized all sorts of resources in order to be able to self-regulate. When self-regulation through interest and talent seemed insufficient, he used alcohol to keep him further apart from his abandonment depression and from others. He viewed other people as potentially depriving, devaluing, harmful, or threatening. As a child, he had often lain in bed at night frightened by shadows on the walls; he still felt, he said, "People were like those shadows. Ominous, unclear. Always threatening harm, but not actually doing it."

Finally, at the age of 30, his drinking was causing medical problems and he began to attend Alcoholics Anonymous (AA). He found such involvement intolerable. Although he could sit quietly and listen to others, he felt unable to participate. Soon just the presence of others became too uncomfortable for him to continue. However, during the brief period he was attending meetings, he met the woman with whom his breakup had inspired him to enter treatment. Mr. X. substituted the relationship with the woman for that with alcohol, and he was thus able to detoxify himself and remain abstinent. The relationship allowed him enough of a feeling of connection that he could hold a steady job, stay free of alcohol, resume some creative art work, and feel safe.

Essentially, he had effected a compromise on his own, one that was better than alcohol, with a woman who seemed to require or demand no greater intimacy than their on-and-off relationship offered. It was a relationship that avoided the extreme of closeness and entrapment and that of endless alienation.

Nonetheless, it was a compromise. While it was better than alcohol, schizoid anxieties still raged. Lovemaking was a typical battleground. Mr. X. spoke of how he found it easier to approach his girlfriend than to allow her to approach him. He could put his arms around her and feel tolerably close and safe, but if she were to put her arms around him, he would immediately feel endangered. It was as if they were not her arms, but chains being wrapped around him. They did not hold him and give him comfort; they trapped him and made him feel imprisoned and hopelessly anxious.

The final breakup was precipitated by the girlfriend's wish to live with him. Mr. X. was not ready for such a move, seeing it as the "final nail in the coffin. Now her control would be total. There was no way I could allow that to happen."

During the initial period of treatment, several issues arose around establishing conditions of safety. Mr. X. made it clear that he did not expect nor would he tolerate being told what to do. He stressed this, he said, because in a previous treatment experience the therapist, as Mr. X. saw it, had felt that he knew more than Mr. X. did and intended to impose his views. Actually, the therapist had suggested to Mr. X. that he make no final decision about his relationship with his girlfriend until he understood better what had happened. This apparently good advice was seen by Mr. X. as the therapist's need to impose his agenda. Therefore, "I had no choice but to end the treatment after three sessions." I understood the danger for Mr. X., and I felt forewarned.

Mr. X. also soon made it clear that he needed to follow me into the office rather than allow me to follow him in from the waiting room. The first time I did that, Mr. X. stopped and insisted that I go first. He explained, clearly and directly, that he felt too uncomfortable with me walking behind him. For a long time, Mr. X. described this as simply feeling "unsafe." It was not, he stated, any specific feeling or thought of danger. I stated to him that it seemed an ideal way for him to know exactly where I was at all times. I suggested that it was also a symbol of his need to know my exact whereabouts at all times. Thus he was able to monitor not being too close to me, and yet not being too far away. I concluded that then he could feel comfortable and in control. He agreed with this initial attempt at interpretation of the schizoid dilemma (and schizoid compromise), and said it felt right to him.

Throughout the treatment, Mr. X. always needed to know where I was, both literally and figuratively. He needed to be able to set the distance from me that he could risk, whether it was physical distance or, as it became more evident later in the treatment, emotional distance. These initial opening moves, which reflected his need to control the situation and to set clear boundaries and distances with me, were instrumental in allowing him to take the first steps toward building a safe alliance.

Early in the treatment, he described his relationship with his girlfriend in great detail. He said he was consciously aware of, and surprised by, the extent to which he felt detached from his feelings about her and about the treatment. I interpreted the schizoid dilemma, and I reflected that it seemed to me that he had been threatened by his girlfriend's wish to move in. This was a closeness for which he was not prepared, and he reacted in the way with which he was most familiar: he retreated. He agreed, saying, "For the first time since we split up, I feel sad right now." Then he fell silent. After a few minutes, he commented that he was not thinking of anything and that his mind had gone elsewhere. I wondered if, in discussing his retreat, he perhaps had felt that he had gone too far. Perhaps he felt disconnected, and that was one of the reasons why he had resumed treatment, that is, in order to feel some sort of safe connection again. Further, I wondered if sharing too much about his feelings about this woman with me made him feel trapped in our relationship, and if part of his detachment in the treatment was to protect himself by carefully controlling and titrating his connection to me.

In response to this and other interpretations, he was able slowly to share his feelings of hurt and rawness in his relationship with his girlfriend. Her demands and control had become so intolerable that he felt he wanted to die. It was then that he decided to break away and enter treatment. This was a surprising revelation to him on two counts: first, because he had forgotten the suicidal feelings of despair, and second, because he had not expected to share those feelings with me. This feeling, identified in the first months of treatment, later would provide the door into his early childhood suicidal feelings and despair.

He reported that he had felt disconnected from his girlfriend to a distressing degree throughout the relationship, and he began to wonder how much this really had to do with her at all. He reported that, while growing up, he had had similar feelings about his mother. He said, "Even when we were together, it was like she zigged when I zagged. We never really connected. Never. We were always going in opposite directions." He remembered this as a thought he had had when he was four or five, in the period just prior to the parental separation and his exile.

In the second year of treatment, he would increasingly relate memories and feelings from childhood and the present. While he took more risks, gained more access to feelings, and shared more with me, he also always protected himself. Often he would follow a new communication with the statement that perhaps he should stop coming to treatment, or that it was time to stop, or that he had gone as far as he could, or that he no longer needed treatment. The variations on the basic theme were many. My response was always the same. I would interpret these comments in terms of his dilemma, that he had shared with me important and meaningful information about himself and then the sharing began to feel dangerous to him. At that point, he would feel the pull to retreat, and would contemplate distancing himself from me once more. My comments clearly indicated to him that I understood the terrible anxieties he had and the dangers to which he felt exposed. These interventions would interrupt his defense and allow him to reconnect.

Over time, as the therapeutic alliance grew, the patient would communicate more of how he perceived himself. There was a heavy emphasis on his feelings of badness. He wondered what had been wrong with him that had caused him to be treated and dismissed in such a fashion. He wondered where he had failed in what he had to do in order to be loved by his parents. At points in his reflections, he would stop and wonder whether such bad feelings about himself were in some way meant to "confirm her (mother's) view of me" (resonate with her view of him) or to "take over her fears and make them mine" (resonating with her view of herself). In either case, he said, he wondered if these were the only options left to him in order to feel connected to her. Typically, after sharing this kind of observation, he would follow it almost immediately with the expression of feelings of frustration, confusion, or of wasting time. Interpretation of the schizoid dilemma would promote further working through.

As he gradually began to explore more of his struggle over closeness and distance, he was able to use the therapeutic relationship as an entry point to understanding different perspectives on his past. For example, at the beginning of the third year of treatment, he remembered more clearly the times his mother visited him. He remembered how he would watch her from a window until she drove away. However, by the time he was around seven or eight years old, he had stopped looking for her and would ignore her when she approached. He commented that somehow this seemed connected to his need to keep me in sight at all times. It represented both his fear that I would not be there as someone on whom he could count and his wish to get closer and to feel more connected.

Later in the third year, as the therapeutic alliance continued to strengthen, the patient would report more intense struggles to remain connected to his feelings and his memories. He remembered that around the age of five or six he would consciously and repeatedly say No to himself: No to his own feelings, No to allowing himself to feel any hurt, No to allowing himself to feel despair or hope. No was his mantra, his signal to disconnect. In the session following the sharing of his mantra, Mr. X. reported a dream. At various stages in the working through, certain dreams occur that seem to signal that the patient is at a crossroads where he or she must decide once again whether to go deeper into memory and feelings, or to strengthen new defenses and new, better compromises. These two therapeutic pathways are not mutually exclusive. In fact, a period of strengthening defenses is often a necessary and vital preparation for deeper and more painful exploration. The capacity to work through should never outpace the capacity to defend in a timely and appropriate fashion. Yet there are critical points in the treatment process where the schizoid patient must decide *either* to continue the working through *or* to defend.

MR. X.'S DREAM. In his dream, Mr. X. was in the basement of a house with a man whom he thought might be me. We were preparing to dig up the floor of the basement. The sense he had was that we would dig until we reached China. All of a sudden, he begged me not to start digging. He felt there was so much pressure under the floor that if I were to start to dig, it would blow up, perhaps killing both of us. After yelling for me to stop, still uncertain as to what I would do, he raced away and flung himself out of a basement window to safety.

MR. X.'S ASSOCIATIONS TO THE DREAM. Mr. X. commented about the obvious distrust that was manifest in the dream, which he still felt consciously much of the time. In addition, he reflected on the fact that he continued to stop his own creativity and potential by becoming frightened, unwilling to dig, and then trying to escape. Throwing himself out of the basement window (safe escape) became a metaphor in the treatment for his distancing to get away from the unthinkable anxieties of his schizoid conflict.

At the same time, the therapeutic relationship increasingly became a window through which to view the past. The very fact of his coming and going from treatment led to more memories and feelings from the times when his mother had picked him up and dropped him off after visits. He felt she had little regard for either his safety or his feelings. He recalled feeling torn apart, agonizing, hating every moment of being with her, as well as those of being without her. He began to both experience and remember the volcanic rage within himself that he had "capped off" at the age of seven or eight, and which he was reexperiencing for the first time (this was the pressure under the floor in the basement).

The schizoid patient's seeming detachment from feelings should never be accepted as the real state of affairs. As Mr. X. dramatically began to demonstrate, once he was able to move closer to his feelings and become less distant from himself, the full volcanic nature of these feelings became obvious to both of us. The more he experienced the force of his feelings, primarily overwhelming sadness and rage, the more he was driven to want to drink again or to retreat into fantasy (especially) in order to gain some distance from himself and from me. However, rather than act, he would usually talk—and feel. Although I expressed clear interest in his fantasies, especially as they might involve me, he seemed unwilling to elaborate in any way, and I waited patiently for him to be willing to do so.

At times he would become preoccupied with his work or his art, both outside and inside the sessions. Sometimes these activities seemed to re-fuel him. At other times, they seemed clearly to function as escape hatches, or compromises. When they felt like compromises to me, I would identify them as such to him, suggesting that they were a way to stay connected, but at a safe distance.

Not infrequently, he would become upset at these interpretations because they made him feel boxed in. If healthy defenses were compromises and unhealthy defenses were no longer acceptable to him, then the only path to follow was further working through. Once he exploded in uncharacteristic anger at me following an interpretation, and he said that what he was doing was not a compromise or a distancing. In fact, he argued, he felt like he was being "sucked in" by me and was losing himself. It took all his energy not to succumb to me. I interpreted at this point that identifying and interrupting his efforts at compromise left him feeling momentarily in danger of precipitously and prematurely being sucked into a closeness that felt intolerable and overwhelming, a resurrection of his master/slave fears. He nodded in agreement, fell quiet, looked at me, and said that he was struggling to stay present.

More and more, I was able to identify aspects of experience as residing in the realm of schizoid compromise. These included compromises, particularly around brief relationships with women, that lacked any sense of closeness, depth, or commitment. Remembering one of his childhood fears, I interpreted that he seemed tempted to settle for the shadow of a relationship rather than continuing to take the real risks necessary in sharing more, whether with friends or with more intimate partners.

As compromises slowly fell away, painful and intense feelings increasingly emerged. Fantasies took on a more central role in his life. These fantasies appeared to function less as an avenue for escape and more as a vehicle for expressing feelings. He began to be aware of new and unusual physical sensations, which he imagined and interpreted as physical manifestations of feelings. For example, on one occasion he described the sensation of wanting to press his mouth against his hand in order to alleviate the aching or pressure he felt in his lips. He described this as a sensation of wanting to suck, of wanting to see how it felt to do so. As he reflected on this, the very thought made him salivate. He associated this reaction to very early memories of the only person for whom he had allowed himself to feel as a child—his grandmother, who had cared for him from the time he was two years old until he was four. When this memory arose, he began to feel incredibly sad and started to cry. He paused only to say, "It seems so strange to have been so young and to have had all these feelings. I never remembered feeling like this. I never thought I could." After a few minutes of silence, he looked at me and said that he had blocked again. I commented that he seemed involved in an enormous emotional tug-of-war: to feel or not to feel, to feel or to stop his feelings. He responded, "It must have been an overwhelming experience all those times when I was young. What were the feelings? It's all still too much in my head. I can't get to them." After another period of silence, this time for almost 10 minutes, he continued, "The closer I get to these feelings, the more terrified I feel." Then he started to weep loudly, murmuring, "Oh my God, oh my God!"

After many minutes of crying, he paused and reflected, "This does not make sense to me. It is stupid what I am doing." I responded that his characterization of "stupid" again seemed to be a compromise and a settling, and that, and only that, seemed to me to make no sense. He cried again.

More and more, he expressed feelings of sadness, anger, longing, and loneliness that he no longer could avoid. At times, he expressed feelings of being extraordinarily helpless and weak, which were not usual feelings for him. I understood these feelings to be genuine concerns about whether he could handle the intensity of his emotions or whether they would overwhelm him. At times his mind would go blank, and he would stop feeling; I would then reflect that this was his place of refuge.

He seemed to be going around in emotional circles. I began to feel impatient. Finally, this impatience expressed itself in a misattuned interpretation of his flight into refuge, which, because it originated in my countertransference acted-out feeling of impatience, was experienced by him as a confrontation. He replied, "I don't want either my mother or you too near to me. I brought myself up and did a damn good job of it, and I don't need either of you now." He retreated further: "I feel totally detached." Then, "Even as an infant I seem to remember having been detached. I can remember even then lying in the crib feeling numb, totally numb."

I wondered if he did not feel so detached, remembering the numbness at this moment, because he had once again experienced my words as too intrusive. This was an intervention that I was accustomed to giving and he was accustomed to hearing. This time he laughed, and said it was not my words but my very breathing that felt intrusive to him. He became serious again and started to cry. He commented that his whole body seemed to ache: "This seems to be the way I experience it whenever I imagine mother trying to hold me. There was no way that she was ever able to comfort me. She just hurt me." His crying continued. He went on: "To be here, to be truly here, I will have to feel and totally feel." He paused for several minutes. Then he said, "It feels like I'm a dead dog coming back to life and I'm just starting to pet the dog again."

Well into the fourth year of treatment, the patient began to share with me the extent of his fantasies about me that had been operating throughout the treatment. The spontaneous sharing of the more intimate nature of the fantasies followed the spontaneous emergence of his feeling life. This is the usual sequence. Access to and sharing of feelings more generally should precede the sharing of fantasies related to the therapist. If the reverse occurs, the sharing of such fantasies will usually be in the service of resistance. As discussed previously, such revelations will be used as a means of avoiding or circumventing the feelings associated with the abandonment depression.

The fantasies about me revolved around the theme of failing and then succeeding in connecting to me in ever closer and more intimate ways. A typical fantasy early in treatment that produced excitement was of sitting in my office with me but separated from me by a raging river. In this fantasy, we were both dressed as Chaplinesque characters performing an elaborate pantomime. The pantomime enabled us to communicate across the expanse of the river and make our needs known. I had a huge ladder that extended across the river, with which I was trying to reach him. Once the ladder was in place, one of us could crawl across it to the other side. At one point in this fantasy, he started to race across the river, jumping from one slightly exposed rung to another. All of a sudden, he discovered that the rungs onto which he was jumping were really the submerged heads of alligators, and he was scarcely able to scamper back to safety on his side of the river.

Exposing and sharing many of his fantasies about varying degrees of closeness and intimacy seemed to remove a final obstacle or compromise to the challenge of working through the abandonment depression. His fantasies now changed to an ongoing play or drama that took place over a series of months. In this drama, both parents were placed on trial for crimes they had committed against him. Much of the sessions' content seemed to be a transcript of the proceedings of the trial that was taking place in his head, in which his parents were accused, prosecuted, defended, and finally convicted. The affects that accompanied this drama were terror, depression, and rage as the evidence unfolded, and Mr. X. would report as exhibits the memories and feelings he had had throughout his childhood.

The entire experience of the trial scenario seemed to represent the deepest and most profound aspects of working through the abandonment depression. For a period of weeks at the conclusion of the trial, Mr. X. seemed particularly distant and lost in his own thoughts. Finally, he reported that he had been spending much time in recent weeks staring at inanimate objects for hours. "I guess," he said seriously, "I have attached myself to inanimate things." I responded that, after all this time and very difficult work, it seemed to me to be one hell of a poor compromise. He then put his hand to his head and said that he felt nauseous, as if he were about to faint. It was like the old feeling of spinning off into empty space. After a few minutes of silence, I commented, "But now you have a choice, and what will you attach yourself to now?" "Mars," he replied. I asked him, "Why so far?" He paused for a moment and said with dramatic clarity, "I am more aware at this moment than I have ever been in my life of how truly alone I have really been. I am also aware of something else that perhaps I have only been aware of in the past. Maybe I knew it and maybe I didn't, but now I know with certainty. I have always wanted someone to be with. I have always wanted someone to love me and for me to love."

For my part, I realized, after almost five years of treatment, the extent to which he had worked through his abandonment depression and had discovered something at his core, woven into the fabric of his existence. He had found a way of being, a fundamental way of feeling and experiencing himself, his feelings, and his need for another.

Now the final stage of treatment began. The working through of the abandonment depression heralds the beginning of the separation process for the schizoid patient. All the disorders of the self share one feature in common in the separation process—the wish to hold onto a fundamental fantasy that governs the work until the separation phase begins. This notion or fantasy is that ultimately the relationship to the therapist can be preserved intact, intrapsychically, as the fundamental preserver of attachment experiences. It cannot. The fantasy is not an anchor; it is a distortion and a final obstacle to the emergence of the real self.

What is at stake again relates to the fundamental dichotomy between spontaneity and reactivity, that is, whether the person will be primarily a spontaneous and creative actor or a reactor to the impingements of others. The fantasy or distortion that remains in the last stage of treatment, and which the previous working through has now prepared the patient to face, is not a communal accommodation made by the patient's healthy public self; rather, it is the final vestige of the participation of the patient in the kind of false-self structures that heretofore dominated the patient's life.

This distortion is present in all the disorders of the self at this stage of treatment. It just looks different in the different disorders. For the borderline patient, the fantasy is: "When all else fails, or in situations of enormous conflict or uncertainty or fear, I am afraid that I cannot just rely on another, but must inevitably collapse into the arms of another." The distortion is not in the borderline patient's need to rely and depend on another person when his or her own capacities or skills are unavailable, overwhelmed, or taxed to exhaustion, but that, at critical moments, one not only *may*, but *will*, need to be taken care of by another. Initially in treatment, the other is often anyone and everyone. In the last stage of treatment of the borderline patient, the other is the therapist. Delimited though it might be, this is basically a remnant of a helplessness in which one surrenders to another's caretaking or impingements.

Similarly, the distortion or fantasy operating for the narcissistic patient is the preservation of the need for the gleam in the therapist's eye as fundamentally crucial to the patient's experience of himself or herself as a stable, cohesive, valued individual. Holding on to such a fantasy is not an expression of healthy or mutual interdependence with a self-regulating other, but is a fundamental overinvestment in and dependence on needing others as a primary component of self-regulation. Such an overinvestment, early or late in treatment, with many others or with only the therapist, is not a spontaneous act as part of the experience of sharing between self and other, but is an involuntary act of surrender.

For the schizoid patient, the particular nature of the fantasy has a different quality from those of either the narcissistic patient or the borderline patient. Mr. X. provides a striking example. In following the course of Mr. X.'s therapy, the interrelationship between working through the abandonment depression and the exposure or sharing of fantasies about the therapist has been noted. Once again, Mr. X.'s fantasies about me took on a dramatic and increasingly intense quality. The sharing of these fantasies and the working through of their meaning became the task and challenge of the final separation stage. This is the key to being able to manage the separation phase. If these fantasies are understood as the final effort at compromise, then the working-through process can be finally and fully completed. When separation involves the schizoid patient's reluctance to invest in mutually shared experiences with truly available others, then the healthy emergence of the real self will be frustrated and impeded.

Throughout the trial phase of working through, Mr. X. had cast me alternately in the roles of prosecutor, defense attorney, and judge. But the therapeutic relationship itself seems to have taken a back seat in the drama. Now, with the trial's having concluded and Mr. X.'s having acknowledged the core aspect of his nature, what was coming to the fore once more was his relationship with me.

At this time and throughout much of the working through, Mr. X. continued to take important strides in his efforts at relatedness and connection outside the therapy. As suggested earlier, this risk-taking behavior should be continuously monitored as a helpful barometer of self-activation, as opposed to compliance. Throughout the treatment, I implicitly and explicitly encouraged exploration and experimentation in the world outside treatment. The pace and intensity of these explorations had varied, but Mr. X. had managed to make some significant progress toward relatedness, both at work and in his personal relationships. Of the two, the effort to build a supportive and gratifying network of colleagues and friends in general had outstripped his effort at establishing a mutual, intimate, personal relationship. There was a sense that he was holding back from progress in this area. I brought this to his attention.

At that point, he slowly shared the full extent of his fantasies about our intimate connection. These fantasies, which for so long had served as the catalyst for his motivation to do the painful work required, now served as the ultimate compromise. I was his rescuer, protector, companion, and source of his power when he would grab hold of my erection in his fantasy and feel invulnerable. Of all these fantasies, the most important and consistent theme that was emerging was that it was with me alone that he could ultimately experience the most profound sense of being attached and connected. After listening to the uncovering of these fantasies and discerning their meaning, I gradually began to interpret the compromise aspect. Mr. X. repeated his previous cycles of initial anger and upset at this interpretation of the compromise, followed by renewed feelings about my sadistic rejection of him, and finally by steps down old, well-worn paths of retreat.

All of this, however, was done in a much more muted fashion than previously.

Gradually, the fantasies involving me began to thin out and then diminish. They became less colorful, gratifying, and exciting. Concurrently, he slowly began to be more willing, even eager, to experiment with other relationships. He expressed surprise at the degree of pleasure and pain that he felt.

Two other aspects of the separation process with a schizoid patient are the issue of setting a termination date and that of follow-up appointments. The setting of a termination date is not just a therapeutic afterthought, but is a vital component of the separation process. It is the therapeutic strategy or intervention that shifts the final stage of treatment into high gear. A definitive termination date should be set, and sufficient time must be allowed for the meaning of the termination to be understood and for the patient's feelings to be fully explored. This brings to the patient's attention his or her investment in holding onto the distorted fantasy of pathological reliance on the therapist. Generally, at least six months are necessary to explore the issues of termination with the schizoid patient. A shorter period will allow the patient to keep any fantasies and feelings hidden, either through a precipitous flight into health or through a final withdrawal of affect and refusal to acknowledge and mourn the loss of the last pathological tie to the therapist, as well as the loss of the real relationship with the real therapist. This latter emotional shortcut may be subtle and unrecognized by a therapist who does not have sufficient time to observe the patient. However, a period longer than six months makes the setting of the termination date largely meaningless to the dynamic of the treatment. At worst, it may convey to the patient the therapist's conscious or unconscious countertransference anxieties about termination.

With regard to the issue of follow-up appointments, it should be noted that, unlike the recommendation to plan a specific follow-up appointment in shorter-term treatment, no such recommendation need be made at the termination of intensive therapy with a schizoid patient. Such a planned appointment would defocus the issues surrounding termination. In a successfully terminated treatment, the schizoid patient assumes that should further treatment be necessary, the patient can contact the therapist. When a schizoid patient finds it necessary to ask whether he or she can call the therapist, the therapist should respond with an exploration, once again, of the meaning of the question. Why should the patient feel it necessary to ask permission of the therapist to make a request for future sessions? The exploration of the motivation for such a request may promote further working through of unresolved pathological fears, fantasies, or wishes in the final phase of the treatment.

Mr. X. terminated treatment after nearly six years of therapy. Working through the abandonment depression of a schizoid patient can be a painfully slow process, owing to the nature of the communication deficits present initially, as well as to the extraordinary anxiety and fear about fundamental issues of relatedness. The benefits of working through are obvious: freedom from the trauma of the abandonment depression, freedom from the vulnerability to schizoid anxieties and agonies, freedom from the impaired self-in-exile. In its place, a real self holds center stage, a self capable of experiencing its essential nature and real relationships.

REFERENCES

Masterson, J. F. (1972). Treatment of the borderline adolescent. New York: Wiley.

CHAPTER 8

Safety First: Approaching Treatment of the Schizoid Disorder of the Self

Stephen Silberstein, M.D.

In contrast to borderline and narcissistic disorders of the self, until recently relatively little attention has been paid in the professional literature to the schizoid disorder of the self. It was almost as if mental health professionals were resonating with schizoid patients' fears of the dire consequences of their being seen or heard. This lack of interest has changed with clinicians' growing awareness that, with adaptations of technique, patients with disorders of the self can be treated successfully with psychotherapy. This success has enhanced the interest in and recognition of the schizoid disorder of the self.

The title "Safety First" is meant to emphasize the heightened awareness that persons with a schizoid disorder of the self have of the potential danger to themselves of relationships with others, as well as the psychological defenses they then employ to manage these dangers.

Because they experience relationships with others as dangerous, most persons with a schizoid disorder of the self never consider seeking psychotherapy. If they do come for treatment, often it is because a particular life circumstance caused them to feel their loneliness and isolation to the point of suicidality. Once in treatment, problems will arise if the therapist is unaware of the diagnosis and the unique defensive structure of the schizoid patient. Such a patient, for example, can experience almost any intervention by the therapist as manipulative or intrusive and defensively distance for fear of being controlled. Unless the therapist recognizes this dynamic, the patient may terminate, or the therapy can become stalemated as the patient uses a variety of distancing defenses to ward off experience of painful affect. This therapist was recently consulted by an experienced clinician who was stymied as to how to deal with such an impasse with his most troublesome patient.

Case of Mrs. X.

Mrs. X., a married, middle-aged professional woman, initiated treatment to deal with growing anxiety and depression seemingly brought about by a new supervisor who was monitoring her work more closely.

Inexplicably, after a year of weekly psychotherapy, Mrs. X. had become virtually mute in her sessions. Her therapist was anxious and confused, because initially his patient had been quite verbal in discussing herself and her life; but now she was silent from the moment she entered the consulting room. When the therapist, to manage his feelings of helplessness and isolation, asked questions or introduced a topic for discussion, as the patient suggested he do, she would reply briefly and lapse back into silence. If the therapist, feeling inadequate, inquired whether she were dissatisfed with treatment, she would reply that, on the contrary, therapy was quite helpful and she felt less depressed than when she began. Her actions were consistent with her words, for not only did she always pay her bill punctually, but she came to her sessions every week even if it entailed her driving through snowstorms that kept many more talkative patients at home.

There were no external circumstances to account for the patient's silence. She worked at a job she had had for over a decade, spending the rest of her time peacefully at the home she shared with her husband of many years. They had no children. To an outsider, her life would seem safe and secure, although monotonous; if one were introduced to her at a party, one would soon move on to more engaging company.

Mrs. X. and her husband rarely exchanged angry words, but neither did they speak of their emotions or of their inner lives. On one of the rare occasions that they did, Mr. X. observed to his wife that she told him only 5 percent of what she thought; Mrs. X. did not answer her husband, but did confirm the accuracy of his statistic to her therapist. Most of her time at home was spent in a room separate from her husband where she read or engaged in hobbies. She alluded to frequent daydreams about people at work, her husband, and the therapist, but was vague as to their specific content; because she became anxious when he did so, the therapist felt reluctant to press Mrs. X. for details. The extensiveness of her fantasied interpersonal relationships contrasted with their paucity in reality. She had acquaintances at work, but for years had no friends. Of her marriage, she volunteered that she was surprised that anybody would want to marry her and would want to stay married to her.

Curious as to why Mrs. X. had become mute, the therapist inquired what she was thinking about during her silences. Often, she said, she did not know, and when she did know, it concerned things she felt too uncomfortable to talk about. Mrs. X.'s response to other endeavors by her therapist to get her to talk about herself were brief and equally undisclosing.

At the onset of treatment, when Mrs. X. readily complied with the therapist's recommendation to talk about herself, the therapist felt competent and needed. Now he experienced painful affect in sessions. He was frequently aware of feeling helpless and controlled by Mrs. X.'s silence. If he said nothing, he felt inadequate because the therapy seemed to go nowhere, but if he took action by asking about her life or her silence, her evasive responses left him feeling confused, incompetent, and isolated. Sometimes he felt so alone in the room with Mrs. X. that he found himself daydreaming. His fantasies had sadistic themes, such as images of shaking her to make her talk. Occasionally, he felt he was being psychologically tortured by Mrs. X., but he denied this experience to himself upon observing her frightened or pained expression, or when he recalled her avowals of being helped by therapy.

What was being enacted by the patient and experienced by the therapist were manifestations of the intrapsychic object relations world of the schizoid disorder of the self; in particular, this patient's use of projective identification to manage the painful affects of the sadistic object/self-in-exile part object relations unit.

Mrs. X.'s therapy became unstuck once her therapist abandoned his countertransferential response to her silence of trying to make her talk. He instead interpreted her silence, saying it represented her compromise solution to the dilemma she increasingly felt in therapy: when she revealed herself and her feelings, she felt exposed, as if under a spotlight, and anticipated that this would only lead to her being verbally attacked and having to submit to overwhelming and interminable demands and expectations of her by the therapist. If she tried to escape this servitude by not coming to therapy, she would lose the relationship in which she felt most listened to and understood, and consequently would feel alone and alienated. Her solution to the dilemma, he pointed out, was what she so frequently ended up doing in relationships—she would seek safety through compromise between being too close and being too far away: she would come to therapy, but once there, she would use silence to keep herself at what she felt was a safe distance from being attacked or exploited.

Mrs. X. acknowledged that the observation seemed accurate. She again began to talk about herself while the therapist limited his interventions to how and when Mrs. X. used distancing defenses, such as silence, to manage painful affects in her sessions.

Case of Ms. A.

The first patient this therapist recognized as having a schizoid disorder of the self while still in treatment was Ms. A. Rather than using silence, as Mrs. X. did, as a distancing defense to manage her schizoid dilemma, she employed a visually striking and memorable distancing defense—she would disappear behind a pillow when she felt she was entering dangerous territory in therapy. Ms. A. thereby vividly enacted Fairbairn's (1941) observation of patients with a schizoid disorder of the self: "It is at once fascinating and pathetic to watch the patient, like a timid mouse, alternately creeping out of the shelter of his hole to peek at the world of outer objects and then beating a hasty retreat."

At the outset of therapy, Ms. A. had only distant friends. She had never married. She was successful only at jobs where her contact with other people was almost exclusively over the telephone. Her most satisfying and closest relationship was with her dog. Her emotional life was like Fairbairn's timid mouse, or, as Ms. A. put it, she lived in the safety of a cave from which she only rarely and briefly emerged. Until the age of four, she was repeatedly abused physically and sexually by her father and grandmother. Later, she was adopted by a foster mother, who was critical, controlling, and abandoning.

Early in therapy, whenever Ms. A. would haltingly allude to wishes for recognition from or anger toward the therapist, she would hold a pillow in front of her. The more explicit her wish for recognition or direct the expression of her resentment, the larger would be the pillow. On one occasion, she tucked her feet under her so that only her eyes and forehead were visible above the largest pillow available. The more she exposed her emotions, the more she needed to hide her body, perhaps reflecting childhood physical abuse.

Ms. A. experienced her schizoid dilemma as "like being stuck between the devil and the deep blue sea." Usually she acted in therapy in the master/slave part object relations unit. She reported that she was apprehensive of being found a boring or unmotivated patient and felt she needed to fill the sessions with interesting talk. She was the slave, who, to remain connected with me, felt she had to keep me entertained lest I become an impatient and demanding devil. In this mode of relating, she had only a distant recollection that she also could relate in a very different way.

In the master/slave unit, Ms. A. experienced the object world as dangerous, and to make herself safe, she holed up in a cave. She watched constantly and carefully for any inconsistencies that for her signaled dangerousness. She was especially sensitive to discrepancies between the content of what I said and my tone of voice. Should this occur, her splitting defense was activated and she was behind a pillow, figuratively or literally.

After splitting, however, she experienced me as the sadistic part object representation who was attacking and devaluing her or else was totally indifferent to her. Thereupon she would become silent. She was now in the self-in-exile part self representation where she felt quite safe, as well as secure in her ability to maintain herself totally without any assistance or recognition. At the same time, however, she also felt alienated, depressed, and silently rageful. She felt all alone on the deep blue sea. Once in this part unit, under the sway of her splitting defense, she had only the dimmest memory of herself and me in the master/slave part unit.

As can all patients with a disorder of the self, Ms. A. could also reverse self and object. In her case, it occurred from the safe distance of a letter or telephone call. She would scornfully devalue me and announce that she was going to quit therapy. She became the sadistic object and it was I who felt fear of the sadistic and/or indifferent object, as well as the loneliness and isolation of the self-in-exile.

Ms. A. could also reverse the master/slave part unit. This occurred on a few occasions when she wanted something from me, such as a change of appointment time, which she feared might trigger my deciding to abandon her. She would present her request in a manipulative way that left *me* feeling coerced and victimized.

Ms. A. acted out in the transference based on projections onto the therapist of self and object representations of both the master/slave part unit and the sadistic object self-in-exile part unit. Later in therapy, she revealed another form of transference acting out by telephoning and writing frequently to maintain a fantasy of intimacy with me. The fantasy served to defend her against her anxiety at developing more intimate relationships in real life. Fantasy is commonly used as a schizoid compromise.

The split object relations units of the schizoid disorder of the self described by the Masterson Approach can be used to understand the schizoid dilemma and compromise. The patient moving toward relatedness activates the master/slave unit. Moving away activates the sadistic object self-in-exile unit. To deal with these dual sources of anxiety, the patient will settle for an in-between compromise, developing a fantasy of self-reliance or a fantasy of relatedness. This compromise of fantasy utilization allows safety, but not the development or expression of the real self.

What are the therapeutic interventions to be utilized here? In the Masterson Approach to the treatment of disorders of the self, the therapist endeavors to convert the patient's transference acting out into transference and the formation of a therapeutic alliance. To accomplish this, the therapist first must maintain a clear frame and therapeutic neutrality with the schizoid patient. Ralph Klein states that the therapist also conveys his or her safety as an object by interpretation of the schizoid dilemma as it occurs in the transference acting out as well as in the patient's external life. For example, the therapist may observe in response to a specific behavior of the patient in therapy, "I understand you can get neither too close nor too far away. When you get too close, you feel danger and anxiety and fear of being controlled and manipulated. When you get too far, you feel isolated and fear exile." The patient's realization that the therapist understands him or her and the dilemma becomes the foundation for establishing the therapeutic alliance. Klein states that once there is consensus about the dilemma and the therapeutic alliance is in place, the therapist then moves to interpreting the schizoid compromise, linking it with the dysphoric affect of the abandonment depression. These affects are depression, rage, loneliness, alienation, fear of cosmic aloneness, and despair.

In interpreting the defensive aspects of the schizoid compromise, the key word is safety. An example of such an interpretation of the schizoid compromise in the case of Ms. A. might be seen when the therapist tells the patient, "Just now you became silent for a long time after telling me how your grandmother beat you. You know you retreat into silence to protect yourself after you feel you've stuck your neck out too far, and in this case, I wonder if perhaps you felt your revelation exposed you to one of two dangers: either I'll become disgusted and throw you out of therapy, or will become critical and impatient and demand that you work harder. To feel safe from either of those two dangers, you compromised by retreating into the safety of silence, but in the process had to pay the price of not exploring any other possibilities and were left feeling cut off and isolated."

Klein notes that the schizoid patient manages the painful affects of the dilemma of either being in the master/slave part unit or the sadistic object self-in-exile part unit by taking an in-between compromise position. This position is described metaphorically as being between a rock and a hard place, or of being between the devil and the deep blue sea. In this schizoid compromise, the patient keeps apart from a life of relatedness.

The Masterson Approach emphasizes that patients with disorders of the self can function at a higher or lower level in their occupations and social relationships depending on the degree of developmental arrest of the ego. A patient with a schizoid disorder of the self at the lower level of functioning would be like Ms. A., who experienced caretakers as overly sadistic. Schizoid patients with a disorder of the self at the upper level of functioning resemble absent-minded professors more than they do trauma victims. They function reasonably well unless there is pressure for relatedness. The childhood caretakers of such higher-level patients seem to have been experienced as more emotionally manipulative or intrusive than as indifferent or sadistic.

Case of Mr. B.

An example of a higher-level schizoid patient is Mr. B., who had a distant, self-absorbed, manipulative father and a mother who was either benignly distant or, when she did notice her son's emotional life, intrusively quizzed him about his feelings. Mr. B. is reasonably productive in his professional work and relates comfortably, albeit distantly, to his colleagues. Were it not for his wife's intense and prolonged anger at his emotional distance, he would not have come to therapy.

Mr. B. initially filled his sessions with complex, abstract, but affectless self-speculations, which served to keep him at a safe distance from the therapist. He was an exemplar of Guntrip's observation (1969) that patients with a schizoid disorder of the self often use talking in analytic therapy as a defensive compromise by which to mark time. Mr. B.'s monologues were his compromise in the master/slave part unit, through which he found a safe distance to be in therapy—not too far in, but not too far out. Early on, he would discourse at length about his feelings, but when he began to experience them in sessions, they came up as an experience of intense amorphous emotion in the form of his suddenly becoming tearful, and then just as suddenly choking off the self-expression. Later, those choked-off feelings were more clearly identified with both anger and affection.

The posttraumatic type of patient with a schizoid disorder of the self is more likely to experience the therapist as the sadistic object and, like Ms. A., defensively retreat into silence, whereas the absentminded professor type, like Mr. B., is more likely to experience the therapist as a manipulative coercive master and will use unemotional, nonrevelatory talk not only to serve the master, but also to keep him or her at a safe distance.

For all patients with a schizoid disorder of the self, having their real selves seen is to risk the extreme danger of being appropriated by the perceived master or of being exiled by the perceived sadistic or indifferent object. One schizoid patient who distanced to an extreme in all relationships, described intense dysphoria experienced from just being looked at while walking from the beginning to the end of a long line of fellow students waiting to register for classes. She was certain the students were staring at her and viewed her with the same relentless impatience and dissatisfaction as her mother had. Throughout treatment, episodes of emergence of her real self were quickly followed by anxiety at possibly exposing herself to harsh attack. Another example of fear of having her real self seen occurred when Ms. A.'s rather self-revelatory artistic creation was praised in class by her instructor as being of professional quality. Although she thought her own work was quite good, and the other students had been congratulatory, she was panicky and felt unsafe for days thereafter whenever she thought of her creation, and thus of herself, as being known to others.

The terror schizoid patients experience, that having exposed any of their needs and feelings is to risk the likelihood of being attacked, controlled, or abandoned, causes them to develop formidable defenses against that eventuality. They feel that to invite attention in any way is to court disaster. Like chameleons, they can become invisible in their surroundings. Unlike the patient with a borderline disorder of the self who invites the therapist to become a rewarding part object, or the patient with a narcissistic disorder of the self who invites the therapist to resonate with the grandiose part self representation, the schizoid patient never experiences himself or herself as safe in a relationship and endeavors to keep hidden. As a result, the therapist can mistake the schizoid patient's devaluing or distancing defenses against closeness as the core character structure, and thus diagnostic of a distancing borderline or devaluing narcissistic disorder. Perhaps the camouflaging defenses of the schizoid disorder of the self against the dangers of being seen have contributed to the difficulty in recognizing and understanding this disorder.

Because of the schizoid patient's concern about safety, it is important that the therapist maintain neutrality. If the therapist maintains neutrality and avoids countertransference acting out in response to projections or projective identifications of parts of either the master/slave or self-in-exile object relations unit, then the patient is likely to stay in treatment. The therapist thereupon faces another dilemma—the risk of the patient's using the therapeutic relationship for years as a defensive schizoid compromise, a safe substitute for real relationships in the real world.

Case of Mrs. Y.

The treatment of patients with a schizoid disorder of the self proceeds slowly owing to the tenacity of their distancing defenses. The case of Mrs. Y. illustrates how one schizoid patient, over a number of years, gradually contained her transference acting out of distancing defenses, and once her therapist contained his countertransference, was able to enter a therapeutic alliance, begin to work through the affects of the abandonment depression and increasingly express her real self.

Mrs. Y. was a middle-aged, married, professional woman who first consulted me nine and one half years previously seeking continued pharmacological management of recurrent depression. The first five and a half years of treatment with me had taken place before I was familiar with the Masterson Approach, and had made the diagnosis of a schizoid disorder of the self.

She had had several courses of psychotherapy for depression while in college and graduate school and after she began working at her career. She noted that her time in therapy had equaled in length time she had spent living with her parents. Six years earlier, after moving to the area to advance her career, she first consulted a psychiatrist at her HMO because of frequent episodes of low energy, crying spells, panicky feelings, irritability, various forms of somatic distress, suicidal thoughts, and self-deprecatory ideation that seemed unrelated to external events. The psychiatrist treated her with an antidepressant, which relieved the symptoms, and saw her briefly every four to six months. She was consulting me because she had lost access to her first psychiatrist as a result of changed insurance coverage.

Mrs. Y. was then single; she had had some brief, casual sexual relationships with men until five years earlier, when she felt a strong attraction to the man who became her lover and subsequently her husband. He was seldom available to her when they first became involved, and although they now lived together, he was often out of town. Since moving to the area, she had made no friends, nor did she have a social life aside from occasional dinners with friends of her lover. She worked a lot of unpaid overtime on her job in order to do it well enough to manage her fear of being criticized by her superiors, who in reality were complimentary and respectful. At home, she preferred to read or engage in hobbies involving artistic expression while her lover watched television.

Her initial appearance was unusual in several respects. She peered through heavy-framed eyeglasses that made her look less attractive than she did when she momentarily removed them at the end of the session. Her clothing was loose fitting and on the dowdy side. She wore little makeup. She was someone one might not notice, except for her unusual quality of trying so hard to see without being seen, much as would a mouse looking out of its hole, to observe if the outer world were safe. Her face was deadpan, and her voice almost devoid of emotional expression.

She told her story in a very deliberate, thoughtful manner; when asked a question, she would think for a moment before replying carefully and coherently. Although I was not aware of it at the time, her behavior exhibited that quality of a person with a schizoid disorder of the self of being both in and out at the same time. For example, she said she did not want to return for four to six months, but she would also like to feel she could consult me sooner if she were to become emotionally upset. I responded by asking how long an appointment she wanted to schedule four months hence—a brief visit to talk about medication or a longer appointment in case there were other issues she wished to discuss. Without hesitation, she chose the latter. I noted at the time that although she appeared controlled and somewhat cold in manner, at the same time she managed not to seem aloof, hostile, or rejecting. I believe I was picking up on her ability to protect herself with distance and yet call as little attention to herself as possible while doing so—a quality I did not then realize was characteristic of the schizoid patient's propensity to be there and yet not to be there.

Mrs. Y. was using medication as a distancing defense. As she gradually found me to be a safe object, she returned at more frequent intervals for fifty-minute appointments. Fifteen months after her initial appointment, she asked to be seen for weekly psychotherapy. She remained on antidepressant medication throughout her treatment, except for two occasions when she gradually discontinued use for several months. After doing so she noted a progressive return of irritability, crying spells, insomnia and self-deprecatory ideation, the intensity of which made her feel suicidal. These depressive symptoms were unrelated to the external events or issues they addressed in psychotherapy.

Mrs. Y.'s history, as it gradually emerged, featured significant early abuse and neglect in a general atmosphere of unsafety. She was the second of four children. Her mother periodically exhibited symptoms of a major psychiatric disorder during which she would either retreat for one to two days to a broken-down shed behind the house where she would pace and smoke cigarettes, or equally frightening, would rage at her husband and children, throw things, or unexpectedly slap the patient without explanation. She could be kind to her younger sons but not to the patient. Not only did the father do nothing to control his wife's rages, they were never talked about in the family.

Also frightening were her mother's unpredictable verbal assaults. Mrs. Y. recalled how, as a young adult, after telling a friend how much she enjoyed an outing in the mountains, her youngest brother volunteered the comment that if the mother heard either of them talk so enthusiastically, she likely would say sarcastically, "Well, la-di-da for you." Although her mother's attacks were unpredictable, they at least were identifiable, and perhaps for that reason, several years earlier, during an angry tirade by her mother, Mrs. Y. told her she would never visit again if her mother ever lost her temper in her presence. Her mother has not done so since.

Toward her father, Mrs. Y. felt a fear that was more pervasive and less identifiable. He would mention disparaging remarks he had heard about her from his friends, and add that he was keeping an eye on her. He would tell her that he knew unspecified bad things about her friends and that she should stay away from them. Mrs. Y. felt that her parents subtly sabotaged all of her childhood friendships, except associations with children at their church. Her father was a vocal advocate of unpopular causes and enjoyed argument. He would invite Mrs. Y. to state an opinion and then argue the opposite point of view. Listening to him as an adult, she found his speech often rambling, fragmented, and illogical. An amateur detective, her father, without anyone asking him to, spent part of several summers trying to track down the ex-wife of a younger brother. Unlike her mother, he could be insightful and funny, and he encouraged Mrs. Y. to participate with him in sports. Most disturbing about her father was a fear, without specific recollection, that early in her childhood he had repeatedly molested her sexually in the middle of the night.

Mrs. Y.'s older brother relentlessly argued with his parents despite repeated beatings. Later, he achieved national prominence in his work. Two younger brothers were passive. She clung to the brother who was closest to her in age, often going to his bed when she was too anxious to sleep during the night. He was the only family member with whom she felt safe. She said they cared for and helped raise each other; they did not engage in any sexual activity.

Mrs. Y. left home to go to college, achieved financial independence quickly, and seldom returned for visits.

During the first five and a half years of treatment, I did not follow the Masterson Approach or keep process notes. During that time, Mrs. Y. married her lover and dealt with several severe depressions following her husband's separating from her for several weeks without warning or a perceptible cause. Because she experienced me as a safe object who was sensitive to her need for distance, she continued with therapy, which diminished her feelings of isolation, and hence her depression. If I continued to serve only in that capacity, however, there would have been no opportunity for character change.

When I began intensive training in the Masterson Approach, I started to question her diagnosis. Mrs. Y. came regularly to sessions, where methodically, with limited affect, she would report her dreams and the events of her week. She made slow progress, and I had taken this compliant behavior in treatment as indicative of a neurotic disorder and the presence of a therapeutic alliance. Her previous years of therapy evidently had helped her to modulate the more obvious signs of a character disorder. Her slow progress and general lack of affect in sessions after years of treatment, however, raised the question of her having a disorder of the self. But which one? Her history of social isolation, self-sufficiency, and an active fantasy life displayed in frequent dreams and artistic endeavors suggested a possible schizoid disorder of the self.

The issues Mrs. Y. discussed in treatment supported this diagnosis. She complained of feeling either ignored or controlled by her husband, intimating that it was too dangerous to let him know about those feelings. Yet it was he who always reached out first to her, and on the few occasions in which she did let him know her wishes, he seemed capable of responding with some care and understanding.

At work, she described never refusing any request of her superiors. She usually brought work home. Her need for perfection was not to support grandiosity, as one might see in a narcissistic patient, or to be the good, special child seeking the approving care of a rewarding object, as might be seen in a borderline patient. Her slaving away 60 to 80 hours a week was the minimal effort she expected of herself to stave off expected severe criticism by her superiors, which never occurred in reality.

With me, as with her employer, she was hard-working and uncomplaining. She was punctual and dutifully brought in a lot of material to fill the hours. She did not become upset or angry with me. She was in the room physically, but at the same time, there was a sense that she really was not present as a result of her extensive use of distancing defenses.

Mrs. Y. usually saw herself as having no choice but uncomplainingly to take care of the unending demands of others lest she be harshly criticized or abandoned. In this regard, she was in the master/slave unit, where she projected onto me and others on whom she was dependent the properties of a coercive master while experiencing herself as an obedient slave.

Mrs. Y. avoided as much as possible sticking her neck out in any assertive way, as she feared she would be attacked. When she reluctantly agreed to teach a class, for example, she was terrified that participants might publicly demean her. When she anticipated such attacks, she would leave the situation as quickly as possible, and if she could not do so physically, would enter a dissociative mental state instead. This fear of attack and the need to distance from it occurred in all relationships and could be seen as a manifestation of the sadistic object self-in-exile unit, wherein she projected the intent to attack or devalue onto others, and experienced herself as being isolated and self-contained. Somewhat later in therapy, when she felt safer with bringing up feelings toward me, she described her schizoid dilemma as she experienced it in therapy as follows: "It's as if I'm on the spot. If I talk of how I'm feeling in here, I'll be criticized in some way. What I say won't be enough or I'll have the wrong feelings. When you're quiet, it's as if you are withdrawing from me—making it more torturous, as if you're getting a thrill out of knowing how to help but not doing it just to watch me suffer."

On the basis of her history and of observing her in therapy, I changed my diagnosis to a schizoid disorder of the self.

I began to take process notes in my treatment of Mrs. Y. and obtained supervision. The first result of this change was seeing how unnecessarily active I had been in offering frequent interpretations. As soon as I shut up and got out of her way, Mrs. Y. demonstrated the capacity to explore herself.

My overactivity was a not uncommon countertransference reaction to patients with a schizoid disorder of the self. In part, it was my defense against Mrs. Y.'s projective identification of her feelings of helplessness in the master/slave unit. I was picking up her feelings of helplessness, and if I talked, I did not feel helpless, and, consequently, neither did she. Another source of my countertransference was her distancing defenses, which elicited in me the uncomfortable feeling that I was not needed, so that if I said more, she would need me more. Finally, to a lesser degree, my talking was in response to her initiating my activity by asking questions. She tended to do this when she was feeling unsafe in the sadistic object self-in-exile unit, and for safety asked questions to get a sense of how dangerous I might be at that moment.

Once my countertransference was under control, Mrs. Y.'s issues became clearer. I was able to interpret her silences. I might say: "Just now I got the feeling you're waiting for me to pull you out of your silence as a way to protect you from your experiencing the angry feelings you just talked about because feeling them started to make you feel unsafe." Note the somewhat tentative way in which I began by observing, "I had the feeling that." Patients with a schizoid disorder of the self are wary of being appropriated or coerced, and thus respond best to tentative interpretations.

Mrs. Y.'s initial response to my being quieter was to feel attacked. She managed this feeling by bringing in descriptions of her many dreams since the previous session. I asked if she were using her dreams as a means of getting control of her emotions in therapy. She acknowledged that this was so, and began to talk about her anger and her fear of losing control of it.

At the same time, she began to express her anger more, increasingly defending herself in sessions by distancing to a silent, dissociative state. This defense had to be repeatedly interpreted as a manifestation of her schizoid dilemma. Within a year of my doing so, there was evidence that a beginning therapeutic alliance was replacing Mrs. Y.'s previous compliance. She would increasingly begin a session at the point where she had left off the previous one. She also began to see me more as a whole object, both good and bad, rather than as split into either the coercive master or the sadistic object. For example, she said she experienced my becoming quieter as painful to her; I was meanly withholding my help, yet, at the same time, she said she knew I was doing this because I thought it would help her.

With my countertransference under control and evidence of a therapeutic alliance forming, I began to interpret her schizoid compromise. Once again, she had come home from work to find a note from her husband saying he was leaving. She described her reactions to this note. I replied, "Earlier you talked about how angry you were at your husband for leaving you and thought of ways to make him suffer the way you are suffering. Then you felt tired and became silent because you may have felt unsafe in talking of how angry and vengeful you feel." Mrs. Y. picked up on this interpretation in the next session, describing what it was like for her to feel abandoned. I was able to point out to her how she often projected her own angry feelings onto others. She began to discuss how angry she frequently felt and how she dealt with it. She said: "It embarrasses me to be so critical. There is something cruel about it. . . . I'm also afraid I'll turn on you the way I have on people at work." Thus she began to take responsibility for the anger she projected onto others and to express her anxiety about losing control of it.

As Mrs. Y. explored her anger, she also began to talk about visual and somatic experiences suggestive of sexual abuse. When she did so, she said she felt dirty and ashamed, whereupon she would become either silent or self-critical. I would interpret her schizoid compromise: "You're feeling anxious, ashamed, embarrassed, and vulnerable to harsh criticism. To manage these painful feelings, you've progressively retreated to a place where you feel safer because you're alone. But when you are alone, you feel there is nothing to live for."

It was necessary repeatedly to interpret Mrs. Y.'s schizoid compromise in dealing with feelings of vulnerability or anger. I would say: "I think the issues you bring up today about feeling exposed at your job was your way of taking a safe distance from talking about feelings of being exposed in here, which came up last session." Or, "I noticed that after you expressed your anger at my not giving you enough help here, you became silent and seemed to sit stiffly to protect yourself from how risky it felt to follow through and explore your feelings about being left in the lurch by me." Mrs. Y. began to have memories with greater affect in therapy. At the same time, she began to articulate fears of being abandoned if she talked about her anger.

With the formation of a therapeutic alliance and my focusing my interpretations on Mrs. Y.'s schizoid compromise defenses, she not only experienced more and deeper affect in her sessions, but also began to look for and identify her feelings on her own. A frequent source of anxiety was her noting that she expected others to abandon her if she expressed any of her anger.

She continued to draw images and to have body sensations suggestive of sexual abuse. She made several drawings to represent pain she was experiencing in different parts of her body. When making a drawing representing the experience of pain in her sacrum, her image was one of being raped with her legs spread apart. The initial images were in bright colors, which she later toned down and blurred with white. Her comments about the revision suggested she may have feared that further investigation of possible abuse would lead her to experiencing feelings of extreme helplessness.

Although she may have backed away from talking of specific incidents of sexual or physical abuse, she was willing to look at emotional abuse. She said, "The cruelest part of the abuse, whether verbal or sexual, is that you take on that abusive role. I don't need my dad around, I do it to myself."

On a number of occasions, Mrs. Y. presented material suggestive of sexual or ritual abuse in the form of dreams involving blood, knives, or torture, or of her oldest brother's approaching her with an erection. After presenting this material, she would back off from exploring it. How should I respond to her presentation? I decided to let her know I was quite open to hearing about sexual abuse if that sort of material began to emerge, but I did not pursue this information by asking questions, nor did I comply with her request that I hypnotize her. I saw her asking to be hypnotized as a test of whether or not I could be trusted to respect her need for boundaries.

After the formation of a clear therapeutic alliance, Mrs. Y. showed the beginning of an emergence of the real self. An early appearance was in the form of a dream in which she ice-skated almost effortlessly over an obstacle course. She felt exhilarated at having fun and mastering something difficult. She had been quite athletic during latency, but gave up sports when the boys began to tease her about being so good at them. Not too long after this dream, she began lessons in a former sport. Later, she found people to play with, greatly improved her performance, and then participated in her sport internationally.

Another sign of emergence of the real self was that she no longer produced artistic creations just for herself, but began to show them to other people—an intimate sharing that formerly would have seemed impossibly unsafe.

Mrs. Y.'s appearance gradually changed; now she has her hair done in a becoming style, tastefully but sparingly uses cosmetics, wears contact lenses, and has a wardrobe of flattering professional attire. Her face is no longer masklike, and she has revealed a sense of humor.

With the development of the therapeutic alliance, Mrs. Y. began to experience and describe affects associated with the abandonment depression. In the following description of her feelings in a dream, there are clear references to feelings about both the indifferent object and the self-in-exile. She said: "The feeling when people started shooting at me is similar to how I feel when my husband leaves me. How frightening, as if he's doing it without any feeling for me. As if he could act without feeling. As I talk about this dream, I have trouble breathing. As in the dream, I feel like going outside by myself to get away from the depression inside me." Or later: "I think I'll die without him. I'm so sensitive to feeling I've been left. It's a bodily reaction; it hurts and it's chilling from being so frightened. I'm losing my grasp."

Mrs. Y. experienced many of her childhood memories in the form of bodily sensations, (perhaps a dimension of her athletic propensities). Noting a pressured feeling of wanting to bolt from the consulting room, the sensations of which reminded her of being with her parents, she commented, "I'm always frightened when I'm with them. I feel I always have to come up with something to make them feel safe in order for me to feel safe. So I'm always on the spot." I think this is a poignant description of her self-experience in the master/slave part unit.

Parenthetically, this patient was quite creative in using visual imagery, dreams, and writings to explore and express herself. When she talked of her feelings, she was often poignant. In my experience, this capacity for and use of artistic expression is not uncommon in patients with a schizoid disorder of the self. (This artistic sensitivity in schizoid individuals is vividly portrayed in *An Angel at My Table*, Jane Campion's film based on the life of New Zealand author, Janet Frame).

As therapy continued, Mrs. Y. used more adaptive defenses than before. For example, several years earlier, she would often distance by spending almost half a session in a silent dissociative state. Now, without my saying anything, she often will catch herself beginning to dissociate and then talk about the feelings that triggered this defensive reaction. These often are fears that she will be attacked and humiliated if she expresses her feelings or needs. She related that saying what she feels is experienced by her as feeling as if she is parading herself naked.

As Mrs. Y. controlled her use of dissociation, she increasingly experienced the affects from which her dissociating defended her. Often the affect was anger. Acknowledging the anger, she began to see how she also managed it by attributing her anger to others. She then expected hostile criticism for expressing herself. She also discovered that she used self-attack as a way to contain her anger in situations in which she would be justified in expressing it, but felt unsafe in doing so.

The longer Mrs. Y. engaged in working through the affects of the abandonment depression, the more her real self emerged and the less I needed to direct my interpretations just to manifestations of the schizoid compromise. Many times now in treatment, my interpretations are not much different than they would be if Mrs. Y. were a neurotic patient rather than character disordered.

Mrs. Y. continues to be in therapy.* I believe, however, that the outcome using the Masterson Approach has made a difference for Mrs. Y. in allowing her to experience and begin to work through the painful affects of the abandonment depression. As a result, Mrs. Y. feels much less unsafe with experiencing her anger. Consequently, she now has much less difficulty in

---

*The lengthy duration of her treatment in part reflects the generally greater caution of schizoid patients in modifying their defenses in comparison to patients with borderline or narcissistic disorders.

delegating work to others and making her feelings and needs known to her husband, as well as to supervisees and superiors at work. She has developed a small circle of colleagues with whom she enjoys having lunch, and she occasionally invites them to her home. In addition, her life has been enriched by the emergence of her real self in terms of artistic creation, athletic accomplishments, and an expanding capacity for self-expression and intimacy in relationships. As she recently put it, "It's as if my heart were opening."

REFERENCES

Fairbairn, W. R. D. (1941). A revised psychopathology of the psychoses and the psychoneuroses. In *An Object Relations Theory of the Personality*. New York: Basic Books, 1952.
Guntrip, Harry. (1969) *Schizoid Phenomena, Object Relations and the Self*. New York: International Universities Press.

CHAPTER 9

Narcissistic Defenses Against a Schizoid Disorder

Barbara L. Short, Ph.D.

Ms. V. was referred by her therapist, who said he was retiring, and who also wanted to know whether I was accepting new patients. He was calling to check because he did not want her to be turned down by someone he recommended. He had been seeing her for several years, and said he felt very concerned about the way she might react to his retirement.

The first information I received about Ms. V. that helped with diagnosis was that her previous therapist was concerned about the referral. In fact, he was rueful, chagrined, uncomfortable—as if he were dreading Ms. V.'s reaction when he told her about his retirement. I felt as if he were lining me up as an offering to appease her, like a lion tamer entering a cage only after the lion is busy with dinner.

HISTORY

The next information about Ms. V. was her behavior with me and my feelings about her. My first session with Ms. V. was strained, and I recall thinking that she probably would not continue therapy with me very long. She was 55 years old, attractive, white, and dressed like a successful business person. She was openly disappointed in me, my way of doing therapy, and was angry and resentful that her previous therapist was retiring. She was contemptuous or disdainful of, or disappointed with, almost everyone and everything in her life, and she often sneered openly when talking about others. She reported that she wanted more out of life, was disappointed about the way everything had turned out, and had little hope that therapy with me or anyone else could do anything for her. However, she said she was desperate, because her life was running out, and she believed that therapy should help her attain a better life. Ms. V. seemed to feel entitled to "get" me to do something to make her life better. It was clear she was not in therapy to explore and understand herself in order to bring about the changes she wanted.

I had a strong countertransference reaction to Ms. V. I was immediately apprehensive that she would turn her contempt more directly on me, and I felt stuck, helpless, angry, and defeated. My awareness of these feelings shifted from background to foreground many times in my work with Ms. V. It seems to have significantly influenced my initial diagnosis.

I began to suspect that Ms. V. had a middle-level to low-level exhibitionistic narcissistic disorder of the self. Persons with a higher-level narcissistic disorder often are able to develop their talents and abilities successfully, and may be capable of great achievements in their chosen fields. Those with lower-level disorders have severe difficulty in object relations, and are less able to achieve the status and success to which they believe they are entitled.

The narcissistic disorder has characteristic split object relations units: the false defensive unit, consisting of a fused grandiose self/omnipotent object, and the empty self/aggressive object fused unit, which contains the affects of the abandonment depression. It appeared to me that Ms. V. attempted to live in the false defensive unit, but owing to the fragility of her defense, was unable to sustain a connection of any duration. I saw her display of contempt, superiority, entitlement, and cold perfectionism (directed even toward her son) as characteristics of her grandiosity, although, at the time, those features somehow seemed more porous and fragile than the ubiquitous, global, and airtight defense described by Masterson (1981). However, I ascribed this quality of porosity to her having a low-level narcissistic disorder. Similarly, I believed that genuine efforts at self-activation, which should precipitate activation of the abandonment depression, were largely absent and that she devoted herself to performance designed to elicit admiration and approval from others. She seemed ceaselessly to search the world for mirroring to maintain her fragile sense of self-esteem, and was extremely vulnerable to the slightest failure of others to reflect what she needed (and felt entitled) to experience.

When her previous therapist announced his retirement, it appeared she had experienced it as a massive disappointment, and lost her experience of being mirrored. This loss activated the empty self/aggressive object fused unit. In order to restore her sense of self-esteem, she projected the fragmented, empty, worthless part self onto others, and acted out the aggressive part object with unrelenting devaluation. I was aware of some of my reaction to this projection—the experience of fearing her contempt and devaluation—but I was not aware of having received the projective identification through which I experienced her futility, helplessness, anger, and defeat. During the first months of treatment, I was largely immobilized by my apprehension, so I said very little. Much later, I came to understand I was probably acting out a projective identification.

I should note that her feeling of futility about therapy had some basis in reality. Prior to spending several years in supportive therapy with the therapist who referred her to me, she had read "tons" of self-help books and had sought help from many other therapists over more than two decades, including various types of groups and weekend workshops, all of which had, in her words, "done no good at all—nothing ever changed." She was referring to their failure to make her life better by changing others, not herself. In a way, therapy had failed Ms. V. In another way, she had defeated therapy with the constant transference acting out of her false, defensive self.

The next information about Ms. V. emerged from her history. This case is a good example of how initial history is filtered through the defensive structure of the self and object representations. For example, Ms. V. first presented herself as having a behavior problem of such severity that she had to be sent away from home—a story she had often been told by her mother. Much later in treatment, a different picture of her history emerged as Ms. V. began to shift from her lifelong identification with her mother, and explore what her own experiences had been.

In evaluating historical material for diagnosis, the therapist also must think in terms of the kind and degree of attachment the infant/toddler was able to negotiate with his or her caretaker during the critical stage of the arrest. Ralph Klein refers to this as the negotiated contract for connection, for attachment, for survival. Persons with a narcissistic disorder negotiate a contract to get approval, acknowledgment, and affirmation in exchange for resonating perfectly with the caretaker's idealizing projections. Those with a borderline disorder negotiate a contract to get these resources in exchange for resonating with the caretaker's needs for them not to separate or individuate. And those with a schizoid disorder negotiate a contract to have no needs, to be totally self-reliant, in exchange for having at least a tenuous connection that would not result in being appropriated or treated with total indifference. In addition, Klein suggests that understanding the quality, as well as the nature, of the negotiated contract is a major factor in determining whether the disorder of the self is high level (open to interpretation) or low level (airtight).

Ms. V.'s initial history was sketched with a few stereotypical descriptions. Her mother appeared to have had a narcissistic disorder. She would occasionally do things for Ms. V. that had little to do with her, sometimes attack her verbally, but mostly ignore her or send her away. For example, her mother spent "hours" making her "beautiful" clothes that Ms. V. later said she did not like, sacrificed financially to pay for music lessons on an instrument she later admitted she had not liked, and then would turn on her with rage, derogation, and distancing for failures, or for no reason at all. She remembered trying to do things for her mother "to get her to like me— even just to look at me." Later, she transferred these efforts to teachers whom she seemed to idealize.

Her father was described as nicer, but passive, hated by her mother, and seldom at home. At times her mother enlisted her in deprecating the father, and at other times equated her with her father as being "worthless, dirty, and vile." (Additional details about her father did not emerge for years.) Her family was, in her words, working class, of which her mother, and later she herself, was ashamed.

Ms. V. characterized her relationships with others in two ways. She blandly reported that she had not been popular as a child or as an adult, had never had many friends, and was always the last to be chosen, if chosen at all, for activities in school, socially, or at work. With a little laugh, she said that even her mother found her too difficult to deal with, and had to send her to boarding school from the second grade to the 10th grade. This, she explained, was because she was "too difficult to handle" and "a spoiled brat." She reported this, as she did most of her self descriptions, in a bland, offhand, detached manner. She appeared to have completely accepted her mother's rationale for sending her away, reporting that she was lonely at first, but rapidly adjusted. "You can get used to anything," she observed.

However, she also described almost anyone with whom she associated as being inferior, stupid, and even contemptible. This included her son, from whom she had been estranged for nearly 15 years, and both of her ex-husbands. She had remained friends with her second husband after a marriage of less than one year, although she was angry at him for what she scornfully described as his "marshmallow" passivity. Nevertheless, she was able to tolerate seeing him for an occasional dinner, and grieved when he died in 1990.

Other than her second ex-husband, the only person with whom she had an ongoing relationship was her employer, a successful professional with whom she worked for about 20 years until his death in 1990. It seemed that she felt gratified by his status and mirrored by his careful treatment of her.

For the most part, however, Ms. V. would complain about not having a better relationship with her son, co-workers, and people she met who might be friends, and, in the next sentence, would describe them (including her son) as stupid, inferior, or contemptible. She joined innumerable groups, such as Parents Without Partners, travel groups, and singles groups; would attend briefly; and then would withdraw in anger, describing the other members as boring, stupid, ugly, and so on. Although she owned her own home, a condominium, she felt her community was beneath her. She wanted to move back to a county where she had lived with her first husband, noting that it was where "more interesting and intelligent people lived."

Ms. V. excelled academically, and described herself as liking school, and later work, "if it wasn't boring." She graduated from high school, moved into her own apartment with no reported difficulty, put herself through secretarial training, and later, at the suggestion of her physician, put herself through college in four years. She married, moved from her home in the Midwest to the San Francisco Bay area, and helped her husband build a successful small business, largely through her efforts.

Her first husband had been an illiterate, itinerant laborer when she met him. She taught him to read and keep books, and worked as his staff to build their business. When he left her for another women after six years of marriage, she returned to secretarial work and night school to train for a paraprofessional position. She was able to separate from her family with little difficulty, and pursued goals that would elevate her above her "embarrassing" working-class beginnings. Ms. V. described each of her significant separations with the same blandness or anger as she did the rest of her social history. Her descriptions of leaving home to go to boarding school and later, at 17 years of age, to get her own apartment, had the bland offhand quality of all her self descriptions.

However, separations from her husbands and her son were reported with anger and contempt. I believed that her identification with her narcissistic mother enabled her to leave her original home, and later, each of her marital relationships, with little separation anxiety. She transferred her idealization and search for mirroring to teachers, employers, supervisors, and, later, her husbands. It seemed mirroring by others enabled her to have the fleeting experience she must have felt when her mother enlisted her collaboration in being special, unique, and superior to others in their working-class neighborhood, and even to her father.

THERAPY

According to the Masterson model, therapy with a disorder of the self progresses through three stages: testing, therapeutic alliance and working through, and separation. During the first or testing phase, the patient is engaged primarily in transference acting out, and attempts to pressure the therapist to resonate with his or her false defensive self in order to avoid affects of the abandonment depression.

The second, or working-through, stage is characterized by the patient's no longer engaging primarily in transference acting out, being able to experience and contain affect, and to work internally through the transference. In other words, in stage 2, patients are somewhat aware that they are splitting, projecting, denying, avoiding, and so on, and that the source of their repetitive self-defeating experiences and interpretations of reality is largely internal. Later in this stage, the patient relinquishes the protective defensive structure, works through the affects of the abandonment depression, and emerges with whole self and object relations.

Ms. V. entered the testing phase testing *my ability* not to withdraw from her provocations or to ally with her false, defensive self through mirroring. She adamantly refused to be in therapy more than once a week, stating that it was probably a waste of time and money. For months, I was caught in countertransference acting out, and I alternated between using supportive interventions and mirroring.

I told myself that her age, prior history, and defeat of previous therapy demonstrated that she would be unable to work toward integration, and that the best I could hope for was alleviation of her distress through supportive counseling. I hid behind this rationalization—which is absolutely contrary to the basic premise of the Masterson Approach, which is that therapy begins with the assumption that every patient with a disorder of the self is capable of self-activation and, ultimately, of whole self and object relations. This is not to say that every patient will achieve these goals. However, a patient's inability to do so must be empirically verified through therapy, not assumed or inferred on the basis of history and the therapist's countertransference.

I was caught in my countertransference, and used these old wisdoms as my shield. As a result, I did not direct her focus to what was happening in the hour. Rather, I would murmur something like "It sounds like that was very painful for you," when she reported being treated badly at work, or note how disappointed she seemed when others—potential friends, groups, dates—turned out to be, in her words, "inferior, a little stupid, and very boring."

Ms. V.'s search for the perfect mirroring environment seemed to be continuous. However, she was vulnerable to the slightest criticism or disappointment, and would quickly experience anger, which she expressed by devaluing and distancing. She was offended when not waited on immediately and with perfect courtesy in stores and restaurants. A loud child in a supermarket or a teenager's loud radio would trigger her rage. It seemed that she felt entitled to not having these things happen "to" her, and complained bitterly that "someone ought to do something" to stop or punish people who did these things.

A few months after she entered therapy with me, Ms. V. saw my name on the faculty list of a nearby college, and appeared to transfer her lifelong idealization of teachers to me. She also said she felt that I understood her, and finally settled on me as an acceptable object for idealization. As she continued to spend her sessions talking about the stupid, incompetent, inconsiderate, individuals with whom she had to deal in her life, I gradually controlled my countertransference, and began to address her entitlement to perfect mirroring and her vulnerability to criticism and disappointment. However, I did not fully bring it into the hour and engage her disappointment in me until I raised her fee at the end of her second year. At this point, her entitlement to perfect caring and consideration by me, and her envy and rage at me (and the world) for failing to mirror her, emerged full blown.

She reacted with fury and contempt to what she called my greed, and said she did not want to continue therapy with someone as insensitive and inconsiderate of her as I was. I acknowledged that she seemed to be extremely disappointed in my fee increase. However, I suggested that it seemed she was doing here with me what she did with other relationships; that is, she felt so disappointed when others displeased her that the only way she could make herself feel better was to withdraw, but that would destroy her therapy.

The discussion continued for three or four sessions, and ended in a draw. I raised my fees; Ms. V. did not like it and was not inclined to explore her disappointment with me or others. However, she decided to stay in therapy, noting that "it was better than nothing."

After about three years of therapy, the content of Ms. V.'s sessions slowly began to change. The shift was so gradual that I did not notice it for months, and later had to go back and review my notes to identify when the shift had begun. I also had my countertransference more under control. I had dealt with some of her projective identification by identifying and processing the feelings of helplessness, defeat, and futility, and, eventually, describing them to her as part of her experience.

Ms. V. continued to respond to interpretations of failure in empathy with a kind of "damned right" agreement that I should have known better, and was insulted when I suggested that it was curious that she would expect that such failures should not occur. She also was offended when I suggested that she was doing with me what she did out there in her work and social life. However, I became increasingly able to make these interpretations in a firm, neutral, interested way, and began to add that this was a lifelong pattern that seemed to thwart many of the goals she had for herself in life—to have friends, a husband, and a good relationship with her son.

As this process continued, Ms. V. did not acknowledge that any problems might originate within her, nor did she explore her vulnerability to disappointments and failures in empathy—responses expected if the diagnosis and interventions had been correct. However, the change in the content of her sessions became more and more evident. For example, Ms. V.'s bland, detached reporting of the "spoiled brat" stories changed as the truth began to be questioned, and to be told with affect and with a change in content. She described how much it hurt her to be told she was spoiled no matter what she did, and that she wondered why her cousins, who had been more disobedient than she, had not been sent away.

She recalled how alone she had always been, and began to experience fleeting feelings of sadness as she described memories of her isolation. For example, she remembered waiting every Sunday for her mother to visit—standing at her window looking down the road long after the last train had arrived, hoping that she might still appear. In the seven years she was away at school, she recalled her mother visiting on two occasions. Her father did not visit at all.

As memories of her aloneness and loneliness began to unfold, she recalled a turning point in her life when she was about seven or eight years old—before she was sent to boarding school. She and her mother had a "terrible argument." Her mother told her she was so nasty and ugly that no one would ever love her. Although this was the kind of thing her mother often said, on this occasion she recalled sobbing for hours and begging her mother to love her, finally going to bed exhausted, knowing with certainty that her mother did not love her and that there was no hope. She awoke from a dream that her mother loved her and was being kind and sweet to her. She had the "most wonderful feeling of warmth for a few moments," she said, and then the memory of the preceding evening flooded in, and she realized that it had just been a dream, and that there was no hope. As such memories began to emerge, her expressions of anger and hostility diminished in intensity and frequency, and moments of sadness and loneliness began to occur, followed immediately by one or another of her defensive maneuvers. The affects of sadness and loneliness seemed to be the first genuine expressions of affects of the real self, but when I addressed her defenses by mirroring interpretations of her vulnerability to experiencing and expressing these feelings, she typically responded with blandness, laughter, and some offhand remark, which I later recognized was her camouflage—her way of staying hidden.

DIAGNOSIS RECONSIDERED

Ms. V.'s therapy seemed to be taking a direction that I could not explain based on my diagnosis. I had assumed that the basis for her inability to have a long-term relationship with anyone was that she drove people away with her aggressive devaluation following failures in mirroring. However, interventions directed to vulnerability to failures in empathy had not had the effect expected with a narcissistic disorder. That is, they had not helped her explore her need for perfect mirroring and the affects of the abandonment depression it defends against.

The painful memories now emerging had much more to do with feelings about loneliness and alienation than the "empty, despised self." As I listened to her, I began to wonder whether she attacked people and drove them away in the service of staying safe to cope with an underlying schizoid disorder. In addition, it was becoming increasingly clear that her constant expression of hostility masked the degree to which other expressions of affect were unavailable. I also noticed that although her memories and affect were gradually shifting during her sessions, significant portions of her behavior had not changed. Her behavior with others outside therapy was still characterized by variations of the old, familiar approach–disaster–avoidance sequence.

Her behavior with me had been stable for years, and, in retrospect, seemed to be far more careful, cautious, and circumscribed than I would expect from a patient with a narcissistic disorder. For example, she would never call me to ask to change appointments, preferring to inconvenience herself rather than ask me for anything.

When I quizzed her about this, she reported that she did not want to bother me—a reply inconsistent with the diagnosis of narcissistic disorder. She was scrupulous about observing the rules. She was always early for appointments, never missed one, and had her payments ready before they were due. Increases in fees were occasions for anger at me, but mirroring interpretations did not lead to exploration of her feelings of disappointment.

As she became more able to describe her reactions to fee increases, it was clear that rather than feeling entitled to getting therapy at a low fee, she felt controlled—that I had the power to do something to her, and that it always came as a surprise, which she "really hated." She would not consider more involvement in therapy by increasing her sessions per week, using finances as her reason. However, I noticed she was able to afford an expensive computer, printer, and a continuous series of classes in computer use—one endeavor she really enjoyed.

In addition, characteristics I had earlier identified as part of her grandiosity now appeared to be less well articulated than a full narcissistic defense. For example, her air of superiority and perfectionism seemed to be a way of maintaining and rationalizing her need for distance rather than a display of the grandiose self of the narcissistic disorder.

I considered the possibility that she might have a narcissistic defense against a schizoid disorder. However, as she continued to disclose new information about her history, I discarded this notion. Masterson (1981) noted that if a child transfers his or her symbiotic relationship with the mother to a narcissistic father before the rapprochement crisis, the child's grandiose self will be preserved and reinforced. However, if there is a transfer after the formation of a split self and object relations unit is established, the child develops a narcissistic defense against the underlying disorder—in this case, a borderline disorder. As I learned more about Ms. V.'s family, it seemed likely that both the mother and father may have had schizoid disorders. The mother I was now learning about was alternately indifferent, sadistic, and appropriating. With this mother, there was no safe way to form a negotiated attachment to receive nurturance. The father was described as being more benign and able to have some attachment with Ms. V. when she was very young. However, he was seldom in the home and made no special effort to be with her.

It seemed increasingly clear that, except for her hostile presentation, she had a quality of wanting to be not noticed, which I had never noted. I began to wonder whether the anger and hostility of her presentations had been a camouflage for her not being present in her sessions—a "there but not there" quality more characteristic of the schizoid personality disorder. R. D. Laing wrote about not knowing and not knowing that you do not know. Perhaps, in this instance, I had not noticed, and not noticed that I had not noticed.

Klein (Masterson, 1993) has characterized the schizoid disorder as mimicking other disorders of the self. This is true of all personality disorders, but perhaps most of all of the schizoid character structure. Fairbairn (1950) noted that those with a schizoid disorder avoid real emotional contact with others by playing roles, efforts that often leave them feeling exhausted and depleted. Similarly, in his review of the literature regarding the schizoid disorder, Salman Akhtar (1987) noted that while there was considerable disagreement about diagnostic criteria, virtually "all authors note the discrepancy between the outer and the inner worlds of the schizoid individual, and emphasize the 'divided self' of such a person" (p. 501). The chimerical quality of the schizoid disorder appears throughout the analytic literature. Wilhelm Reich (1950) noted that schizoid patients have a strong wish for and against involvement; they keep people away and then draw them in by evoking curiosity and interest. They strike a balance or, as he called it, a compromise, by developing a kind of psychic contactlessness. Fenichel (1945) described schizoid characters as having pseudo-emotions and pseudo-contacts, and as responding to slights with narcissistic withdrawal.

Understanding the hidden nature of the schizoid disorder was greatly enhanced by the British object relations theorists Klein, Fairbairn, Winnicott, and Guntrip. Fairbairn built on Melanie Klein's ideas regarding early splitting of good and bad objects (the paranoid position), and later, regarding splits in the ego (the schizoid feature of this early position), and concluded that when early relations with objects are depriving or damaging, the infant establishes internal objects that act as substitutes. Guntrip elaborated on Fairbairn's theory, describing the schizoid disorder as being characterized by a dilemma: If one moves toward others seeking human companionship, one is in danger of being swallowed or absorbed. If one moves away from others, one feels totally insecure and lost. The only way to resolve this dilemma is to retreat from object relations, to become emotionally inaccessible. Guntrip listed the characteristics he believed identified the schizoid personality: introversion (including the final regressed ego unique to Guntrip's theory), withdrawnness, narcissism, self-sufficiency, a sense of superiority, loss of affect, loneliness, depersonalization, and regression.

The Masterson Approach provides a unique synthesis of object relations theory, developmental theory, and attachment theory for understanding the schizoid disorder.

Ralph Klein has described the origin of the schizoid disorder of the self as arising out of a very tenuous negotiated attachment to the caretaker formed during childhood. He suggests that the difference between a higher-level and a lower-level schizoid disorder is probably based more on the quality and quantity of the attachment than on the exact time of the arrest. A kind of final severing of attachment is often reported by these patients as occurring at about the age of eight or nine, when they finally gave up hope of relying on parents to provide emotional nurturance; they realized that any fundamental network of attachment as a source of nurturance and support was never going to happen.

It is generally recognized that persons who develop a schizoid disorder have experienced severe abuse, neglect, and especially appropriation and indifference at the hands of their early caretakers. This treatment results in the uniquely schizoid picture of an individual who, as an adult, maintains a careful internal and external emotional detachment, and, in most cases, a physical distance from others.

They long to be attached, to be in relationships with others, and to receive the affirmation, acknowledgment, and approval of which they were deprived. However, this longing evokes an intense anxiety about being in danger of being appropriated, used, and discarded as they were by their original caretakers. The only way to control their anxiety, to feel safe, is to withdraw internally as well as externally.

When they withdraw, they feel alone, alienated, and, finally, a kind of cosmic loneliness—as if they have lost the capacity to communicate with other human beings. This is the schizoid dilemma as developed by Klein within the Masterson Approach.

Unlike the borderline and the narcissistic disorders, the schizoid disorder of the self does not have a way of maintaining emotional attachment with an internal or external object; both attachment and unattachment carry danger for the patient with a schizoid disorder. Attachment in the master/slave unit results in appropriation and domination. Attachment in the sadistic object/self-in-exile unit results in a sadistic attack or indifference. Only through developing a false-self compromise of withdrawal of affect and self-reliance can the person with a schizoid disorder strike a balance that allows the person to be safe and still have a functional connection to the world. This part of the compromise can be thought of as a kind of evenly hovering or equidistant position through which the individual tries to stay at a safe distance from both the controlling master and the sadistic-indifferent split objects. The other part of the compromise is the final sanctuary for the schizoid disorder, a life of fantasy. In an often richly elaborated inner world, persons with a schizoid disorder experience relationship, and hold alive the hope of emotional connections too dangerous to attempt in their external world.

THERAPY RECONSIDERED

Ms. V.'s later disclosures about her past, her circumscribed behavior with me, her continuing approach–disaster–avoidance patterns with others, and especially the use of distancing from affect, led me to reevaluate her diagnosis. With the new information emerging in her sessions, it seemed increasingly clear that whenever she attempted to move toward being close to others or tried to really belong to a group, she would experience two distinct kinds of apprehension. On the one hand, she would describe ways they took advantage of her, or "drained me dry," as she would say. On the other, she reported feeling she was not perceived, that they did not know she was even there, and would give up in defeat and fatigue and go home.

This could be thought of as the schizoid disorder of the self triad: self-activation or trying to move toward attachment (the real-self task of the schizoid disorder) evoked the fear of being appropriated or treated with indifference, which, in turn, led to defense—in this case, anger, withdrawal, and "going it alone." For Ms. V., self-reliance meant becoming more educated at a level that did not require her to perform outside a highly circumscribed (safe) arena of accomplishment. She did, however, use her intellect—a typical schizoid pattern—to create a world that allowed her to be self-supporting and safe. (On one occasion, she observed that "education is one thing they can't ever take away from you.") Her primary source of connection with others was through reading, watching television, and daydreaming about the kind of life she would like to have.

The Masterson Approach identifies the schizoid dilemma as the primary defense to be addressed in work with the schizoid disorder. Klein has observed that once there is a consensus about the dilemma, the schizoid compromise can be addressed by linking it first to the dysphoric affects of the schizoid dilemma and later to the affects associated with the abandonment depression. The compromise of self-reliance and attachment through fantasy is the person's way of staying safe, and interpretations directed to this sanctuary must be based on the patient's clear readiness to explore it.

Patients with a schizoid disorder believe that in order to stay safe, they must be totally self-reliant and keep their "real self" hidden. To be known is to invite being appropriated, dominated, and treated with indifference. Therefore, initial interventions must be couched in terms of the dilemma— the danger of revealing oneself or moving toward attachment in therapy, having to withdraw, and feeling unsafe.

When real affect-appropriate content emerges, patients with a schizoid disorder will experience and express a wide variety of defenses to return to safety both internally and externally. Among these defenses are withdrawal of affect, denial, projection, projective identification, and intellectualization. In addition, since a major concern of these patients is being appropriated, Klein suggests that interpretations be couched in the most tentative, least intrusive terms, and presented as hypotheses for their consideration.

With this in mind, I began to observe to Ms. V. that it appeared that she had experienced a lifelong pattern of moving toward getting involved with people, and then withdrawing from them, and I wondered whether her anger had kept her safe by keeping people at a distance, keeping them from getting too involved. Ms. V. seemed startled at this new intervention, but then readily agreed.

Gradually, over many sessions, she began revealing this aspect of herself. The following are portions of sessions that followed my beginning to use the interpretations of the schizoid dilemma and her fear of revealing herself.

> I seem to be two people. One sits down and says, "These things are possible. You can do this (go out and be with people)." Then the other person takes over and says "I'm too tired, no energy, I want to be by myself, stay put and be by myself. I'm too tired." Then that person takes over for a long, long time . . . [laughs] Maybe I'm just a loner. [*therapist*: it seems that you began to talk about how you really feel, and maybe began to feel that you revealed too much, and then you kind of distracted yourself and me.] Yes, it's the way I always do it. (silence) I go to Lyons (restaurant). I can be among people and be alone. I can be with people and be by myself. But when I go there, I can't wait to get home . . . I just have no energy.

Here Ms. V. talks about her experience of attempting to move toward others, which triggers affects of the abandonment depression and leads her to withdraw "for a long, long time." She remains alone until her longing for a "real" relationship draws her back to repeat the same pattern again. My intervention called to her attention this dynamic that was occurring in the therapy hour, and she was able to return to her self.

Ms. V. began to wonder about her past relationships, and ways that her need to protect herself had destroyed her chances to have the relationships for which she longed.

> I never felt there was any real connection with V. (her first husband). We never really touched each other inside. There was never any real intimacy. It was that way with any man. I would turn against them and not want to be touched. That's the way my mother was. She used to talk about my father as though he were dirty scum. I tried not to do that, but I went right ahead and did it. I always found something. I could never engage in real intimacy, sexual or any other way. I was always afraid because if I did get involved, I wouldn't be able to fulfill my commitment because I'd get too frightened. Like the last time I thought I had a relationship. I had turned off to him, but I didn't want him to leave me completely. Sometimes, when he'd come over, I couldn't wait for him to leave. He wanted to leave his pillow here. I wouldn't let him. To me it represented something—I don't know—like it was an invasion of my space, of me. In a way, anybody was better than nobody, yet when he was here, I wanted him to go.

In this case, Ms. V. described her inability to tolerate having anyone move into an intimate relationship with her. The possibility of being close evoked her fears both of being unable to please (unable to be a good slave) and of being appropriated. To get away from this anxiety, she had to withdraw again and use anger to distance. This segment also vividly illustrates Ms. V.'s growing awareness of her identification with the aggressor, her mother, and her activation of that part object to achieve distance, probably very much as her mother had done.

Ms. V. also began to talk about her fantasy life, and the ways in which it had sustained her through times of retreat from contact altogether. She had begun to report her dreams, conspicuous by their absence from her first years in therapy, and told of one in particular that seemed to illustrate her feelings of isolation and longing.

> I always dreamed of a wonderful relationship with a man. We would have a beautiful home, go dancing, have a warm, close relationship. We would feel really close, no matter what. That's what I was looking for. That's what I couldn't achieve with anybody.

I had a dream that I was on one side of a big glass—like Plexi-
glas—divider. Everyone else was on the other side, having a party.
I was going to be executed and I was screaming, but no one could
hear me. I could never get anyone's attention.

When I was very little, I'd daydream about a wealthy man giving
me money so I could do things for my mother and father and they
would see I was a nice girl.

Ms. V. spontaneously revealed her fear of being controlled and its source
in her past experiences. Interventions calling to her attention that movement toward revealing herself made her feel unsafe enabled her to stay
with the anxiety and begin to explore it.

It's sort of like when you're little and people can do things to you
and you have no control. That's the way I've been feeling. I'm so
tired. I don't make any sense. I'm rambling. [*therapist:* you reveal something about yourself and then stop yourself. I wonder
if it could be that you don't feel safe to know or have me know
these things.] Yes! I was always afraid of people. They could do
anything they wanted with me. I have a terrible tearing back and
forth inside me. I've always been afraid. I was always alone, always lonely. I'd go home for holidays, and be alone, and go back
to boarding school and be alone.

Finally she began to explore the function of her anger in keeping her
safe and, in a paradoxical way, from being controlled.

When I get scared, I get nasty. Like at the condo meeting last
night. I didn't know about the new rule (about parking). I didn't
know and felt like I couldn't control what they were going to do
to me. I felt real hostile. That's one of the important things I want
to get over. My fears are out of proportion, and then I get angry.
I cry a lot now, and I'm not sure why. I get so frightened. I feel
like I'm babbling, and I'm frightened. I want to get to the bottom of this anxiety. It seems like I'm feeling it so much these
days. . . . , I've been avoiding people—I stay disengaged so I don't
mind so much when things go wrong.

Ms. V. continues to work in therapy. Her affect is emerging, and her contacts with others are becoming more prolonged and more satisfying. She has been able to spend holidays with her son and his girlfriend for two years, and has actively participated in three groups for over a year. In addition, she is considering running for the board of directors at her condominium. However, she still lives alone, cannot tolerate others in her home, and maintains her careful "need-less" connection with me.

CONCLUSION

In evaluating the early work with Ms. V., one would wonder why anything of lasting value happened given that I made the wrong diagnosis and was using inappropriate interventions. I now believe she did not have a narcissistic disorder or a narcissistic defense against a schizoid disorder. Rather, I believe the features I mistook as indicating the presence of a narcissistic disorder were an acting out of the sadistic/master part objects of the schizoid disorder, projecting the slave/self-in-exile part selves, and retreating behind a cloud of contempt and anger. I believe I absorbed this projection, and remained at a safe distance from her for several years. My struggle to stay neutral enabled me eventually to process the projective identification of these self parts, coming out of *my* hiding, and engage in an effective therapeutic alliance with her.

I can only speculate that she felt that I was committed to my work with her, and that my continuous struggle to stay neutral and nondirective (once I gave up supportive interventions) allowed her to feel safe enough to begin revealing herself and exploring her fears about being in relationships with others. Even though I was suggesting to her what she might be feeling by using mirroring interpretations of narcissistic vulnerability, she did not experience this as so intrusive and controlling that she had to withdraw from therapy. I suspect she had begun to make a real attachment to me and to therapy long before I realized it.

REFERENCES

Akhtar, S. (1987). Schizoid personality disorder: A synthesis of developmental, dynamic and descriptive features. *American Journal of Psychotherapy*, 41: 499–518.
Fairbairn, W. R. D. (1986). *Psychoanalytic studies of the personality*. Boston: Routledge, Chapman & Hall.

Fenichel, Otto. (1945). *The Psychoanalytic Theory of Neurosis*. New York: W. W. Norton & Co.

Masterson, James F. (1981). *The Narcissistic and Borderline Disorders*. New York: Brunner/Mazel.

Masterson, James F. (1993). The emerging self. New York: Brunner/Mazel.

Reich, Wilhelm. (1950). *Character Analysis*. New York: Farrar, Straus and Giroux.

PART II

Early Trauma and the Developing Self

In recent years, emotional problems related to early abuse—physical and/or sexual—have increasingly come to the center of the clinical stage through such diagnostic categories as posttraumatic stress syndrome and multiple personality disorder. Many controversies have arisen, such as the validity of recovered memories. There are disagreements over what is the best therapeutic approach. Some argue that all one has to do is access and abreact the traumatic material.

Dr. Orcutt has constructively applied the Masterson Approach to this area, and she emphasizes a different point of view: it is necessary to titrate the abreactive work on the trauma with work on the character defenses for the patient to recover fully.

In Chapter 10 she describes the effects of trauma on the developing self. In Chapter 11 she describes a posttraumatic syndrome in a patient with a borderline disorder of the self, and in Chapter 12 she details the treatment of multiple personality disorder incorporating the Masterson Approach. In Chapter 13 Dr. Clark reports on the effects of early sexual abuse.

J. F. M. & R. K.

The Influence of Early Trauma on the Developing Self

Candace Orcutt, Ph.D.

Personality disorder may also be complicated by the presence of
other disorders. . . . Posttraumatic stress disorder based on physical
and/or sexual abuse may also coexist. Sometimes the posttraumatic stress
disorder is obvious, and at other times, it can be quite hidden, not
revealing itself until well into the psychotherapy.
Masterson, 1993, p. 63

The self manages trauma in childhood by hiding it in closed-off places in the psyche that remain dormant as the operational self matures. I propose that traumatic events experienced in the formative years affect the development of the self through the following psychic processes.

1. When the child is threatened by physical/sexual events that may exceed the protective capacities of the self-and-other dyad of the formative years, the perceived danger may be split off and dissociated, and this may produce posttraumatic stress disorder if the input is sufficiently intense or chronic. If the physical/sexual transgression of the child's "world" is traumatic, the sensory, emotional, and cognitive processing are interrupted and suspended in a defensive cold storage. Because of this lack of integration, a memory is not established, and may never be. A part of the self is, in effect, left behind in time; it is unable to grow. And to compound the dilemma, the knowledge of this situation is not available to the conscious self.

2. When significant misattunement in the self-and-other dyad of the formative years leads to the creation of a personality disorder, the resulting rigid patterning of primitive defenses further reinforces the posttraumatic disorder.

3. The institution of the repression barrier—a developmental phenomenon that sets a seal over the processing and structuring of the formative years—acts as a reinforcement of the psychically internalized model of the self-and-other and their unique relationship, whether that model is healthy or dysfunctional. The model then becomes a fundamental assumption, and conscious awareness is freed to address the tasks of later childhood and beyond. The inner model resembles a computer program that continues in automatic effect unless it can be accessed and changed through another unique dyadic relationship—the relationship created through dynamic psychotherapy.

Even when the repression barrier can be established only in a rudimentary fashion (due to the extensiveness of early developmental damage), the persistence of primitive splitting as a major organizing defense of the self guards the psychic inner model of being from healthy change and growth in disorders of the self.

4. To reach the place of abandonment depression in the treatment of some disorders of the self that have also been exposed to trauma, it may not be enough to complete what appears to be a competent level of character work. In addition, it may be necessary to resolve the primitive dissociation, based on trauma, that further stopped and distorted the growth of a part of the self. The lost part of the self, recovered by trauma work, is integrated into the conscious, maturing character, and the whole self is then available to work through the abandonment depression.

TRAUMA, POSTTRAUMATIC STRESS DISORDER, AND DEVELOPMENTAL TRAUMA

Trauma as it affects the psyche is defined as follows in the fourth edition of the *Diagnostic and Statistical Manual of Mental Disorders* (*DSM-IV*, 1994):

> The essential feature of Posttraumatic Stress Disorder is the development of characteristic symptoms following exposure to an extreme traumatic stressor involving direct personal experience of an event that involves actual or threatened death or serious injury, or other threat to one's physical integrity; or witnessing an event that involves death, injury, or a threat to the physical integrity of another person; or learning about unexpected or violent death, serious harm, or threat of death or injury experienced

by a family member or other close associate. . . . The person's response to the event must involve intense fear, helplessness, or
horror (or in children, the response must involve disorganized or
agitated behavior). . . . The full symptom picture must be present
for more than one month, . . . and the disturbance must cause
clinically significant distress or impairment in social, occupational,
or other important areas of functioning. (p. 424)

The manual describes three "characteristic symptoms arising from the
exposure to the extreme trauma:"

1. Persistent reexperiencing of the traumatic event.
2. Persistent avoidance of stimuli associated with the trauma and
   numbing of general responsiveness.
3. Persistent symptoms of increased arousal.

It is interesting to note that "inability to recall an important aspect of the
trauma" and "dissociative flashback episodes" are listed under the manual's
diagnostic criteria for PTSD, but do not have to be present to make the diagnosis (p. 428).

Wilson (1989) in reviewing the origins of the theory of traumatic stress
reactions observes:

Freudian influences postulated a model of traumatic neurosis
based on *intrapsychic* mechanisms in which the "protective
shield" of the ego was overwhelmed by an excessive influx of stimulation produced by a stressful life event. Once the ego was traumatized, however, other stimuli could function to become equivalent to the original stressor. Freud's model . . . is interesting
because his original theory (i.e., seduction theory) was an early
formulation of post-traumatic stress disorder. (pp. 3–4)

In reviewing *Studies on Hysteria* (Breuer & Freud, 1895), it is interesting to see that Freud and Breuer perceive the presence of psychogenic amnesia and its uncovering during flashback* episodes as intrinsic to the def-

---

*Flashback—a term referring to the literal experiencing of a past traumatic event as
if it were occurring in present time—tends to be used interchangeably with the more
formal term "abreaction." There also seems to be a tendency to use abreaction to describe the therapeutic process of guiding the traumatic experience into full conscious
resolution.

inition and treatment of hysteria. In hysteria, the trauma is out of awareness, "like a foreign body which long after its entry must be regarded as an
agent that is still at work" (p. 40). Furthermore:

> We found, to our great surprise at first, that *each individual hys-*
> *terical symptom immediately and permanently disappeared when*
> *we had succeeded in bringing clearly to light the memory of the*
> *event by which it was provoked, and in arousing its accompany-*
> *ing affect, and when the patient had described that event in the*
> *greatest possible detail and had put the affect into words.* (pp.
> 40–41; original italics)

They make the famous statement that *"hysterics suffer mainly from remi-*
niscences" (p. 42), and conclude:

> It will now be understood how it is that the psychotherapeutic
> procedure which we have described . . . has a curative effect. *It*
> *brings to an end the operative force of an idea which was not*
> *abreacted in the first instance, by allowing its strangulated affect*
> *to find a way out through speech; and it subjects it to associative*
> *correction by introducing it into normal consciousness. . . .* (p. 52)

As Freud adds later in "Remembering, Repeating and Working-Through"
(1914), in unresolved neurosis "the compulsion to repeat . . . replaces the
impulse to remember." It is to be understood that this repetitive behavior, as the analysand's way of remembering, will become manifest inevitably
in the analysis, and will persist until the working through brings the meaning of the behavior into consciousness (pp. 150–151).

At this historical juncture, Freud emphasized the necessity for the integration of "forgotten" *inner* experience (which has its inception in unresolved oedipal fantasy, with a minimizing and ameliorizing of actual physical and sexual events in childhood). This integration of the analysand's
conscious narrative history is accomplished in the process of working
through, in which the analysand consciously and affectively resolves hidden childhood conflict by understanding how distortions in the relationship
with the analyst repeat this old, unfinished business. Steadily, memory para-
doxically preserved and denied in symptoms is translated into conscious
recollection. Feelings and perceptions that had been kept from awareness
are released, mastered, and transformed into a continuous, autonomous
sense of identity moving responsibly through time. The neurotic symptomatology lifts, but not because of a single dramatic experiencing of a traumatic event. The abreaction of the earlier cathartic method gives way to

the many less devastating "aha" moments of insight (about misattuned or misapprehended relationship) that incrementally build toward a coherent sense of self.

Freud's concept of working through is an indispensable contribution to psychotherapy with all forms of psychic disorder, since it shifts the work from emphasis on a rapid, almost magical cure to engagement in a process that respects and combines with the natural process of psychic growth itself.

However, when Freud largely abandoned his early seduction theory, he effectively dismissed an important reality factor in the creation of many psychic disorders. In addition, he rejected the technically valuable tool of hypnosis and the clinical phenomenon of abreaction. Freud, whose mind is at its most brilliant when arguing dialectically, abandoned his usual style in the matter of hypnosis versus evenly hovering attention and abreaction versus working through. These are not mutually exclusive concepts, but have their own place and time with the appropriate patients. Freud also lost track of the concept of dissociation during the problematic years from 1896 to 1899 (the period that brought him from *Studies on Hysteria* to *The Interpretation of Dreams*). Colin Ross (1989), who rarely minces words, writes: "When Freud repudiated the seduction theory, he abandoned dissociation and led psychiatry astray for much of the 20th century" (p. 138).

It is important to know that even a man with Freud's mind and professional courage can be carried from the mark where so many social and psychological tides intersect. To make Freud the focus of these issues is valid to a point, and then becomes a diversion. Freud was dedicated to understanding the dynamic operation of human psychopathology. Freud developed a constantly evolving theory of this dynamic, and proposed numerous ways in which to schematize and work with it therapeutically. He rejected or modified many of his theories and techniques, but rarely seems to have proposed a way of working or understanding that could not be used by another, if not himself. However the field of dynamic psychotherapy moves on, we are still indebted to Freud's belief, which he never compromised, in the inner world of the psyche, its base in biology, and its conflict with the emerging, conscious, civilized self.

APPLYING FREUD'S CONCEPTS TO DISORDERS OF THE SELF

Masterson: Transference Acting Out and the Working Through

While Freud focused his theory and practice on the neurotic patient, other early analysts, notably Jung, devoted their work to preoedipal pathology. Since the 1970s, concern with personality disorder (a concept more theoretically evolved than is character disorder) has been of special interest in the field. Masterson's concept of disorders of the self (in turn, a theoretical expansion of personality disorder) draws on fundamental Freudian ideas in particular.

Masterson finds an explanation of the dynamic of his concept of transference acting out in Freud's work. Citing "Remembering, Repeating and Working-Through" (Freud, 1914), he writes: "We have only to substitute the words 'transference acting-out' for the phrase 'expressing what is forgotten in behavior' " (Masterson, 1981). He continues:

> Freud highlighted the following: the patient remembers nothing, but expresses it in action. He/she reproduces it not in memory, but in behavior. He/she repeats it in his transference acting-out. The compulsion to repeat an action which replaces the impulse to remember is activated in treatment through the transference relationship. (p. 148)

It should be recalled that Masterson is not describing an oedipal phenomenon that results in neurotic symptomatology; he is defining a pre-oedipal happening that has its origins in the years in which the sense of self, other, and their interrelationship is formed, and contributes to the style and expression of the personality. In conjunction with the use of object relations theory, he follows Mahler's developmental model, with its emphasis on the mother–child dyadic interchange that when healthy fosters the infant's growing capacity to separate and individuate, and when unhealthy, arrests these tendencies.

The behavior repeated in transference acting out reenacts the "event" in the infant's stage of development when the learning of adaptive relationship is arrested by significant dissonance in the mother–child dyad. As a result, the infant learns that an exercise of autonomy is met by a withdrawal of love, and this is sufficient to skew the formation of the self away from the independent goal. Instead, a false self is defensively constructed to accommodate to the mother's emotional requirements, and so to secure enough positive response (or lack of negative response) to permit psychic survival. Forms of defensive false self take their characterological coloration from the particular conditions imposed by the particular mother–child dyad.

The defensive false self acts repetitively and maladaptively to avoid any interpersonal situation that may suggest, and so perhaps invoke, the intolerable past threat to the infant self: "The aim of the repetition compulsion [in the disorders of the self] is not to master conflict, as in the neurotic, but to avoid separation anxiety and abandonment depression" (Masterson, 1981, p. 136).

As the patient perceives the relationship to the therapist as significant, subliminal fears of separation/abandonment begin to be activated, and the patient demonstrates characteristic defensive behavior:

> To avoid the pain of depression . . . the patient frequently defends against the emergence of each segment of it by acting it out in the transference. . . . The patient is impelled to "replay" his conflicts using the therapist as mother and/or father, thereby relieving his inner tension without having to face the suffering of the original conflicts that remembering and working-through imply. (Masterson, 1976, p. 102)

It is the goal of the therapy to address the primal defenses (denial, avoidance, and so on) that support the defensive false self, and especially to interrupt their rigid and indiscriminate use. The interruption of the false defensive self style prevents the discharge of feeling through acting out, and leads "to the awakening of memories, setting the stage for working-through" (Masterson, 1981, p. 149). The working-through phase of therapy allows the patient to understand the existence and power of the repetition resistance, and to come to grips with the memory of the interpersonal history that necessitated the formation of such resistance. Masterson concludes in this synthesis of Freud's theory and his own: "Theoretically, one may correlate the working-through with the 'abreaction' of qualities of affect pent up by repression that has been manifested in hypnosis" (p. 149).

Masterson's work gives full weight to the significance of psychic fixation in early childhood, and synthesizes Freud's ideas with concepts from object relations, developmental, and self models. This not only restores important insights revised or discarded by Freud himself, but uses them as a cornerstone for the construction of a theory of the self and a method for the healing of its pathology. This, like all creative approaches, generates new ideas in turn. I believe that Masterson's refocusing of Freud's work to inform our understanding of the emerging self further encourages us to take a new look at Freud's original trauma theory and its implication for the formation of the self in the developmental years.

Developmental Trauma

In Freud's original trauma theory, the stressor impinges from the outer world. In his later theory of neurosis, the stressor becomes a psychic phenomenon primarily generated from the inner world of the individual (the Oedipus complex). Neurotic patients are fixated at a preoedipal stage for reasons based on fantasy, which may or may not be supported by real events. The neurotic person is able to transcend the fixation, however, until the perceived threat of the oedipal phase sends the person back regressively to the earlier period of fixation. That regressive conflict expresses itself in a symptom or character trait that takes on the coloration of the fixation.

Masterson (together with other theoreticians and clinicians concerned with preoedipal states) has shown how preoedipal fixations in themselves shape the individual. Freud was primarily concerned with fixation of the libido. Ego psychology and developmental theory extended the concept of fixation to developmental arrest of the ego; and the failure of internalized object relations to progress normally would now be considered intrinsic to the dynamic concept of personality disorder. Masterson (1993), who pioneered this synthesis, has expanded the concept of personality disorder to disorders of the self: "[*The Emerging Self*] . . . continues to reflect the shift in my perspective on the personality disorders from a developmental object relations approach that included a notion of the self indirectly . . . to one that considers the developmental arrest of the self as primary" (p. x).

Suppose, following Masterson's direction, one examines the concept of fixation, or developmental arrest, in terms of its impact on the formation of the early (preoedipal) self. And suppose one then restores the original Freudian component of trauma to this construct. It might then follow that significantly acute or chronic physical abuse and sexual abuse might create childhood PTSD that might impinge on the growth of the self. This form of PTSD, especially if accompanied by psychogenic amnesia (as Freud and Breuer described it), would be harmful in a way difficult to diagnose, especially if the PTSD were comorbid with a disorder of the self.

For the purposes of this inquiry, developmental trauma is defined as PTSD that occurs in the developmental years. It is based on physical/sexual abuse sufficient to cause psychogenic amnesia and is likely to be a condition comorbid with a disorder of the self, in which case it may contribute to overall developmental arrest of the self.

Since the inquiry ventures into many areas being newly explored in the field of dynamic/biological psychotherapy, the conclusions—and even some of the basic assumptions—have to be tentative and reliant on anecdotal findings. For instance, it is tempting to make the assumption that developmental trauma will always be found in conjunction with a disorder of the self, but the evidence to support this idea is yet to be examined.

Since the 1970s, there has been a growing understanding both of personality disorder and traumatic states. There has been a lesser tendency, even some resistance, to examining the two phenomena in conjunction. It is difficult enough to accept the mounting evidence that much of the maternal unavailability and chronic misattunement that lead to the creation of personality disorder may be reinforced by severe physical/sexual abuse. It is harder still to speculate that the same mother–child dysphoria may be conducive to a practical/emotional environment in which developmental trauma may occur, be unknown, be ignored, or otherwise be removed from the possibility of communication and resolution.

Sometimes it seems that the need of the patient to be objectively understood is overshadowed by the therapist's need to separate an abused child, or formerly abused adult, from a label that suggests that a degree of pathology may exist in the victim. This is often demonstrated by the question: "How can you say someone has a personality disorder when the person is really a victim of abuse? You're blaming the victim!" Ongoing abuse, especially in the formative years, leaves its mark, and we neglect the victim by minimizing the lasting effect of this kind of trauma. Survival does not guarantee emotional health. The false polarization between victim and patient diverts our attention both from the prevalence of child abuse and from its affect on the formation of the self. Where developmental trauma exists, the situation is painfully compounded by the absence of conscious, corroborating memory of abusive experiences, and the patient is victimized not only by the original event, but also by the disruption in the formation and continuity of the self as the patient defensively refuses to accept the full impact of what has happened. It is unfortunate when the original victimization is further compounded by the reluctance of others either to allow for the possibility of severe abuse, or to link it with the pathology that may result from it.

Experience with numerous cases has led me to believe that developmental trauma, when it exists in conjunction with a disorder of the self, begins to emerge as a patient starts significantly to dissolve that disorder. As defenses become more adaptive, the therapeutic alliance is forming, and the working through of the abandonment depression has begun, the patient may become disoriented; be subject to fugue states; experience flashbacks or episodes suggestive of flashbacks; revert to old, maladaptive defenses; experience unexplainable (and sometimes undiagnosable) bodily pain; or be haunted by a sense that he or she cannot remember something important. As the self has become stronger, the necessity for keeping traumatic material out of awareness is less, and the drive toward mastery and self-actualization supports the therapeutic process. However, recovered traumatic experiences must be incorporated in the working through of the abandonment depression if the self is to be made whole.

Work with the personality disorder and therapy of developmental trauma meet in the working through of the abandonment depression. The abandonment depression is the powerful residue of mother–child psychic misattunement that must be acknowledged, grieved, and transcended if the real self is to come into being. If, in the formative years, the child is physically or sexually abused by the mother, a direct link exists between developmental trauma and abandonment depression. However, the importance of the mother as the unquestioned perceived protector of the child's first years of life cannot be minimized in understanding the child's emotional development and the inhibition of that development. If the abuse is protracted, and the mother withholds the minimal soothing that comes with the acknowledgment of the reality of the situation and reassurances of her concern, the perception will be that the mother, even if she herself is not the abuser, somehow permitted the abuse to happen and condoned it.

In addition, if a child in the formative years is physically or sexually abused, whether or not the mother is the abuser, or even if the mother fails to rectify or acknowledge the abuse, the child receives a destructive double message about the nature of relationship. This messages adds to the depth and fixity of the abandonment depression.

REPRESSION, SPLITTING, AND DISSOCIATION: A NEED FOR A DEFINITION OF TERMS

Repression

There is a confusion over the use of terms such as repression, dissociation, and splitting that began with Freud, and persists in ways that affect both theory and clinical practice.

Initially, Freud (working from the topographic model) used the term "repression" as a specialized definition of dissociation:

> Psycho-analysis . . . accepts the assumptions of dissociation and the unconscious, but relates them differently to each other. Its view is a dynamic one, which traces mental life back to an interplay between forces that favour or inhibit one another. The process is known as "repression." (Freud, 1910, p. 213)

Freud was concerned with establishing a psychodynamic concept, and with distinguishing it from Janet's view of dissociation as a "[failure of] mental synthesis resulting from a congenital disability" (Freud, 1913, p. 207).

The use of repression as a dynamic synonym for dissociation essentially eliminated the latter term from Freudian psychoanalysis. It is interesting to note that such useful reference works as *The Language of Psycho-analysis* (Laplanche & Pontalis, 1973) and *A Clinician's Guide to Reading Freud* (Giovacchini, 1982) do not include the term "dissociation" in their indexes.

The shifting from dissociation to repression became more complicated when combined with Freud's replacement of the seduction theory by the oedipal construct and his introduction of the structural model. As he noted in his monograph "Repression" (1915): "Psycho-analytic experience of the transference neuroses . . . forces us to the conclusion that repression is not a defence mechanism present from the very beginning, and that it cannot occur until a sharp distinction has been established between what is conscious and what is unconscious. . . ." (pp. 85–86).

The vicissitudes of Freud's definition of repression, through *Inhibitions, Symptoms and Anxiety* (1926) in particular, is a complex theoretical matter that can only receive superficial explication here. Giovacchini (1982) sums up some of the critical turns:

> As Freud repeatedly stated, all neuroses are based on repression. Can repression exist before the formation of the superego? . . . It is unlikely, however, that there are no repressive forces operating before the age of 3. . . . He once again divided repression into two types, primal repression and . . . secondary repression. . . . Primal repression, he believed, occurs very early and represents an attempt to deal with . . . primitive states of terror. (pp. 206–207)

By 1915, Freud acknowledges that a direct equivalence between the unconscious, repression, and defense can no longer be made. In *Inhibitions, Symptoms and Anxiety*, he notes that "repression is only one of the mechanisms which defense makes use of" (p. 40). Finally, he opens the way to the contemporary division of oedipal and preoedipal defenses with the following statement: "It may well be that before its sharp cleavage into an ego and an id, and before the formation of a super-ego, the mental apparatus makes use of different methods of defence from those which it employs after it has reached these stages of organization" (p. 90). In effect, repression is defined as a more evolved, postoedipal defense. This leaves the defensive operation of the preoedipal disorders of the self open to further exploration.

Splitting

The contemporary interest in preoedipal issues, personality disorder, and disturbed self states has sought to name the predominating archaic defense that precedes the institution of repression. Splitting has been the defense most frequently accepted in this regard.

However, the concept of splitting has suffered its own vicissitudes.

Pruyser—in his exhaustive study, "What Splits in Splitting?" (1975)—argues that the term "splitting" is too imprecise, overused, and faddish to be valuable. Among the many difficulties it presents, he points out that it has been employed by numerous major models of psychoanalytic and psychiatric thought in different ways, and as different parts of speech: noun, verb (transitive and intransitive), and adjective. He concludes: "Elevated to a psychological concept, the words *splitting* and *split* create more problems than they solve" (p. 44).

I propose that if we retain the definition of splitting as it is used in Masterson's Approach to the disorders of the self, the concept becomes pertinent in understanding and resolving the destructive effect of developmental trauma, as well.

Masterson uses the Kleinian theory of the maturational split between concepts of "good" and "bad" to explain the divided inner world of the patient caught in a developmental arrest. In addition, he describes how the self may also use the capacity for dividing aspects of the inner world in a defensive way.

Developmental trauma, certainly as it relates to disorders of the self, reinforces the arresting of the good/bad split. In cases where the patient sees the world in opposing camps of victim and perpetrator, and especially when these roles are acted out repetitiously, a history of early physical/sexual abuse should be considered as a possibility.

When splitting is used defensively, there is a rupture in the integrity of the self. As Masterson (1985) reflects: "Because early subjective experiences may be organized by multiple self representations, the 'I' of one state of mind may not necessarily be the 'I' of another state of mind" (p. 21).

The self may defend against threatening experience by splitting off a subordinate part of the self attached to that experience, and then dissociating it. The most dramatic evidence of this use of defensive splitting is found in multiple personality disorder, where subordinate aspects of the self take on quasi-independent lives of their own.

Dissociation

Dissociation has reemerged as a psychological concept, but in a way that even now is somewhat sidetracked from the highway of psychoanalytic thought. The term has returned, by popular demand, via such grass-roots movements as 12-step programs, veterans' groups, feminist causes, and the growing concern with the abuse of children. In the past two or three decades, however, an increasing number of theory-building clinicians have delineated the effect of trauma on the individual, and its connection with dissociative sequelae is finally receiving establishment recognition. And PTSD and multiple personality disorder have found a place in the DSM nosology. DSM-IV (1994) defines the dissociative disorders as "a disruption in the usually integrated functions of consciousness, memory, identity, or perception of the environment. The disturbance may be sudden or gradual, transient or chronic" (p. 477).

Putnam (1989) summarizes the nature of dissociation as follows:

> What emerges is a near-unanimity of opinion by authorities that the dissociative process occurs along a continuum ranging from minor "everyday" examples (e.g., daydreaming) to psychiatric disorders (e.g., multiple personality). Pathological forms of dissociation are characterized by a profound disturbance of memory and a profound disturbance of the individual's sense of self, and are often a response to overwhelming physical and/or psychological trauma. The dissociative responses may initially be adaptive, but becomes pathological when its persists beyond the trauma context. (p. 25)

Dissociation, like splitting, would seem to be an archaic defense (perhaps preceding repression culturally as well as developmentally). Like splitting, dissociation—in addition to its defensive aspects—may have its origins in an unfolding developmental process. As Ludwig (1983) notes:

> Dissociation represents the fundamental biological mechanism underlying a wide variety of altered forms of consciousness. . . . This mechanism has great individual and species survival value. Under certain conditions, it serves to facilitate seven major functions: (1) the automatization of certain behaviors, (2) the efficiency and economy of effort, (3) the resolution of irreconcilable conflicts, (4) escape from the constraints of reality, (5) the isolation of catastrophic experiences, (6) the cathartic discharge of certain experiences, and (7) the enhancement of herd sense (e.g., the

submission of the individual ego for the group identity, greater suggestability, etc.). (p. 93)

Splitting and dissociation, it would seem, interoperate early in life to defend the self not only from the disorders of the self based on dyadic misattunement, but also from the physical/sexual abuse that may contribute to the disorders of the self and even threaten psychic survival. When the two defenses combine, a self state can split off from the supraordinate whole and be "lost" from the available life "story." Insufferable pain can be suspended in storage, although at the expense of the sense of identity (the result of splitting) and the loss of conscious continuity (the effect of dissociation).

The Repression Barrier

If splitting and dissociation may be defenses that we learn from our initial experience of them as innately unfolding developmental mechanisms, it might be interesting to speculate that repression could have a similar dual nature. Perhaps infantile amnesia, the forgetting of childhood memories Freud attributed to repression, is a developmental phenomenon. Perhaps our acquisition of repression as a defense is based on the successful institution of the repression barrier (which, in turn, is affected by many variables that impinge on it). If this might be so, the patient suffering from a disorder of the self might to some extent implement childhood amnesia as a seal over childhood misattunement and trauma, in addition to splitting, dissociation, and the other early defenses already in play. Thus, although repression as a defense proper is not available to disorders of the self, an overall capacity to store disruptive conflicts of the formative years may act as an additional fail-safe mechanism against later dysfunction.

THE RELATIONSHIP AMONG TRAUMA, DISSOCIATION, SPLITTING, REPRESSION, THE FORMATION OF THE SELF, AND PSYCHOTHERAPY

In the foregoing, I have tried to sketch how psychodynamic theory has taken shape around ideas about the impact of trauma on the formation of the self, and, subsequently, how this has influenced the new science of psychodynamic therapy. The theory has been concerned with the interaction of the inner and outer worlds of the individual, and demonstrates a fluctuating theoretical opinion as to where the emphasis belongs, what the nature of the trauma might be, how it is managed, and what the clinician might do to help.

Here I would like to describe my own professional experience that has drawn my concern to the specific issue of traumatic abuse, and present three cases that elucidate the clinical relevance of that concern to the treatment of some disorders of the self.

Connecting the Disorder of the Self to the Developmental Trauma

My training and practice have impressed me with an unexpected outcome of rigorous character work. The systematic working through of characterological issues has at times led to a central impasse that could only be resolved by work with a heretofore hidden level of childhood trauma that had been split off and dissociated. These patients had PTSD and a disorder of the self. I found this to be especially true in my work with patients suffering from borderline disorder of the self, but I have encountered this same impasse in the schizoid and narcissistic disorders of the self, as well—in extensive consultation and in my own caseload.

To reconstruct these disorders of the self from the inside out, my impression is that the patients' formative years were beset by events sufficiently severe and ongoing to create a disorder of the self. This disorder of the self, by Masterson's definition, is created when either the infant is abnormally sensitive, or the mother's attunement and protectiveness are inadequate, or the mother herself is unavailable (or a combination of variables may occur). Concomitantly, physical (including sexual) abuse, in addition to the more global dyadic dysfunction, also intrudes into the sheltered interpersonal space, where child and mother are creating the child's internal model of self, other, and interrelationship. Dyadic misattunement leads to the developmental arrest and rigid configuration of defenses that form the basic disorder of the self. Physical/sexual abuse destructive to the fundamental formation of the self is dissociated—it is stopped before it can enter a system that cannot integrate it—and its physical, perceptual, and cognitive components are held separate and encapsulated, producing PTSD.

Dissociated trauma in the formative years presents another specialized problem. When significant abuse occurs, the idea of mother as destructive or nonprotective must be denied, in order not to risk increased evocation of the abandonment depression. It is imperative in infancy to perceive the mother as a source of protection, not as a threat.

The child thus makes use of an impressive array of early defenses to avoid these central, threatening dilemmas, and the use of primitive defenses (dissociation, splitting, acting out, and so on) shapes the character around the avoidance of the abandonment depression that detours the establishment of the real self.

Working outward from the core of the child self, past the dissociation that encapsulates developmental trauma and the early defenses that act as character armor, there may still be another seal that protects the self from psychic overload. In *Three Contributions to the Theory of Sex* (1905), Freud puzzles over the phenomenon of infantile amnesia, "the peculiar amnesia which veils from most people (not from all) the first years of their childhood. . . ." (p. 581). Freud posits "an ultimate connection between the infantile and hysterical amnesias," saying: "We conclude therefore that we do not deal with a real forgetting of infantile impressions but rather with an amnesia similar to that observed in neurotics for later experiences, the nature of which consists in their being kept away from consciousness (repression)" (p. 582).

At some point near the close of early childhood (the exact age seems to range quite a bit in the literature, but probably could be given as somewhere from three to five years old), a putting away of early experience occurs that makes use of a mechanism akin to the defense of repression. The difference would seem to be that the repression barrier that creates infantile amnesia is not selective (as is defensive repression), but covers the entire range of the early years. One wonders again (as Freud intimated) whether the repression barrier is not a manifestation of normal development that allows the growing child to set aside conscious concerns with the developmental process itself, and so to free energy and awareness to deal with a wider range of social tasks.

What is the role of *defensive* repression in this layering of protective barriers around the core self? Repression is generally understood to be a higher-level defense that permits us to deeply forget experiences or fantasies that could impede our progress into psychic maturity. These experiences are, in effect, buried, unless they are so conflictual that they must be brought into full consciousness to be resolved. From Freud's work on, repression has been conceived of as a defense critical to the self's ability to transcend the oedipal challenge, rather than as a defense needed to build and preserve the structure of the developing self. Repression concerns itself with memories and concepts that are already formed within the self. Dissociation, on the contrary (in conjunction with splitting), interrupts the processing and integrating of experience into the self, leaving an aspect of the self in a potential, divided-off state, and so profoundly affects the nature of the manifest self. The defense of repression, therefore, does not come into play where disorder of the self is comorbid with developmental trauma.

Approaching the Hidden Trauma Therapeutically

Working clinically from the outside in, one must first deal with the characterological fortress set up by primal defenses determined to protect the self from any shift in belief or experience that would challenge the inner model. Such a challenge might open the way to recognition of abandonment depression, the impact of which is still perceived by the impaired self as intolerable.

Any attempt to work with the dissociative level that guards early physical/sexual trauma should be avoided or minimized, if possible, until the character work is relatively in order, and the abandonment depression is accessible to the working through. Following the guidelines of resistance analysis, ego work should precede the expression of deep feelings, especially those originating in childhood, to assure relatively sound containment of those feelings. As Fenichel (1941) notes in his book on psychoanalytic technique: "The surface first of all, the defense before the instinct" (p. 73). As the ego becomes more realistic and adaptive, feelings and perceptions that once would have been unmanageable now can be dealt with, and even have a tendency to float up with the improved readiness of the patient.

I do not find, however, that the dissociative level of the work always floats up with regularly predictable spontaneity. Sound character work brings the patient to the beginning of the dissociative level, but the therapy may be stalemated at that point. This may happen in part because the treatment has encountered the repression barrier, which will tend to block further change, or even gradually restore old, maladaptive character patterns, until it is dynamically breached.

Clinical experience suggests that it may be necessary for the therapist to use hypnotic technique to pass through the repression barrier and enter the dissociative level of the work. The goal is then to proceed with care and respect for resistances, in order to bring through the abreactive material in a safe way, and assist its transformation into a conscious verbal narrative.

At this stage, the therapy no longer moves from the outside in, but significantly begins to move from the inside out. The character work and trauma work lead to the discharge of the abandonment depression, and so reveal a changed perspective on the formative years (basically, on the view of the nature of the self, the mother, and the relationship). This brings its own emotional crisis, which must be dealt with by the reintegrating of the self in a healthy way.

It should be stressed that a misunderstanding of the cathartic method of psychoanalysis suggests that conflict is something to be ejected from the self. But Freud and Anna O., herself, stated that the "cure" came from conscious verbalization—from the *integration* of conflict into an aware, narrative sense of self.

Here, the divided pathways of psychodynamic technique meet. If therapeutic work with dissociated self states is to have lasting value, it must be made part of the building of mature character structure. And if psychotherapy with disorders of the self complicated by dissociated states of consciousness is genuinely to be worked through, it must reclaim the parts of the psyche that have been dissociated for the sake of individual survival. I believe it is this integrative work that reclaims the whole self and releases it to be and to grow.

THREE CASE VIGNETTES

Ms. A.: Emergence of Emotional and Physical Trauma

Ms. A.'s case demonstrates the coherent emergence of childhood traumatic material as the patient's ego strengthens.

Ms. A. was just 30 years old when she came to the Masterson Group with a history of chaotic relationships, a minimal and sporadic work record, an incomplete college education, a failed marriage, a sequence of psychiatric hospitalizations, and a continuing role as the family scapegoat. Her diagnosis was one of borderline personality disorder. Treatment then (and, to some degree, now) focused on her independent functioning—holding a responsible job, maintaining her own apartment, and beginning to look and act like her potentially sophisticated self. Her psychotherapy required undaunted confrontation of an alternately clinging and hostile aggressive false self: Ms. A. either telephoned incessantly for reassurance or went on emotional rampages. Insight into anything other than a here-and-now grasp of the consequences of her behavior was irrelevant, even undermining, compared with her learning to manage her feelings more adaptively.

During the first seven years of her therapy with me, Ms. A. began to make her life work. She modified her chaotic defenses, strengthened her observing ego, held a high-functioning job, settled down with her cats in a good apartment, and paid her own way. (This phase of her treatment was described in *Psychotherapy of the Disorders of the Self,* Masterson and Klein [Eds.], 1989, pp. 140–143; pp. 231–240.)

During the last three years of her therapy, Ms. A. has become increasingly aware of periods of depression and sometimes disorganizing panic. These episodes existed before, especially at times of separation stress, and were sometimes mistaken for transient psychotic states. However, as these episodes emerge in a life no longer characterized by indiscriminate confusion, they become more observable as traumatic fragments from childhood that begin to piece together coherently as they surface.

Typically, Ms. A. has little recall of her childhood years, although she remembers her adolescent rebellion: fighting off her father with a chair and threatening her mother with a knife. She has often protested that she does not wish to recall anything worse than her adolescence, since she has formed a positive relationship with her parents in recent years and is afraid to damage it. (I try to reassure her that genuine gains made in present time are likely to benefit from the lifting of past fears.)

The traumatic narrative is emerging as follows: The disapproval of a male authority figure in present time acts as a trigger for a state of disorganizing panic, followed by a sense of terrifying isolation and an overwhelming need for reassurance and approval (in the transference, she becomes frantic to know whether I am still there). As she has separated her feelings from present-time events, she has begun to remember how frightened she was of her father's violent anger, and how her mother, who was also frightened, failed to protect her and covered the family discord with a thick veneer of denial.

This childhood reconstruction was confirmed by her elder brother, who remembered the father's outbursts, when he would suddenly ragefully pursue a terrified child into a corner and slap the child around. Home movies also supported Ms. A.'s abandonment reaction, as they clearly pictured the mother's turning away in cold disapproval from her small daughter, who was not opening her birthday presents for the camera in the way the mother wished. The movies also showed Ms. A. as consistently frightened, and the patient had night terrors after viewing them.

As a result of this work, the patient has steadily come to grips with an unexpressed level of rage and hopelessness—related first to the father, but then more profoundly to the mother. This level of feeling is no longer being exclusively acted out, but appears in dreams, the transference, and verbalized insights.

Ms. A. asks me: "Am I becoming who I am?"

I believe that the emergence of Ms. A.'s traumatic material relates directly to the openly chaotic way the family has functioned until quite recently (the parents' aging and Ms. A.'s emotional maturing now have calmed the family situation to some degree). I would speculate that Ms. A. has never been able to establish a consistent repression barrier because the family's traumatic behavior was ongoing during her developmental years and long after, not only creating a developmental lag, but repeatedly evoking her early overwhelming experiences. I would additionally speculate that where the barrier exists, it has "thickened" to preserve the patient's psyche from an overload in childhood that, I believe (from the disorganized and paranoid nature of her abreactions), otherwise might have led to a psychotic break.

Ms. B.: Emergence of the Dissociative Level

In the case of Ms. B., the unfolding of the defensive layers was more clearly shown, but the introduction of hypnotic technique was required to facilitate the emergence of the dissociative level. Again, I can only speculate about the nature and function of the repression barrier. I would hypothesize that, since Ms. B.'s disorder of the self was on a minimally pathological level, and since her abuse occurred during her developmental years only and was of relatively brief duration, developmental lags in her psyche were less entrenched than in the case of Ms. A.

Ms. B.'s dynamics were essentially borderline—shifting from a need for reassurance to aversive forms of anger, and with a deep susceptibility to separation and an inhibition of self-assertiveness. However, she functioned on a high level of competency that disguised this underlying dynamic.

Ms. B., in her late 20s when she came to the Masterson Group, applied herself to seven years of intensive character work, making dramatic changes in her professional and social life. She also began to separate emotionally from an enmeshed and crisis-prone family.

However, the therapy came to an impasse marked by the appearance of a public-speaking phobia, and continued detachment from some deeper levels of feeling.

Ms. B. felt that she was blocked by an early, painful experience she could not access. Aware that hypnotic techniques sometimes prove useful in resolving this type of therapeutic impasse, she asked to be hypnotized to explore the experience. Dreams and associations tended to support the possibility of a "forgotten" pathogenic experience. At the point where I found the working through clearly repetitious, I agreed to try a hypnotic approach to the impasse.

Careful hypnotic establishment of a sense of inner safety and control, followed by age regression, led to the accessing of scenes of savage sexual abuse by an uncle when the patient was four years old. The mother had left her with the uncle at a point when the mother was depressed and overwhelmed, and never seemed to notice her daughter's distress at any time during the episode. As the patient painfully pieced together the memory, she was validated by her sister. The sister had witnessed the abuse and dissociated it, but began to have flashbacks when the patient turned to her for support.

Ms. B. experienced a time of direct anger and a sense of sureness and freedom she had not felt before. Then, frustratingly, the public-speaking phobia refused to lift, and the feeling of unfinished business returned.

We resumed the hypnotic work, but uncovered nothing more. I then hypothesized that the remaining impasse might relate to her need to synthesize the trauma memory and the abandonment depression associated with her separation work with her internal mother. This proved to be the case for, as the patient focused on her deep wish for her mother's approval, as well as on her mother's neglect of her personal needs, she began to acknowledge realistically the mother's weakness and, finally, her own strength. The speaking phobia lifted, and the patient, approaching termination of treatment, significantly let go of the intellectual detachment that had remained a transferential barrier to the growth of the real relationship between us.

It seems to me that this patient's abandonment depression (maternal unavailability reinforced by sexual abuse) not only was guarded by dissociation and a rigid character pattern, but also was sealed off by a strong repression barrier. A major reason why it was so difficult to overcome the repression barrier, I believe, was that the family (especially the mother) maintained a consistent (if false) pretense that their household was an ideal household.

In this case, also, it was evident that the whole self could not be healed until the trauma work and character work were integrated, a process that took two years.

Ms. C.: Emergence of Multiple Personality Disorder

Ms. C.'s case showed a clear layering of resistance similar to Ms. B.'s case. Ms. C., 15½ years old, had entered therapy in a crisis, having overdosed following a brutal rape in a parking lot. Her borderline self style emerged as the crisis attenuated; she alternated clinging with avoidance and hostile outbursts, could find no middle ground, and displayed much sensitivity to separation.

After three and a half years of character work, Ms. C. had modified her defenses, and had graduated from high school with high grades. As she left for college, I had the sense that there were unresolved sexual issues with the father, but believed Ms. C. was now well prepared to exercise her creative intelligence and social skills with sufficient psychic freedom. (This phase of the patient's therapy has been described in *Psychotherapy of the Disorders of the Self,* [1989, pp. 185–196].)

Partway through college, the story changed. Ms. C. began to evidence unusual symptoms, experiencing jumps in consciousness, where she would light a cigarette, only to find it burned down to her fingers after what seemed seconds. Her blood pressure fluctuated with no medical explanation, and she was unable to sleep.

She returned to therapy and completed college as the symptoms increased. She began to lose consciousness abruptly, and had some serious falls in the street. Since medical findings still were negative, I wondered if she might be experiencing some kind of fugue state. I thought of my hypothesis of possible paternal incest.

Working through got us nowhere; it only seemed to intensify the patient's altered states, so that she began to reinstate old dysfunctional character defenses (such as bulimia nervosa) to control them.

At that time, I had never used hypnosis in conjunction with dynamic psychotherapy, but began to wonder if the course described in *Studies on Hysteria* might not be the one to follow. Consequently, I accompanied the patient for a brief sequence of visits to a hypnoanalyst. As I had speculated, a dissociated layer of trauma emerged.

The patient began to abreact paternal rape when she was four years old. I incorporated the hypnotic work into the regular sessions and, over a period of weeks, the complete memory was reconstructed. However, the story was told not by one, but by three "inner children." It soon became clear that the dissociative level contained innumerable abuse events held by multiple subpersonalities.

To make matters still more involved, continued trauma work revealed complex groupings and layerings of internal personalities created by years of ritual abuse. Not only had the repression barrier given way to dissociated material, but to a whole dissociated side of the self.

It would take two more years of intensive work to access the part of the self closed away in an inner world created by trauma, and then to continue the character work as the dissociated part of the self integrated into the conscious part.

In all, psychotherapy with Ms. C. covered a span of 10 years. During those years, I was repeatedly amazed by the hidden resources of the self—the degree and amount of suffering that can be endured, even in childhood, and how the self can divide (and subdivide) to contain trauma and protect the practically functioning part of the self from psychic overload. And it became clear to me that real healing of the self cannot take place until the lost part of the self that guards developmental trauma is recovered to create an integrated whole person.

REFERENCES

American Psychiatric Association (1994). *Diagnostic and statistical manual of mental disorders* (4th ed.). Washington: American Psychiatric Association.

Breuer, J. & Freud, S. (1895). *Studies on hysteria* (J. Strachey, Ed. & Trans.). New York: Basic Books, 1955.

Fenichel, O. (1941). *Problems of psychoanalytic technique* (D. Brunswick, Ed.). New York: Psychoanalytic Quarterly.

Freud, S. (1905). Three contributions to the theory of sex. In J. Strachey (Ed. & Trans.), *The standard edition of the complete psychological works of Sigmund Freud*, Vol. VII. London: Hogarth Press, 1953.

Freud, S. (1910). The psycho-analytic view of psychogenic disturbance of vision. *Standard edition*, Vol. VI.

Freud, S. (1913). On psycho-analysis. *Standard edition*, Vol. XII.

Freud, S. (1914). Remembering, repeating and working-through. *Standard edition*, Vol. XII.

Freud, S. (1915). Repression. In E. Jones (Ed.), *Collected papers*. New York: Basic Books, 1959.

Freud, S. (1926). *Inhibitions, symptoms and anxiety*. (A. Strachey, Trans., & J. Strachey, Ed.). New York: Norton, 1959.

Giovacchini, P. (1982). *A clinician's guide to reading Freud*. New York: Aronson.

Laplanche, J., & Pontalis, J.B. (1973). *The language of psycho-analysis* (D. Nicholson-Smith, Trans.). New York: Norton.

Ludwig, A. M. (1983). The psychobiological functions of dissociation. *American Journal of Clinical Hypnosis*, 26, 93–99.

Masterson, J. F. (1976). *Psychotherapy of the borderline adult: A developmental approach*. New York: Brunner/Mazel.

Masterson, J. F. (1981). *The narcissistic and borderline disorders: An integrated developmental approach*. New York: Brunner/Mazel.

Masterson, J. F. (1985). *The real self: A developmental, self, and object relations approach*. New York: Brunner/Mazel.

Masterson, J. F. (1993). *The emerging self: A developmental, self, and object relations approach to the treatment of the closet narcissistic disorder of the self*. New York: Brunner/Mazel.

Masterson, J.F. & Klein, R. (Eds.). (1989). *Psychotherapy of the disorders of the self: The Masterson approach*. New York: Brunner/Mazel.

Pruyser, P. W. (1975). What splits in splitting? A scrutiny of the concept of splitting in psychoanalysis and psychiatry. *Bulletin of the Menninger Clinic, 39*, 1–47.

Putnam, F. W. (1989) *Diagnosis and treatment of multiple personality disorder*. New York: Guilford.

Ross, C. A. (1989). *Multiple personality disorder: Diagnosis, clinical features, and treatment*. New York: Wiley.

Wilson, J. P. (1989). *Trauma, transformation, and healing: an integrative approach to theory, research, and post-traumatic therapy*. New York: Brunner/Mazel.

CHAPTER 11

Uncovering "Forgotten" Child Abuse in the Psychotherapy of a Borderline Disorder of the Self

Candace Orcutt, Ph.D.

At a 1990 Masterson conference, I presented an ongoing case that appeared to exemplify the Masterson Approach to the diagnosis and treatment of an upper-level borderline disorder of the self. The patient, referred to as Diana, was very bright and highly functioning. She had been intensely motivated to pursue the nearly five years of psychotherapy (increasing after two years from one to two sessions a week) that helped her to correct maladaptive defenses, and dynamically to resolve deep problems of separation and individuation with her internalized mother from the past as well as with her real mother in the present.

But just as Diana seemed ready to end a successful process of therapy, a new level of conflict emerged, as though the character work—the resolution of the false self defense—had strengthened the patient's real self to face some previously hidden part. It appeared that the borderline character structure not only had protected her in childhood from the abandonment depression, but it overlaid a dissociative response to an early traumatic experience. Once the character defense had been essentially resolved, her real self became strong enough to face and reclaim the part of the self encapsulated in the dissociated response to the trauma, and to manage the pain of accepting that "lost" part.

This led to a period of intensive work focused on recovery of this traumatic material (two to three sessions a week for seven months). The final working-through stage required management of residual character work; the experiencing of early, buried trauma; and the integration of both into a reconstruction of her life story and sense of self that was perceptually convincing and emotionally transformative. After two additional years of this working through, she was aware that her sense of self was healing, that she believed in herself and her reality.

Diana entered psychotherapy at the age of 29. At 34 years of age, she began the uncovering of the early traumatic experience, and successfully terminated treatment at the age of 38.

ISSUES RAISED BY DEPARTURES FROM CLASSIC DYNAMIC TECHNIQUE

The shifts in technique required by this case raise questions regarding the role of the therapist and therapeutic neutrality, and relate to the skills, judgment, and flexibility useful in meeting the appropriate needs of the patient at the right time.

For the initial character work, the therapist had to be active, confronting the transferential acting-out distortions of the patient from a position of therapeutic neutrality. In the working-through phase, as the patient took on more responsibility for feeling and insight, the therapist became less active, limiting interventions mainly to interpretations intended to raise transference distortions to conscious awareness.

In the working through, it is the neutral, nondirective attitude of the therapist that provides the even ground that, by contrast, accentuates the patient's transferential reactions. However, in therapy with disorders of the self, it is usual to revert to active, ego-oriented interventions at times (especially as the abandonment depression emerges) to help the patient resolve regressions to old, maladaptive defenses. It is the building of an inner, dynamic structure that allows the patient to manage this technical shift in a constructive way. As Masterson (1976) has described:

> The developing alliance between the therapist's healthy ego and the patient's reality ego brings into existence, through introjection, a new object relations unit: the therapist as a

positive (libidinal) object relations who approves of separation-individuation + a self representation as a capable, developing person + a "good" feeling (affect) which ensues from the exercise of constructive coping and mastery rather than regressive behavior. (p. 64)

I suspect that this strengthening of the ego and the therapeutic alliance, together with the internalization of maturing object relations, is also a critical condition for the introduction of hypnotic technique in work with dissociated events. When an isolated instance of posttraumatic stress disorder occurs in an adult with a relatively mature psyche, good basic ego strength and object-related intactness may provide a sufficient foundation for hypnotic work; in fact, the issue of transference may be a minimal one. But when the "forgotten" trauma has occurred in the developmental years, issues of arrested development need to be dealt with first, to provide the self with the capacity to "remember" that which once had to be "forgotten" so that the impaired self could survive. Perhaps still more important, issues of transference and countertransference have to be sufficiently understood and resolved so that hypnotic techniques do not contribute to antitherapeutic fantasies.

In a case that has unfolded therapeutically as the patient's real self has grown stronger, the need for varied techniques may be called for—in response to the unfolding of the real self, and to facilitate it.

Ideally, it seems, work with forgotten trauma, or posttraumatic stress disorder, should be approached only with patients who have reached a high level of interpersonal differentiation and a sense of the real self. Unfortunately, we are too often faced with the patient whose traumatic reactions exceed his or her capacity to contain them effectively.

It might be helpful to draw a comparison between the use of medication and the use of hypnosis. The use of hypnosis as an anesthetic is a relatively accepted medical procedure, especially in the practice of dentistry and in the modification of chronic pain. Hypnotic techniques are used in these instances much as medication is used. Indeed, they are sometimes understood as a way of stimulating the brain's own self-medicating skills (for example, the production of endorphins).

The introduction of hypnotic techniques into the process of dynamic psychotherapy also raises questions reminiscent of those evoked by the administration of medicine.

The use of hypnosis as an anesthetizing, containing technique is also finding acceptance in the mental health field, especially in work with phobias and other anxiety states. In addition, ego-building hypnotic techniques that support self-confidence are coming into use, along with hypnotic techniques that reinforce dissociative barriers.

The use of hypnosis to anesthetize, desensitize, and contain may not have reached the level of acceptance achieved by medication, but it is relatively uncontroversial as compared with use of hypnosis as an opening-up technique, especially in conjunction with dynamic psychotherapy.

As an exploratory, experiential technique, hypnosis is being refined, scrutinized, and questioned. The case presented here is an anecdotal example of the benefit that hypnotic work can bring to a patient who has dissociated an early traumatic experience. The case also raises questions for the thoughtful clinician about the nature of memory (which to some extent is always a reconstructed, narrative phenomenon).

The presentation describes a persevering woman who was able to work selectively with hypnosis to unblock the emergence of her real self. The foundation of her endeavor was the character work and working through she pursued rigorously with the Masterson Approach. With this foundation, she believed she had the strength to hold and integrate the impact of the abuse memories she perceived to be gradually surfacing.

I do not think that hypnosis is a shortcut to revealing a disarmed impaired self in any way. However, it can be a method of supporting the unfolding of the real self that has gone through a process of strengthening its containing, observing, managing, and integrating capacities.

CHARACTER WORK OR EGO REPAIR

Initial Consultation

Diana came to the Masterson Group because of a separation crisis. She told me she had been "in an unhealthy relationship with a married man." She said: "I had such difficulty ending it that I was frightened. I couldn't cope with things because I was so preoccupied with my feelings." She had been depressed, with persistent fears that she would go crazy. She had experienced something similar when she graduated from college—an "overwhelming feeling of not knowing what to do." She had broken off the relationship, and she was determined to know what had happened to her.

Underlying the presenting problem were deeper separation issues. She described herself as a strong-willed and independent person, and had clashed with her father when he opposed her going away to college. She argued ferociously with her mother, who was aggrieved because Diana refused to confide in her about the affair she had just ended. But she also spoke protectively of her parents. She said that her father had eventually supported her independence, and that they were just getting to know each other in an adult way when he died suddenly of a stroke when she was 19 years old and away at college. She said that her mother always had been "really good," and that she felt close to her, and depended on her for support and approval. Although Diana had been essentially on her own for the past six years, there had been occasional periods of living with her mother.

Diana is intelligent and attractive, with golden-red hair that sweeps around her face. She combines fashionable poise with a vulnerable prettiness, and directs herself with a clear, analytical mind. In talking with her, I was interested in her paradoxical combination of childlike appeal and intellectual matter-of-factness, and mentioned this to her. She replied that people often brought this to her attention. She added that, although she looked to others for moral support, she was "critical of people—I don't give them a chance." This longing for relatedness, paired with aloofness, became a consistent indicator of her central conflict over intimacy.

History

Diana was the third of four living siblings. There were two older sisters, who both struggled with physical and marital problems. A third sibling, a boy, died soon after birth. Diana, born next, was a favored child who took the place of the dead brother until a younger brother was born into the family when she was four years old.

The mother, an active, opinionated woman, ran the family. All the siblings looked to her for support, and used her as a confidante even as adults. The father was somewhat more emotionally available than the mother, but less influential.

Diana described her family as ideal. Her childhood memories were vague and rosy. She thought her problems had begun with adolescence, when she became headstrong and rebellious. She had expected to float through a debutante adolescence, but felt that the magic had run out when her turn had come.

Although she fought to have her own way, she clung to romantic attachments to carry her across the transition points in her life. In her work situations, she was effective, but took a second-in-command role. As a result, she frequently was hurt and frustrated by superiors who seemed less perceptive and organized than she was. She still had not found work that truly satisfied her, although her position as a private school administrator was challenging. She dedicated herself to working with children because, as she said, she was disgusted with adults who act like children.

The diagnostic impression was of a high-level borderline disorder of the self, with separation-individuation issues and a characteristic oscillation between clinging and distancing defensive positions. Unless one paid attention to this preoedipal dynamic, it would have been easy to mistake her for neurotic, thus stalemating the treatment in some falsely compliant or hostile form of acting out.

Observing Ego

During the first year of her therapy, Diana's observing capacity strengthened. Intellectually, she set herself to work immediately, exploring patterns in her life. She noted that she felt like a teenager, dependent on her mother, but trying to be independent. She resented the sense of obligation she connected with dependency, and wryly remarked: "My sisters have their husbands, and I have my mother."

She began to play out her character patterns in the therapeutic relationship. She wanted me to guide her, but resisted my inquiries. I noted that she seemed to want to lean on me, but then pulled away. She told me that, after our second session, she dreamed that a woman cab driver had taken her to Trump Tower. Diana had liked her until it was time to pay, when she realized that the woman planned to shoot her. This was followed by another dream of being shot in the back by a woman friend.

The dreams were associated with trusting her feelings to a special other person. She told me that she had resisted my inquiries about her love affair, because she knew she would cry and she was afraid to let it happen. She thought relationships changed once a partner showed feeling, and remembered her mother's often saying: "Don't wear your heart on your sleeve, or they'll take advantage of you."

She began to see her childhood and her family in a new way. From the outset, I had confronted the discrepancy between her idealized account of her past and her uncertainties about her present self and relationships. It seemed puzzling that such seeming security could produce such insecurity. At first, she had said that the only upsetting event of her childhood was when the dog died. Now she viewed her life "in two places—like day and night." There was the shiny surface that was presented to the neighbors, and beneath it was a dark side marked by arguments, emotional isolation, and rebellion.

She realized that she had been frightened of her mother, who had given her the impression that love is a relationship between a powerful person and a helpless, needy one. She remembered that her mother's disapproval could make her feel as if she had been shot. She recalled her dependency on approval, and how smart and quick she had become in avoiding disapproval (she learned by watching how the middle sister was scapegoated). She also had adopted an emotional detachment that provided some distance to keep her from fears of being engulfed.

As she became more observing and insightful, she expressed herself more directly with her mother and became more assertive at work. She also began to reveal her feelings in sessions. Her real self was beginning to emerge. She choked up when describing how her life had been an illusion, and how she had learned to undermine the closeness she sought.

Tenacious preoedipal issues dominated the oedipal, which often seemed close to the surface. She dreamed that she was searching for her father, who was lost "out in the dark, out in the waves." When she tried unsuccessfully to date, she had dreams of a wave sweeping the man away. The maternal element predominated, reinforced by the father's early death.

Anger and Therapeutic Alliance

In the second year of therapy, Diana's detachment gave way to outbursts of anger at her mother. She also manipulated the treatment frame in a way that suggested avoidance of anger at me. She increased her sessions to twice a week, but interrupted intense sequences with illnesses and vacations. She filled her sessions with accounts of chaotic and genuinely distressing events, which tended to place the emphasis on *doing* rather than on *understanding*, and also took the focus away from our relationship.

I confronted her various ways of distancing from the sessions. I also shared some of my own induced countertransference feelings. I puzzled over my contradictory impressions of her intense dedication to the therapy and the opposite sense that she might walk away any minute, or somehow was not even there at all. She responded with both consternation and interest. She felt I had criticized her commitment, and yet she knew that she only wanted to present her efficient and intellectual side to me. As she divided her family memories into night and day, so she was dividing her therapy into superficial compliance and covert resistance.

When I asked about this double therapy, she replied that she had no clear sense of herself and was afraid of being robbed of what she had left. She recalled a recurring dream, in which she was about to be married and realized it was a terrible mistake. "Are you concerned that this therapeutic relationship might be a mistake?" She answered by telling another dream: She was trying to find her way to me through a crowded, chaotic store. We then met in my waiting room, with people coming and going. At one point, she walked out on me; at another, I took someone else into my office. In the transference, fears of engulfment and abandonment alternated.

At last, she said, she had come to terms with a transferential conflict. She had been angry that I had not given her wise advice and led her to better feelings. She was beginning to understand what psychotherapy was about, and that she was using me as a guide through a process of self-change—that I could not prevent her from feeling this process was sometimes painful, but I could support her through it.

After this acknowledgment of anger at unmet dependence, she became depressed. She said she felt that she had no power, that the world was hopeless, and that she was frightened all the time. She also released some of her resentment at having to act as mother to her own family and at having to fill the father's place as the problem-solving family member as well.

Diana was more open and ready to reach out. She reported that her friends found her more receptive, and I felt the same way.

Emergence of the Real Self

Diana had protested: "There is no room in my life for me!" During this third year, she began to change. She wanted to let go, but asked: "How can I let go without a sense of self to hold onto?"

Her dreams about water continued, and she told me that she was a capable and fearless swimmer. But, she said, she was fearful of swimming at night and did not know why. As we talked about this, the metaphor "swimming in dark water" became a way of talking about her unconscious.

As she showed more concern for herself, her interest in others increased. Her interest in men also revived.

I wondered why she dated so little when she appeared to have every advantage. She acknowledged that friends had said the same thing, but that she did not see herself as others did. She had no sense of her impact on others and described having a false self, created to comply with the family need for social approval. Inside, she felt inadequate, frightened, and absent. This inhibited self pulled away from romantic contact.

Once she identified this hidden self behind the false *façade,* she was amazed to discover how all-pervasive her anxiety actually was. The "night" side of herself was diffusely, ubiquitously afraid of everything.

Self-activation and Emergence of Phobia

In the fourth year of therapy, she initiated a search for a new job, and she also found a lover. He was a corporate executive who had been a silent admirer of hers for a number of years. However, he had a tendency to remain distant emotionally, even when their relationship became close, and I expressed my concern that she might be repeating her relationship with one or both parents. I wondered whether she was putting herself into the same kind of situation that first brought her into therapy, perhaps as a defense against the deepening of the process. But the couple seemed genuinely devoted to each other, and they worked hard to clarify their relationship in long, soul-searching talks.

At first, she tended to react to his unavailability with alternate clinging and rageful distancing. She recognized her acting out in time, and took a realistic stand. She told him that they would have to separate until he went into therapy to address his conflicts with relationships. Although this assertive move evoked a dream of being cut down her entire body, she held to the separation until, several months later, he entered treatment.

During this year, she also made an assertive job change. She took an executive position in which she was in charge of developing a groundbreaking program.

A dynamic change took place. Her pervasive anxiety, which had emerged when she set aside her old character defenses of avoidance and denial, now became focused in a symptom. She developed a public-speaking phobia. As she explored the phobia, it seemed to symbolize a condensation of oedipal and preoedipal issues: of forbidden self-assertion and dangerous competition with the mother.

Technically, I found myself relying more on interpretation. Earlier in the treatment, my interventions (primarily confrontation and here-and-now interpretations) had been more directed toward ego strengthening. Now I found myself dealing more with the patient's unconscious.

Impasse

During the fifth year, Diana developed a more separate, mature relationship with her mother. She also visited her father's grave for the first time (she is the only one in the family to have done so). She seemed substantially to have resolved inner-world issues with both parents. In addition, her view of her childhood, although disillusioned, was more real and more consistent with her understanding of her adult life. She seemed to be moving steadily to a resolution of her character issues, except that the phobia persisted.

Then she began to feel that she was carrying a terrible secret. The perception did not appear like a sudden insight, but more like vestiges of a dimly remembered dream that steadily became clearer and more convincing. She wondered if she had been sexually molested as a child, and discussed this with her sisters. The middle sister expressed a similar anxiety, but was unable to find any basis for it in memory. Diana's lover also had intuited that she might have been molested. He observed that she had a "scared and angry look" when by herself, and tended to have childlike reactions when upset: she would shiver and her teeth would chatter.

She had dreams of trying to rescue children, while her family went from room to room trying to kill them.

It was clear that the resolution of Diana's character work was releasing a deeper level of conflict. But the nature of the conflict was not clear. Diana was increasingly convinced that she might be able to access some childhood trauma through hypnosis. I thought that the speaking phobia might indicate an emerging oedipal conflict or a deeper level of conflict with the mother, and pursued both possibilities, but with poor results.

Did this impasse represent an earlier abuse or an oedipal—or even pre-oedipal—fantasy pressing toward consciousness? Nearly five years of solid character work had opened the door of the self, only to find another door beyond.

TRAUMA WORK

In the sixth year of therapy, Diana became increasingly dissatisfied with the therapeutic process—she was no longer moving ahead. Her physical symptoms also increased: swollen lymph nodes, ovarian pain, and weight losses of five pounds at a time. Her body seemed to support her verbalized request for help. She said: "I'm trying to remember what I don't remember. I feel there's something there—inside of me—and it's blocked. It makes me have thoughts about being molested—something like that."

Neither logic nor free association could move the process. She reasoned that something might have happened to her when she was four years old, her age when the brother was born and the family was relocating. Her mother had been emotionally overwhelmed at that time, and the patient and the middle sister had been sent to stay with an aunt and uncle. But no further thoughts came, only her sister's dream that terrorists had broken in while she was sleeping at her aunt and uncle's home.

Recollection evaded her, but her painful physical and emotional states increased. She developed sinus trouble and a cystitis-like irritation. Her legs hurt, her skin hurt. "Everything feels sensitive," she said, and then began to develop nausea and intestinal pains. She was given antibiotics for her sinus infection, but could find no other medical relief (or definitive diagnosis). She would become angry with her lover, and then with me, but the anger refused to focus. She hated everything.

As the work remained static, she turned more to her spiritual life for relief, trying to find consolation in a private world of meditation. I believed that my hesitation to explore hypnotically for deeply dissociated material was countertransferential. I wondered if I might not have assumed the role of the mother who would not make the extra effort to look at her daughter's problems, while the daughter detached herself and tried to find her own means of solace. At that point, I decided to incorporate hypnotic technique into her therapy.

The Preparation Phase

Contemporary hypnosis, like other current approaches to the treatment of the self, is not authoritarian; the skill of the therapist is used to facilitate the emergence of the capacities of the patient. The extensively reported work of the hypnotist Dr. Milton Erickson has revolutionized modern trance work in this way. Using the Ericksonian approach, I assured Diana that I recognized her ability to hypnotize herself—that she had developed an unconscious expertise for shifting into protective states of mind—and that I would be helping her to access this ability on a conscious level.

I began by inviting her to try a simple relaxation exercise to demonstrate that the trance state could be a pleasant one. Next, I asked her to choose a calm environment, such as a beach, and to create it clearly in her mind, using all five senses. This, I explained, was to show how resourceful her mind could be in constructing sheltering places to return to whenever she wished. After that, I suggested she explore a deeper trance state, where she would be amazed to find that she could separate her arm from her conscious will, so that it would move by itself, even though her conscious thoughts tried to hold it steady. I assisted the induction of this state by counting down from 10 to zero. When the arm moved independently, she had confirmation of her capacity for dissociative states. Last, I proposed that she return to the beach to enjoy her feelings of relaxation and discovery before coming back to full awareness of my office. I counted from one to five to help her pace this return. (The counting, to facilitate entrance into and exit from altered states, also was to help her begin to use my voice as a reinforcement at times of heightened resistance.)

Diana came to the next session feeling "terrible" and complaining in an unfocused, repetitive way. I assumed that this was a defensive resurgence of the old character work, and confronted her: "You've just taken the initiative to approach your problem from a new angle, and now you're back to waiting for someone to make things right for you." She centered herself around the confrontation, and acknowledged that she was acting out her anxiety, rather than trying to understand it. She said: "There's always something in the back of my head all the time—something that makes me afraid of exposing myself to people." She thought for a while, and then added: "I have to focus more on what *I* need. Basically, I just have no self-esteem."

I suggested that we work together to create a safe place, uniquely hers, that would be a haven in her inner world. (The safe-place induction is a standard procedure for therapy with trauma survivors. It is described, along with other containing techniques, by Brown and Fromm [1986, pp. 279–281].) She chose a hilltop for this inner haven, patterned after a place to which she had gone to meditate during a retreat that had been deeply meaningful to her. The hilltop had a view across farmlands to the sea. In the induction, she would walk thoughtfully to the hilltop and sit at the feet of the great stone angel that stood there.

As she began to reinforce the inner reality of the safe place, she said emphatically: "I *want* to keep going." She did this despite the increasing pressure of sleep disturbance, and awaking from what sleep she was able to get feeling disoriented and wanting a target for unfocused feelings of anger. The establishment of a more containing structure, cognitively and in her inner experience, offered an increased sense of safety, and so seemed to give permission for dissociated material to draw closer to her conscious awareness.

Crossing the Repression Barrier

There still was no spontaneous appearance of lost events. I think that when abuse and posttraumatic stress disorder have occurred during the formative years, they not only are handled by dissociation layered over by character development, but are hidden further from reach by the institution of the repression barrier. Freud equated the idea of the repression barrier with the concept of infantile amnesia, a widely observed but not altogether understood phenomenon that marks a stage of psychic growth at which memories of the first years of life fade or are forgotten. He believed that information obscured by the repression barrier became unconscious, and only tended to return if strong psychic conflicts could not be resolved. In psychoanalytic theory, that which is repressed, or is unconscious in the psyche, is accessible by a different language than that which is consciously available. Freud developed his concept of free association to help the analyst "hear" the analysand's unconscious more distinctly: the nonlinear associations of the analysand's talk—the apparently random remarks that are joined by some common denominator—constitute the primary process language that conveys the message of the repressed.

Can Freud's way of listening to the unconscious be reversed into a way of talking to it? Much has been said about Milton Erickson's use of metaphor to access a part of the mind not reached by linear, secondary process communication. I think there is more involved here than telling a story indirectly (and more pleasurably). When Erickson (1966) strengthens the physically ill gardener by making random references to the growth of a healthy garden (pp. 510–520), he is bypassing logical talk and using associative language to address the unconscious part of the mind. It seems he is using what he called the interspersal technique (1966), or what might be described as reverse associations, as a way to talk to that part of the mind that thinks in terms of space and images, and is in profound contact with feeling.

Watzlawick (1978) has described Erickson's interspersal technique in the following way:

> This intervention is essentially a dream "in reverse": What Erickson says could just as well be reported by the patient as her dream, in which consciously unacceptable material camouflages itself into the language of images in order to bypass the censorship of the left hemisphere. Of course, the important difference here is that the dream is usually the *passive* expression of inner conflict, while Erickson's use of dream language represents an *active* intervention. (pp. 62–63)

I am learning to be concerned with reverse associations when helping a patient across the repression barrier. Before using the more logical, but still unique, language of dissociation, I try to talk to the unconscious, to request passage to the inner world.

In Diana's case, I wanted to send a message to the unconscious that crossing the boundary from the hidden to the open, from the dark to the light, could be accomplished as a natural process; that, no matter how things might seem to change, all still had a safe and natural point of reference. Here is an example of how I incorporated that message, together with her personal image of safety, the stone angel, into the safe-place induction.

> *You follow the familiar path to the hilltop. The earth is solid beneath your feet, while the trees cast a changing shadow that gives way to sunlight, back to shadow and to sunlight again. And, at the hilltop, the path opens to a comfortable area where you can brush away the pebbles and twigs, and settle yourself at the feet of the angel. A line can move imperceptibly as the shadow of the angel moves over the clearing, and the shadow of the mountain moves across the valley. The earth shifts like a dial of shadow and sunlight, and you know it moves as it has to; as the dial of seasons always moves as it completes itself. Just as the far-off tide rises clear on the coast, and the fishing boats float free to turn on the anchor line. You can see through the clear water, down to the bits of shell and fragments of ancient cargoes, and all the sea keeps or may bring in with the tide, or carry back to its depths. Just as you see through the depths of the clear sky, where your mind wheels with the flight of the birds that see and travel far, but always carry with them the unthought knowledge of return.*

Over a period of weeks, the patient seemed to wander in a region of fragmented images. These images related to childhood, and flickered by momentarily, or seemed to form the beginning of a narrative, only to fade again. There were early images of being in her crib: lonely, and sometimes drawn into a corner, seeming to take refuge in a solitude that was more reassuring than the distracted presence of her mother. There were brief impressions of driving somewhere with the family. There were recollections of the sound of a motorcycle going by at night, of falling out of bed more than once.

At first, this response seemed random and frustrating. But there was a sense of nonlinear scanning that made me wonder if the patient's images were sorting their way toward a common theme. The lonely child, the night fears, the family trip somewhere—all might be information communicated to me in the spatial, imagistic language of the unconscious. If this were so, the patient might be making her way across the repression barrier.

In the hope that I was making some contact with my patient's unconscious, I then introduced age-regression techniques. She tended to linger in the area of ages three to four: "I was four when we moved. There's some underlying thing of my mother's being there and not really paying attention to me. . . ." My dolls are around the table for a tea party; I was happy creating things for myself. . . ." With the intensification of feeling, Diana shifted dissociatively into the use of the third person: "I'd like to take her and put her someplace else—a place to play, a place that's happy."

There followed recollections of being by the water in the summer; picking raspberries; being outdoors much of the time, and not home; feeling a distance between her parents. An image of changing her bathing suit in the summerhouse—the intrusion of a smell she did not like—the image of a face in the window.

At this point, she became frightened: "I feel like something happened in that room, but I don't know if I'm making it up." Respecting her protective withdrawal into denial, I no longer asked her about her "own" experiences. I called on her capacity to dissociate to modify her feelings: "Tell me about the four-year-old. Is there anything else you would want me to know about her on that day in that house?" "She's scared to have anyone touch her. She's afraid. She wishes somebody would hold her."

Diana had been "permitted" across the repression barrier by the internal "censor," to be in touch with a hidden, frightened child part of her self experience and self organization. It would take more than seven months incrementally to retrieve the experiences of that early time, but the door stood open.

Evolution of the Traumatic Experience

As we returned to the experiences of the four-year-old, coherent pictures began to form in Diana's mind, accompanied by intense, almost intolerable emotions. She said: "I feel scared and panicky. It's hard not to cry. I want to say 'Stop! I don't want to do this any more!'"

I steadily encouraged her to describe the child and the summerhouse: the quality of the light, the wallpaper, the position of the doors and windows, and the child's perception of another's presence.

She became aware of the man at the window, and his subsequent entrance through the door. She was unable to "see" his face. Realizing that increasing anxiety was reinstating dissociation, I encouraged her to use dissociation in a way that would modify the image she sought without obliterating it. "You are seeing this as if it were a photo in an old family album. The picture is very faint. It is faded with time. But you can probably make it out." As we reviewed the family album in her mind, she found a "photo" of her uncle that matched the summerhouse and the terrified feeling that was associated with it. This identification was further validated by a sense of anger and relief at the end of the session.

Session after session, the narrative moved forward incrementally, like a film strip examined without a projector. The four-year-old put her hand to her face. The man moved forward, his face was close to hers: "When I saw his face, I felt dizzy. Things started to spin. I can't stand his face near my face!"

Increasingly, however, the scene at the summerhouse was interrupted by flashes of another episode—the uncle entering the bedroom where four-year-old Diana and her sister were sleeping.

In successive sessions thereafter, her mind scanned back and forth between the two episodes. When she was able to recall his hand on her vagina in the summerhouse, she remembered his pulling down her pajama pants in the bedroom. Her increased tolerance for one memory seemed to open the way for the next. And, as both episodes moved to the moment when he exposed his penis, a third episode began to unfold, in which she was going down the basement stairs in her uncle's house, and he was there.

"He starts coming down, and closes the door behind him at the top of the stairs. He's talking. He says we're going to play the game again. And it's like she knows what's going to happen. It's the day after the night he came into the bedroom. He takes her arm. Pulls her down the stairs. I think he hits her. [Diana puts her hands in front of her face, and her voice becomes higher pitched.] I feel like I'm crying. Horrible, scared, panic feeling. It's worse than before, because now I know what will happen."

Her mind scanned back and forth among the three episodes as if each evoked the other, and also as if the shifting modified the escalating intensity, as she began to tell how the uncle had raped her vaginally and anally. At first, I was confused by this scanning, thinking it might be avoidance, and then began to realize that it was an unfolding process with a nonlinear logic of its own: the uncanny signature of the unconscious.

Throughout these abreactions, Diana sat opposite me, as she did in sessions generally, but in a trance, with her eyes closed. She was self-contained, holding the work largely in her mind's eye, although she was visibly in conflict and pain. Her hand often reached up to protect her face. She reported alternating disbelief and emotional pain so intense that, at times, she could not continue. Her physical symptoms corresponded to the details of the abuse, and tended to intensify and then lift as she constructed her recollections.

She was consumed by mental preoccupation and physical reaction to the work, but continued to function normally, although she said she felt as if she had to force herself to do every small task.

The impact of the work on her perception of her life was becoming significant. She said bitterly: "The worst part is to have a mother who doesn't know or understand. I can't believe it! I don't know how she didn't know!" And then: "It's a terrible sadness to realize I never had a family. I feel sad for what my mother never was, and how we all had to live in this false world."

She recalled going home as a changed person, and her mother's never noticing the difference. "I was so afraid someone was going to say something. I think that's when it started—when I started going inside my head. Where all the distancing started. I thought everyone else had those things in their heads that they didn't talk about."

External Validation

As Diana began to move from the uncovering of trauma to the integrating of it into her conscious life experience, she began to tell her story, first to friends, and then to her family.

When she related what had happened to the middle sister, she received a startling but confirming response. The sister responded emotionally: "I know what happened in that bedroom. I was in the bed to the right, and you were on the floor." The sister was caught up in a flashback, and sobbed uncontrollably for 15 minutes.

Telling the Mother

The abreactions subsided, but Diana continued to feel tense: "It's something I'm controlling. It feels like the withholding of emotion."

She hesitated about revealing her memories to her mother, concerned that it would only cause more pain and distance in the relationship. A weekend with her family brought home the futility of trying to get close; they seemed cold, and she experienced the old feelings of vulnerability and isolation. "They're such a helpless lot!"

Using energy freed by the abreactive process, and perhaps also trying to offset her own feeling of helplessness, she followed through on practical goals for herself. She applied to resume her studies for a doctorate, and bought the condominium she had longed for and could now afford.

But the momentary lift in energy subsided, and finally she made the decision to break the years of silence and talk to her mother. She was pleased and perplexed by the results. Her mother was sympathetic, distressed, even angry on her behalf. She supported Diana's revelations: "I know my child. To see you in a state like this, I know it's true."

Diana was astonished at the difference that time had made in the relationship: "It's hard separating her now from who she used to be." Who the mother "used to be" was clearer, too, now that past and present could be sorted out: "I really haven't wanted her to get that close to me as an adult. I felt as if she possessed me, could take over my entire being, especially if it had to do with some kind of disapproval."

The old mother still lingered, though, as her present-time mother ruefully reflected: "But you were always so happy!"

INTEGRATION OF TRAUMA AND CHARACTER WORK

Cathartic abreaction retrieves memory, but, alone, does not restore the self. It would take an additional two and a half years for Diana to reconcile her abuse memories with her remaining character issues of present-day identity and relationship.

The first challenge was simply to reperceive her own history. She was angry that, unknowingly, she had had to shape her character to cope with her developmental conflicts, and this, also outside of her conscious awareness, had been complicated by childhood trauma. "It's bad enough to have a problem, but worse not even to know you have it. I feel I wasn't me my whole life."

Past and Present Anger

On the level of dissociation, resolving her early trauma had reclaimed the lost part of herself, but also had released the last, dammed-up reservoir of abandonment depression into her consciousness. She struggled to understand and to integrate this outpouring of hopelessness and anger without letting it slip into behavior, but she could not resist some reinstatement of the old, inadequate, defensive self: "I have a feeling of regret about my life. I feel as if everything's too late; too late to fix it."

The stuckness persisted. Her ability to grieve and let go was blocked by her defensively anchored disbelief in her own worth. Worse still, the public-speaking phobia had returned, flooding her with waves of panic. Facing a resurgence of problems she had fought for years to overcome, she remarked half-jokingly, "I could murder you."

That reaction, I thought, indicated where the conflict remained. The bond of hostile accommodation to the internalized mother of the past (as reflected in the transference) still held her back. She tentatively agreed: "I can't imagine anyone caring a lot about me. I'm just waiting to be criticized. I just hate myself, and expect everybody to tell me how awful I am. I probably don't think I have a *right* to get angry."

She began to understand that "the mother-tie is the crux. That feeling I have that nothing will get better has no real basis any more. But I can't stand the expectation of her anger—it's subtle stuff that permeates things. So I always feel wrong. I'm doing something good and then it turns out to be bad. That's the remaining problem—my fear of being intimidated. My mother's anger blows away who I am."

She began connecting patterns differently, finding past origins for feelings that seemed attached to the present. In the here and now, her anger sometimes focused on me, but especially on a female colleague of hers who held a position of authority. She expressed her anger, noted how disproportionate it was, and tracked it back to the past: "I feel like smashing you. It's consuming. Then it wants to go out of my feelings, out of my thoughts, and into my body. I'm trying not to get sick. Why aren't you helping me? And then I realize that this is the anger I didn't feel at my mother for leaving me with my uncle."

Diana, wishing to establish her self-belief by facing the person who had damaged it, tried to confront her mother. She hoped to reach that part of her mother that knew about the undercurrent of violence and victimization in the family, and, by doing so, to free both of them from the pressure of family secrets. But her mother, now not quite hiding from herself, but too set in her ways to change, responded: "Sometimes it's too frightening to know what's in your heart."

Diana told me: "This is the first time I've really felt for her. She's let me feel sorry for her in a strange way."

Anger was giving way to reality, leaving a growing sense of the separateness of her mother and herself, and of grief releasing the past to the realm of memory.

Capacity for Self-Belief

Diana observed that she now could look in a mirror and see what she really looked like, not what she hated. She was amazed to think of the state of absolute terror in which she had routinely lived. Her public-speaking phobia lifted, her relationship with her lover became downgraded into that of a deep friendship, and her career began again to climb.

The old belief system, supported by the mother's emotional unavailability and absence during a critical early crisis, was losing its hold. What would take its place?

The family had used achievement as the only autonomous way to support a sense of self, but Diana was skeptical about that. "You aren't allowed to say things are just fine. The thought of doing something less than spectacular is unacceptable. But I'm not buying this any more. I think I'm finally all right. I used to wait for the time when everything would be perfect. Now I know I'm going to get upset and get over it."

But what was missing? Another family reunion brought the issue into focus: "They're all shouting 'take care of me.' Everyone *needs* so much—and they need to need because needing feels like love! That's why things have to stay messed up, why this one is complaining and that one is rescuing, and why the crisis never stops!"

This insight was self-affirming, and carried her through a stressful series of interviews for a high-level executive position, during which she was repeatedly interviewed before increasingly larger groups. She maintained her confidence until the last interview, which was to be held before the entire board of directors of the organization. She became unsure, and told me: "I'm getting advice about how to talk, move, dress—but people are just telling me who to be. It's not the answer. I need to be believed in for whom I am."

I reviewed all my reasons, based on over eight years of work together, to support why I deeply believed in her capacity to handle the interview, and why, beyond that, I felt I could believe in her as a person. I realized, as I did this, that my reality-based reinforcement of her qualities as a profession and a person was a new experience for her—that the real relationship she had built with me had helped her to reinforce an internal structure that had received little previous support.

She called me to say that an outsider had been chosen for the job and that the position never really had been available to her. However, past the disappointment, she was now in a new stage of growth, spurred on by enthusiastic responses from board members who had been impressed by her and by her own feeling of having done well and having been herself.

Termination

As the nine-year mark of therapy approached, Diana wound down her work with me. She continued to hear from friends and colleagues how her personality had become warmer and more open. She maintained the devotion and support of a group of close friends, including her former lover. She was well on her way to completing her doctorate, and had found that her exceptional handling of the interview had brought her to the attention of a sophisticated job market.

She was amazed to find that she was not living in daily fear: "I remember when I told you I was in an elevator and realized I didn't have to be afraid of the elevator man—not everybody has a gun!"

Another family reunion had focused her emotional separation from them: "The whole *detached* lot was there, but there was no group. Everyone is afraid or angry about what everyone else is thinking. It's bizarre. There's nothing there except serving and doing. Why don't they *see*?"

She felt there was no sense of unfinished business. However, she mused: "I'm being too intellectual about leaving! It's nine years—a long time—but this therapy saved my life. You've been my only consistent anchor point for nine years."

We reflected together over those years and the process of the therapy itself. I talked about the vulnerable self that hides behind one defensive shield after another, and how skillfully she had hidden herself.

"That touches what happened when I didn't get the job! I put myself on the line with nowhere to hide. If I didn't get the job, I'd have to see if I could believe in myself, anyway. And I could. My belief in myself is real!"

With that statement, some barrier between us dissolved, and the emotional paradox of a good therapeutic closing—combined pleasure and sadness—was also real.

EPILOGUE

A few months after the close of her therapy, Diana contacted me with affirming news. She had been appointed to a substantial and competitive position in a major organization. She was pleased with the results of her perseverance, and especially with the loyalty of her friends and colleagues, who had supported her and whose warmth she now felt freer to accept and return.

REFERENCES

Breuer, J., & Freud, S. (1895). *Studies on hysteria* (J. Strachey, Ed. and Trans.). New York: Basic Books, 1955.

Brown, D. P., & Fromm, E. (1986). *Hypnotherapy and hypnoanalysis.* Hillsdale, NJ: Erlbaum.

Erickson, M. H. (1966). The interspersal technique for symptom correction and pain control. *American Journal of Clinical Hypnosis, 3,* 198–209.

Masterson, J. F. (1976). *Psychotherapy of the borderline adult.* New York: Brunner/Mazel.

Watzlawick, P. (1978). *The language of change: Elements of therapeutic communication.* New York: Basic Books.

CHAPTER 12

Integration of Multiple Personality Disorder in the Context of the Masterson Approach

Candace Orcutt, Ph.D.

In *Psychotherapy of the Disorders of the Self* (Masterson & Klein, 1989, pp. 185–196), I described the case of a borderline adolescent who came to the Masterson Group in crisis, and remained to work through important characterological issues. The chapter was subtitled "From Clinical Crisis to Emancipation." When the patient returned to therapy after a two-year absence, I thought I might title any follow-up of the work: "From Clinical Emancipation to Crisis." It seemed that the first two and a half years of therapy had prepared her to uncover a level of conflict that tested both the patient and the therapeutic process itself.

Underlying the character pattern that had acted as a defensive false self from her infancy was a second line of protection—an elaborate dissociative shield of multiple inner personalities that contained and compartmentalized a lifetime of traumatic experience—a fail-safe barrier that prevented the flooding through of devastating information should the characterological defense give way. At the most, this dissociative barrier would permit only a fragment of past experience to emerge, "held" by an inner personality whose presence, even when made known to the therapist, might not be acknowledged by the patient consciously.

INITIAL PHASE OF THERAPY

Gerda (her pseudonym in the earlier volume) was 15½ years old when she first entered treatment at the Masterson Group. She was discharged to the group from a psychiatric inpatient unit where she had gone as a result of two suicide attempts. The attempts were precipitated by a rape in a deserted city parking lot. It was almost immediately evident that Gerda's problems had not begun with the rape: she had lived a life of surface charm and excitement, while feeling essentially uprooted and neglected. Her parents, both of whom were bright and talented, divorced when Gerda was four years old because of the father's physical abuse of the mother. Gerda had lived a nomadic life with her world-traveler mother, and her closest relationships were with the mother and her own world of fantasy. She was creative, highly intelligent, and attractive, but she was an isolated only child. Although the crisis issue was focal in many ways, the main focus of her therapy was her borderline self style. Avoidance and hostile outbursts characterized her approach to relationship, offsetting the clinging she both desired and feared.

Essentially, she recovered from the rape crisis, worked through many of her borderline issues (mainly by discovering that the use of words could have value), and graduated with distinction from high school. I worked with her on a three-times-a-week basis, later diminishing to twice a week, until she left the city for college.

At the time of the initial termination, I believed there was some earlier trauma connected with her father that she was not ready to approach. Her character work had been done so well that I had felt satisfied to see her more in charge of her life and moving forward.

IMPASSE AND TRANSITION

There was a two-year hiatus while she was away at college. These were troubled years during which she developed severe anorexia nervosa and then bulimia nervosa, which resulted in a leave of absence. She returned to therapy when she learned that her father was dying. She resumed college attendance, and commuted six hours (roundtrip) for a weekly double session with me.

The next two years were marked by puzzling symptoms: fugue states, during which the cigarette she held burned down to her fingers; extreme fluctuations in blood pressure that sent her to the hospital, but received no diagnosis; severe ongoing disturbances in sleeping and eating. She was able to graduate, although she was preoccupied with suicidal wishes.

Back in the city, she found an apartment, secured a position as a decorator's assistant, and worked creatively and responsibly. However, her symptoms worsened, She would abruptly lose consciousness and fall down in the street. She reinstituted (deliberately) once-rejected defenses, such as cutting and bulimia, which seemed to relieve the new symptoms. She seemed to be in a terrible dilemma, neither able to submerge some central trauma nor to bring it to the surface. I wondered if she might be helped through hypnosis, and sought a local hypnotherapist to try a catalytic intervention.

The patient herself located a hypnoanalyst who worked with dissociative states. I accompanied her for three sessions, during which she was helped to transcend her anxiety and find an "inner child"—a $3\frac{1}{2}$-year-old—who was deeply intimidated and expressed fear of her father.

At that point, I incorporated hypnosis into my sessions with Gerda, following the hypnoanalyst's initial guidance and seeking regular consultation with a colleague in the Masterson Institute who was experienced in the use of hypnosis. A primary technique I learned helped the patient to construct a "safe place" in her inner world—a containing induction used routinely in the treatment of posttraumatic stress disorder.°

Gradually, "Little Gerda" began to meet with me in the safe place. We took time to get acquainted, as Little Gerda introduced me to the world of the three-year-old and four-year-old. We went for inner walks and had a tea party with her cat and pet rabbit. After several weeks, she asked me cautiously whether I could keep a secret. When I assured her that I would honor her confidence, she began to tell me about Daddy.

I recognized the event from a dream she had told me years earlier, a dream that had made me wonder about the possibility of child abuse. She often had dreams about a particular window, and in this dream she looked out on cold snow shining outside. She watched as her father approached, "like a great bear," and the dream ended with "something frightening" that she could not remember.

Now, Little Gerda kneeled on her bed, watching Daddy in the window, and then was terrified as someone roughly took her arm from behind. She had been watching her father's reflection in the window at night, and he had actually been entering the room behind her.

The traumatic experiencing of a savage rape followed. For the first time, I witnessed the unfolding of an abreaction—muted, but disturbing to see.

°The author wishes to express her gratitude to Robert S. Mayer, Ph.D., and Diane Roberts Stoler, Ed.D., for their tutelage and support during this challenging, often overwhelming initiation to her work with multiplicity.

The patient spoke and looked like a little child in fear and pain; she broke into perspiration, and her body twisted beneath the blanket in which she always wrapped herself during these sessions.

Another eerie thing occurred. In order to complete the experience of the rape, Gerda divided her awareness into three consecutive personalities. The first "went into her garden" (dissociated) when the rape began; the second endured the rape ("that's my job"), but resisted when Daddy tried to force her into telling him she loved him. He burned her hand on the radiator, and would have broken her spirit, except that another child, meek and sad, took her place and reassured Daddy that she loved him, and said she was sorry that it took her so long to say so. When Daddy finally left the room, the tough little child reemerged and smashed the window that had held his reflection.

At this point, I hypothesized that Gerda was using a dissociative defense—diluting the impact of the traumatic experience by dividing it into different segments of her personality. It was clear that the abreaction was not complete until the three inner children had linked their stories, like pieces completing a puzzle. I was too amazed by the revelations of Gerda's inner world to be able also to grasp that I was working with multiple personality disorder (MPD).

I thought at the time that MPD was very rare, and had never observed an overt case in a clinical setting. Additionally, I had known my patient as an apparent nonmultiple for nearly six years, and could not absorb such a different concept of who she was.

Gerda, also, was too disoriented to consider fully the possibility of multiplicity. She was too upset by the revelations of her inner world, especially when they began to involve shattering recollections of abuse by a religious cult.

The multiplicity had to be faced. She began to abreact outside of sessions, to lose time, to find her apartment mysteriously torn up, or to discover herself perched alarmingly on a windowsill or on the edge of the roof. "Someone" managed her job for her an entire day. I knew I would have to check for an internal alter ego.

I "went inside" to ask if I could speak with someone who could provide me with facts and figures—someone who, without stirring up more emotion in the patient, could inform me about the lost time and the other matters.

I felt a shock as Gerda changed before me into a cold, pragmatic person who indicated that she had taken over Gerda's job one day when the patient was too distraught to function. This was Paulina, who had rebelled against conforming to the cult that had abused "us." She was co-conscious with Gerda and "others inside." Through her, I met a group of alters: Penelope, who was socially charming, avoided the negative, and was present for much of early therapy; Meg, who cut the body to "let out bad things"; and others.

"I feel as if I'm living in a grade B movie," said Gerda grimly after she had filled in the blanks in her conscious recollection with the information I retained. If I was shaken as I reperceived my familiar patient as a system rather than as an individual, how must she have felt? At least I had a continuous conscious recall of the session, and did not have to rely on someone else to be my auxiliary memory (a holding function of the therapist, I believe, that is crucial to the therapeutic process—it is internalized by the patient).

WHAT IS MULTIPLE PERSONALITY DISORDER AND HOW IS IT TREATED?

Diagnosis

The *Diagnostic and Statistical Manual of Mental Disorders* (DSM) conferred official recognition on MPD in 1980. *DSM-IV* (1994) changed the name of the disorder to Dissociative Identity Disorder (DID—although MPD remains the internationally used nomenclature). In the 1994 edition, the diagnostic criteria were somewhat expanded:

A. The presence of two or more distinct identities or personality states (each with its own relatively enduring pattern of perceiving, relating to, and thinking about the environment and self).
B. At least two of these identities or personality states recurrently take control of the person's behavior.
C. Inability to recall important personal information that is too extensive to be explained by ordinary forgetfulness.
D. The disturbance is not due to the direct physiological effects of a substance . . . or a general medical condition. (p. 487)

This certainly would suffice to identify such overt multiple personalities as "Anna O.," described by Breuer and Freud in *Studies on Hysteria* (1895), and other pioneering cases, such as Morton Prince's (1905), about a century ago.

The criteria would not have helped in diagnosing Gerda, or any other patient in a less than unmistakable state requiring no reference to any manual. Colin Ross (1989, p. 102) has listed several nonspecific diagnostic clues for the disorder, which, when they occur together, make it by far the most likely diagnosis. They are:

1. History of childhood sexual and/or physical abuse
2. Female sex
3. Age 20 to 40
4. Blank spells
5. Voices in the head or other Schneiderian symptoms
6. DSM-III-R criteria for borderline personality are met or nearly met
7. Previous unsuccessful treatment
8. Self-destructive behavior
9. No thought disorder
10. Headache

These criteria would have been more helpful in diagnosing Gerda's problem. What would have helped the most would have been a capacity on my part to even consider MPD as a possible diagnosis for Gerda, or any other patient.

(Incidentally, Gerda herself reported additional symptoms that seem to occur frequently with MPD patients: periods of dizziness and disorientation; a persistent ringing in the ears. With regard to evidence of physical abuse, well into her treatment of multiplicity, Gerda suffered from recurrent back pain. It was the policy of her treatment to check out physical symptoms medically before attempting to treat them as body memories. In this instance, Gerda underwent a technologically advanced bone scan that revealed startling results. Her neck had been fractured more than once, and her pelvis and limbs showed evidence of breaks dating back to childhood. Some of these breaks appeared to have healed without treatment. In any case, nothing in her medical history provided any record of or explanation for the data that confronted her chiropractor. Toward the close of treatment, when Gerda had become engaged, she worried that her past sexual abuse had made it impossible for her to bear children. She and her fiancé were relieved when the gynecologist reassured her that she would be able to carry a child to term. However, the doctor shocked them with the observation that her uterus had been torn and stitched. Again, there had been no formal medical history of that event.)

Etiology

Richard Kluft (1988) has described MPD as a chronic posttraumatic dissociative disorder characterized by recurrent disturbances of identity and memory. He observes that the condition is no longer thought to be rare, but now is understood to occur in the wake of overwhelming early experiences, usually child abuse. The besieged child who has nowhere to find protection or hide in external reality retreats to the inner world to "establish alternative self-structures that allow intolerable circumstances to be disavowed or otherwise mitigated" (p. 212).

Breuer and Freud (1895) were very clear that disorders such as Anna O.'s were based on trauma. Freud refined the concept, holding that the psychic illness came from a conflict between the conscious and unconscious parts of the self, rather than from congenital weakness. Freud also acknowledged the importance of actual parental abuse in the creation of this disorder. However, "MPD fell into disrepute following Freud's rejection of dissociation, the seduction theory, and hypnosis" (Ross, 1989, p. 147).

Frank Putnam (1989) proposes a developmental substrate for MPD.[*] He emphasizes the work begun by Prechtl and his colleagues in the 1970s, and notes that behavioral states of consciousness have emerged as the essential ordering principle for all infant studies. He hypothesizes:

> I think that the evidence suggests that . . . over the course of normal development we more or less succeed in consolidating an integrated sense of self. . . . At birth, our behavior is organized into a series of discrete states. . . . The transitions between infant behavioral states exhibit psychophysiological properties that are highly similar to those observed across switches of alter personalities in MPD. . . . (p. 51)

As this sequence of normal developmental states is frozen by trauma, it becomes the ground for the development of subselves:

> One can conceive of these dissociated states, each imbued with a specific sense of self, being elaborated over time as the child

---

[*]Dr. Putnam, in addition to writing a major text, *The Diagnosis and Treatment of Multiple Personality Disorder*, is chief of the Unit on Dissociative Disorders, Laboratory of Developmental Psychology, Intramural Research Program, National Institute of Mental Health, Bethesda, MD.

repeatedly re-enters a specific dissociative state to escape from trauma or to execute behaviors he or she is unable to perform in normal consciousness. Each time the child re-enters a specific dissociative state, additional memories, affects, and behaviors become state-dependently bound to that state, building up a "life history" for the alter personality. (p. 54)

Treatment

Freud, basing his approach on the therapy of Anna O. and others, stressed what Anna had described as the "talking cure" as the treatment of choice. He and Breuer developed the cathartic method of therapy, using hypnosis to access a traumatic event, but requiring that the patient fully describe the event, until verbalization and behavioral repetition merged to create an affective conscious experience. With the entry into consciousness, the trauma was transformed into a memory that, like all memories, could be relegated to the past and released.

However, Freud abandoned the cathartic method; his substitution of the Oedipus complex for literal incest led to the deemphasization of trauma as the basis for his neurotica. Free association, interpretation, and working through (incrementally connecting pathology with infantile antecedents) became the hallmarks of psychoanalytic technique.

I believe it would be a theoretical error to dismiss analytic input into the treatment of multiplicity on the basis of this shift. The concepts of the influential inner world, and of working through, are essential to the dynamic therapy of MPD. The lonely and courageous pioneer work of Cornelia Wilbur (Schreiber, 1973) advocated an essentially psychoanalytic framework for the treatment of MPD. The overall work of Braun, Kluft, and Loewenstein stresses the importance of retaining a dynamic basis in the treatment of MPD, synthesizing it with the dissociative techniques that are more familiarly used.

Although hypnosis is surely *a* treatment of choice for MPD, it addresses only the dissociation, without helping the patient to place the enormity of her or his experience in the context of the history of the self. Resolution of the distortions of character that are built on the foundation of dissociated trauma is necessary if the self is to become whole.

As Karla Clark has noted elsewhere in this volume: "Freud's disavowal of his original trauma theory was a necessary precondition, ironically enough, for the development of theories that are comprehensive enough to treat trauma victims" (Chapter 13).

Treatment of MPD by conventional dynamic therapy typically reaches a stalemate, if, indeed, the condition emerges at all. Abreactive work alone, however, floods the patient when little or no attention is paid to establishing the containment good character work provides. Casualties of either one-sided approach are prevalent. As Braun (1986) sums it up:

> Gathering facts or emotions is useless if they cannot be integrated. Abreaction, without cognitive structure, can be dangerous in an MPD patient because it can activate traumatic memories for which the patient has no defense or coping skill. This in turn can lead to an escalation of acting-out behavior and psychological or physical collapse. (p. 14)

MPD and the Masterson Approach

Gerda has told me repeatedly that the initial work she accomplished, focusing on the Masterson Approach to her borderline self style, was essential in finding the strength to face her real self. The revelations that came with trauma work would have been insupportable (they would have retraumatized her, or worse) without the character work and the beginning of the working through of her abandonment depression. In this phase, she began to access and strengthen her real self to grapple with the trauma. The phase was marked by a more observant and adaptive ego, and a strong alliance with the therapist, supplementing areas where her ego still struggled to mature.

The unfolding of the work with Gerda demonstrates a therapeutic phenomenon I have since witnessed numerous times, both in my own work and in the work of others trained in the Masterson Approach: with patients with a character disorder and MPD, the effective resolution of character (personality) defenses opens the self to another level of dissociated conflict, and the working through must then include an additional area of dissociated trauma.

It appears, then, that the self protects itself in ingenious layers of defense. On the basis of my work with patients at the Masterson Institute, I would propose the following configuration of early defensive groupings in the genesis of MPD.

First, there is a defensive operation that deals exclusively with the early and relentless onslaught of traumatic experience. It would seem that, through splitting, the part of the self that experienced the traumatic episode is divided from the main self and dissociated. Since multiplicity is generally conceded to have its origins in early childhood, repression (as it is defined as a major defense of the mature self) is not available as a means of psychic protection. Instead, the primitive defense of dissociation must be utilized. Freud (1915) referred to this level of dissociation as primary repression, saying that its "essence . . . lies simply in the function of rejecting and keeping something out of consciousness" (p. 86). (Freud substituted the term "repression" for "dissociation" to distinguish his dynamic concept from the then more commonly held concept of dissociation as the result of genetic weakness.)

Second, developmental forces and the dyadic interchange begin to shape the emerging early defenses that form the infant's character (projection, projective identification, denial, acting out, and so on). When the interrelationship with the mother (or a consistent caregiver) fails to be emotionally supportive (or is abusive or allows others to be abusive), the pain of this situation is circumvented by a rigid configuration of early defenses. The character (or personality) becomes set and stereotyped in order to evade, as automatically as possible, the kind of self-expression (related to separation and individuation) that is likely to evoke a response from the mother that will trigger the abandonment depression. Acting out, especially, becomes a major character defense, as it permits some lessening of tension by demonstrating in behavior the dyadic impasse, while keeping the actual understanding of it outside conscious awareness. This forms the intrapsychic structure, which is an encoding of the misalliance with the mother and is repeatedly projected onto all subsequent relationships of importance, including the therapeutic one.

Finally, infantile amnesia, or the repression barrier, further seals off the painful experiences of childhood to prepare the psyche for the new learning tasks of latency.

What brings the patient to the therapist is the failure of these protective barriers to withhold the pressure of excessive infantile pain or the defensive system's being so maladaptive that it presents a difficulty as great as or greater than that it defends against. Thus in good-enough character work, the patient relinquishes old ways of being in order to be more adaptive. This releases a front level of defense, and the patient is faced with underlying traumatic issues, whose primitive dissociation had been doubly fixed in place by the character structure.

When the trauma experienced by the infant has been great enough to create multiplicity, the dissociative level is unique and differs from the dissociation found in more encapsulated experiences of physical or sexual abuse. It is a highly elaborate structure that acts to partialize and contain such a degree of trauma that even a moderate rupture in the multiple system could let through enough traumatic material to break down the psyche. This system not only has its own defensive and executive functions, but exhibits other sophisticated specializations that amaze one with the resourcefulness of the self to persevere, and also with the ability of the self to divide into subselves indefinitely, to both the gain of safety and the loss of conscious continuity.

One realization becomes increasingly clear in the work with MPD: this elaborate dissociative work is not with defensive mechanisms only, but is also with a lost part of the patient and, in talking and interacting with the inner alters, the therapist is in touch with a part of the self that has been divided from consciousness since that part's inception. The real self of a multiple can never be established unless this defensively hidden part of the self integrates with the conscious part.

DYNAMIC PSYCHOTHERAPY WITH GERDA AND HER INNER WORLD

Introduction to the Patient's Inner World

Since the time of Morton Prince (1905), representations of the inner world of the multiple have provided diagnostic guides for the therapy. My first tentative entrance occurred spontaneously when I asked Paulina to introduce me to others she knew in the inner world, and when I asked them to tell me about themselves. Since then I have learned to elaborate on that process. I first introduce myself (partly to set a standard of order and courtesy, partly to allow for occasional inner unawareness of my identity), and then, basically following Bennett Braun's guide (1986, p. 19), I ask:

1. *What can I call you?* Giving a name may be considered dangerous, and certainly a sign of trust, so I may settle for "the one who is angry" until enough trust has been established for me to learn the proper name.
2. *How old are you?* This tends to identify the age at which an especially traumatic event or the need to perform some task in order to survive led to the creation of this alter. However, other reasons may determine the age of an alter, or an alter may have a range of ages (reflecting chronic trauma of a state-bound nature over time). So I also ask: What was the age of the body when you were created? And: Do you have more than one age?

3. *What is your job?* Alters exist for specific (state-bound) reasons. If an alter addresses the therapist more or less directly, this is a useful question to ask, since the alter is likely to have a specialized function ("I get the body to the office," or "I keep the records for the system," or "I'm here to deal with fools like you who ask too many questions"). These typical answers, followed by as full a discussion as is allowed, begin to identify the alters who are concerned with functioning and helping, or who guard the secrets of the perpetrators or are identifications with them.

4. *What is your story?* Alters who "hold" traumatic material—most typically (although not exclusively) victim children—may appear in an abreactive state, and need encouragement to tell the event (release the event from dissociation to the consciousness). Because talking is considered dangerous, the story may have to be told through drawing or symbolic play, or even in sign language or by ideomotor signals.

In this initial phase of the dissociative work, I was becoming aware of the dynamic balance of the inner world, and beginning to realize how the dissociative level had its own dynamic principles that required systematic conceptualization and specific approaches. For instance, the principle of containment was critical: the conscious, nondissociated part of the personality had to be healthy enough to manage the no longer divided-off memories and accompanying feelings that were released into awareness by the abreactive work. This meant that characterological work preceded abreactive work whenever possible, and that abreactive work had to be followed by a period of working through, allowing the once-disavowed past to become part of the aware self.

I also discovered that inner victims and perpetrators had to be kept in balance. After the sequence of inner children had told the story of the father's abuse, the inner father emerged to threaten the system, saying that Gerda, or myself, or both would be hurt if any more secrets were revealed. The presence of the internal abuser needed acknowledgment, and the system had to be helped to overcome and contain the terror evoked by the internal abuser before resistance to further abreactive work could be resolved.

Hospitalization

Gerda decided to enter a hospital specializing in treatment of dissociative disorders. The decision was based on concern for her safety and the need for both therapist and patient to understand more about the nature and treatment of multiplicity. We were worried about the increase in her suicidality and about the management of the violent alters (formed through identifications with her aggressors), and looked forward to contact with practitioners experienced in this work.

I visited the hospital weekly, and attended sessions during which Gerda was held in restraints (cf. Braun, 1986, p. 14). Gerda found the restraint sessions a relief, describing them as her first experience of being positively held, no matter how violent she needed to be. These sessions also provided the basis for her mastering of internal (or hypnotic) restraints, a skill we relied on thereafter. (There is an informal consensus in the field that internal restraints suffice when the patient's ego strength and the therapeutic alliance are in place. I would agree, with the added comment that multiples are overcontrolled people who can benefit from a safe surrounding fully to vent a depth of pain and rage that has only been permitted to be turned against the self or channeled into a mindless repetition of abuse. Perhaps a technique can be found that is less suggestive of past bondage.)

Resumption of Outpatient Treatment

After a month, Gerda returned from the hospital. By that time, we had both gained some sense of balance and direction. We relied on a well-established therapeutic alliance to combine the knowledge gained about multiplicity with her therapeutic work in the past, and to evolve a concept and a strategy that would guide her to integration of her real self.

I believed that Gerda could only be healed if I were able to find an overall way to conceptualize the therapy. Incremental abreactive work with each traumatic episode that appeared would be an impossible task; by definition, MPD is created by years of unremitting abuse, and would take years to undo piecemeal. I was also wary of the evoking of alters indiscriminately—what I call a body count. Both of these approaches seemed repetitious and interminable, and threatened to flood the patient. (There is an analogy here with the therapist who countertransferentially attacks a patient with deep interpretations, when the patient's ego is not strong enough to contain the feelings that are dredged up; or to the patient's perpetuation of a crisis state in order to avoid managing accompanying feeling.)

It was clear that the dissociative level had come forward when the character work had strengthened her ego enough to permit the management of a deeper level of conflict. It followed that the synthesizing of the trauma work with the character work, and subsequent inclusion of dissociative material in the working through, was a step toward integration of the real self. Each time this step was taken, the self became stronger and ventured another forward move.

As I have already mentioned, the dynamic principles of resistance analysis could be readily applied to the treatment of MPD. In addition, therapy with Gerda's inner alters in many ways seemed to resemble work with both adaptive and maladaptive defenses. Acknowledging and understanding the alters sometimes seemed analogous to a second level of ego work. The increasing cooperativeness among alters released warded-off perception and feeling about the past, just as the healthier alignment of characterological defenses had opened the way to a similar understanding of individual depth and continuity. Combined, the character work and trauma work led to complementary aspects of the working through.

Richard Kluft, who is a hypnoanalyst, has initiated much valuable psychodynamic guidance to the treatment of MPD. Gerda, by Kluft's definition, was a highly complex multiple with innumerable subselves. According to Kluft's dynamic approach, these subselves could be grouped variously, in levels and in types, and these aggregates often could be treated with collective interventions. Kluft also emphasizes resistance analysis; for instance, he is concerned with understanding the alter who is blocking the progress of the therapy, and who may represent a source of danger if bypassed. In addition, Kluft (1988; following Braun, 1986, pp. xiv–xv) has conceptualized integration in a dynamic, whole-self way. He departs from the old idea of the forced merging of alters (equivalent to an overriding of major emotional issues) and sees the unification of alters as a basically spontaneous process that (with occasional strategic facilitation) takes place as the need for dissociative barriers dissolves. He understands integration within the larger context of what might be called self-actualization, as he describes the synthesizing of the unifying alters into the maturation of the overall personality: "Integration [is] a more comprehensive process of undoing all aspects of dissociative dividedness that begins long before the first personalities come together and continues long after fusion until the last residua of dissociative defenses are more or less undone" (p. 213).

Perhaps the following could sum up the contemporary approach to the understanding and treatment of MPD. Multiplicity is a complex reconfiguration of the self, intensively relying on dissociation to defend the fundamental integrity of the self from the disorganizing effects of ongoing traumata. Trauma originates in the developmental years and is directly associated with the family of origin, so that the infant has no recourse but to utilize inner resources of the psyche. The infant who is able to access these resources has probably found a way not to go mad or not to fail to thrive. Dissociation, and the elaboration of the splitting defense to contain dissociated material in discrete subself compartments, continues to be the defense of choice in subsequent years, particularly when the abuse is unabated. The treatment of MPD, therefore, is especially challenging, since it not only requires the loosening of the dissociative defense, but calls upon the patient to manage pain and conflict in a unified, conscious manner, and to establish a basis of consistent trust with a valued person in the external world.

The treatment of MPD, as I have learned it within the context of the Masterson Approach, involves what Loewenstein (1990) has referred to as an ecology of therapies. Character work, with its ego-oriented interventions, gives place to interpretation and working through. However, in the case of multiplicity, as early childhood material emerges into the consciousness, specifically traumatic issues also surface, and in a highly elaborate form that is best treated with some knowledge of hypnotherapeutic technique.

In addition, adjunctive nonverbal interventions, such as drawing and play therapy, may prove invaluable in maintaining communication with the patient's inner world (the use of sand-tray "worlds" is a specialized form of nonverbal therapy devised for work with MPD [Braun and Sachs, 1986]). A primary skill, in both the assessment and implementation of the therapy, is knowing when to shift technique, and also knowing how to incorporate that shift into a consciously acknowledged and unified approach. This dynamic psychotherapy relies on the most steady therapeutic alliance, and the synchronization of the work, I believe, provides the basis for that desired dimension of treatment—the real relationship.

Resumption of Outpatient Treatment: Inner Alters and Mapping

When Gerda returned from the hospital, she had a working relationship with a number of her alters, and was constructing highly schematized maps (with the assistance of her inner world) that included all known alters, along with their relationships to one another. The maps changed with the progress of therapy.

Putnam (1989) has described such sophisticated mapping as follows:

> In essence, the personality system is asked to produce a map, diagram, or scheme of the alters' best understanding of how they fit together or their sense of their inner world. The exact form of

the map should be left up to the discretion of the personality system. I have received Mercator projection maps, pie charts, architectural blueprints, organizational personnel charts, target-like arrangements of concentric circles, clock faces, lists, and some totally unclassifiable documents. What is important is that all of the personalities be represented on the map in some fashion. (pp. 210–211)

Gerda's alters primarily conformed to the two main types described by Putnam (1989): those created to protect the system from trauma, and those able to supplement the functioning capacities of the normally conscious self (p. 54). Other subselves, or partial subselves, also made themselves known (see Braun, 1986, pp. xii–xiii). These included personifications of defenses, identifications with perpetrators, representatives of a spiritual state, and fragments. The work with Gerda emphasized four fundamental categories: Victim Children, Perpetrators, Protectors, and Helpers.

The inner alters, under ideal conditions, make themselves known to the therapist after a therapeutic alliance has been established with the host personality—the part of the multiple system that represents the system as though it were unified.

VICTIM CHILDREN.   These alters "hold" abuse memories, and are the primary abreactors.

PERPETRATORS.   These alters are mainly identifications with actual abusers. In doing the therapy, it is very important to remember that these alters are not the external abusers, but represent identifications with those aggressors—identifications that had to be made to survive in an environment where someone else held the power. "If you can't beat them, join them," would be an accurate statement of their rationale. Perpetrators can be arrogant, contemptuous, and even violent, depending on the nature of the original model, but they become more accessible as they are acknowledged and the child behind the identification is found. As Gerda said of the Perpetrators: "They are all children with masks on." Perpetrators are really outdated Protectors, whose capacity to coexist with the external abusers may have saved the patient's life. However, the Perpetrators, like maladaptive defenses, live in the world of the past, and are traumatically fixed to reacting in old, self-defeating ways, unaware that new ways have become available.

PROTECTORS. These alters mainly represent adaptive ego states and preserve the impaired real self. Their basis for being seems to lie in a determination of the self to survive, sometimes formed around brief (but deeply significant) contacts with people who showed caring and values. It is often a Protector who is the first representative of the inner world to contact the therapist.

HELPERS. These are highly controversial inner selves, first described in detail by Ralph Allison (1991), and later by Christine Comstock (1989). There is often a sequence of Helpers, and the central one, the Internal Self Helper (ISH) poses the controversial concept. The ISH represents the spiritual aspect of the self, and has been credited with paranormal abilities. Without entering into the controversy, I would like to define my sense of Gerda's ISH as the function of this Helper affected treatment. This alter understood the nature and possibilities of the entire self system, and willingly worked with me to educate and guide me. The ISH did not claim to be a spirit, but protected the unifying spirit of the self. The ISH could relieve other alters from pain, especially through dissociation, but could not effect psychic change in the system without the presence and concern of a significantly allied outside person.

Although the ISH may have extraordinary influence in the entire multiple system, and is able to perform acts that seem magical in the inner world (such as constructing protective force fields), it is interesting to note that dynamic change in the multiple system happens within a therapeutic, dyadic relationship. Again, the form taken by multiplicity is elaborate, but the psychotherapy of multiplicity follows familiar, well-established rules common to the containment and working though of all types of personality disorder.

The Host Personality

This part of the self, named and described by Bennett Braun (1986), is in its own category. The Host personality has the special function of presenting the multiple system to the daily social world as if the system were a conscious unity (that is, a nonmultiple); the Host, apparently to carry out this task more effectively, is convinced of its own oneness. As Gerda's transition to conscious awareness of her multiplicity demonstrated, probably the first major task of integration of the multiple self takes place as the Host begins to acknowledge the inner world of alters. (Since human individual consciousness may be a relatively new achievement in our evolution, and since modern scientific culture demonstrates antipathy toward the concept of the unconscious, the dilemma of the Host personality suggests correspondences with the larger, evolving social self.)

Braun specifically defines the Host as "the personality that has executive control of the body for the greatest percentage of time during a given time period" (p. xiii). The fact that the Host must give place to inner alters that push through, that these alters may be at cross-purposes with the Host or consider the Host inconsequential, and that the Host may not even be aware of having been displaced, but only aware of having lost time, tends initially to create animosity, or at least much anxiety, in the Host's attitude toward the inner world. Well into the last stages of integration, it was my task to encourage Gerda's Host personality to work with her inner world, and to facilitate the cooperation and adaptiveness of the inner alters in supporting the Host's increasingly mature goals and actions. I found it especially important to strengthen an alliance between the Host and the "Front."

The Host, as I understand that part of the self, could probably be described as an outer alter. In Gerda's case (which I have found to be typical, both in my experience and as mentioned in the literature), there had been more than one Host. A child Host had committed "suicide" when she lacked the strength to act as container for an increasingly embattled system. She had been replaced by a stronger Host. During the process of therapy, Gerda (the Host carries the daily name) often came to the edge of despair, and the ISH once quietly remarked: "We may have to make a new one." However, this Host personality was able to maintain herself, and then strengthen herself enough to integrate the younger Host who had "died." (Death, madness, illness, disfigurement, and dismemberment all may be found in the multiple system. These conditions are reversible as long as the body remains alive and intact and the total system is not overwhelmed.) Braun (1986) mentions the importance of finding the "original personality," which "is often difficult to locate and work with, but . . . [this] needs to be done to achieve a stable and lasting integration" (p. xiv). In Gerda's case, the finding of the Host and the integrating of the entire Host line, back to the original personality, who had had the potential to contain a united self, were difficult, but essential for healing.

It is my experience that the Host, when first encountered in therapy, is a type of false, defensive self. The Host keeps up social appearances and carries the personality disorder that initially may bring the patient into treatment. Gerda, the Host, carried the borderline personality disorder. When the character work advanced, the Host was adaptive and strong enough to begin to acknowledge the inner world of alters. As the trauma work and the working through progressed, Gerda held steady enough (although severely tested and often suicidal) to accept into consciousness the knowledge previously held in compartments by the inner alters. (It is interesting to note that the inner alters often had very different diagnoses than did the Host, and had to be addressed by the style of intervention suitable for that diagnosis. The Perpetrators were almost invariably narcissistic, whereas certain of the Victim Children were psychotic. The ISH was normal neurotic, if neurotic at all, and demonstrated conflict only briefly over the acceptance of sexual maturation.)

As the therapy progressed and the personality disorder of Gerda's Host was resolved, the Host gradually became the conscious, adaptive container for the unifying real self. Gerda's impaired real self was inherent in her inner world, but had to overcome seemingly endless inner division, as well as support the Host's struggle with inhibiting defensiveness in order to emerge. The result of Gerda's integration could be described much as Masterson (1985) describes the real self:

> The term real self refers to the normal, healthy, intrapsychic self and object representations and their related affects. It functions along with the ego to effectively adapt and defend in order to maintain a continuous source for the autonomous regulation of self-esteem as well as to creatively identify and articulate or express in reality the self's unique or individuative wishes. (p. 30)

The more the Host was able to become continuously, consciously aware and to manage a full range of feeling, the more the real self was able to find a focus and a container for growth.

The Front

Scattered throughout the literature are references to an inner executive committee or team of specialized alters who are aware of the Host personality's problems and seek to maintain the functioning of the self by supporting, or even temporarily coopting, the Host. This group may be coconscious and constructively cooperative when first met by the therapist, or they may need to discuss with the therapist the advantages of clarifying and pooling their adaptive capacities for the safety and growth of the self. In Gerda's case, the Front, represented initially by Paulina, needed recognition and guidance from the therapist to form a working coalition. Once this coalition was established, the Front was indispensable for creating inner structure for safety, setting up warning systems for inner and outer dangers, shoring up the Host, and offering a rounded assessment of the progress of the therapy. In Gerda's situation, the Front was especially helpful in maintaining her daily functioning, protecting the inner children, and finding ways (especially hypnotic restraints) to modify the destructive impulses of alters who still operated according to past rules of power and abuse.

The Front, when united, operates as a sort of ego within the dissociated part of the self: it facilitates healthy functioning and defense. It is my impression that a number of multiples decide on a good-enough termination of their treatment when the Front operates in a highly coordinated way with the Host personality. This would be the equivalent of the patient who is satisfied to stop psychotherapy on the adaptive level and not venture into the revelations and emotional stress of the working through, and it has its own validity.

The Inscape

I have borrowed a term used by the poet Gerard Manley Hopkins (1918, p. xvii) to identify the geography of Gerda's inner world. This Inscape, depicted through a series of evolving drawings, charts, and verbal descriptions, symbolized the patient's conscious acknowledgment, understanding, and gradual unification of her inner world.

Much of the Inscape was vague and uncharted. Even when the area was fairly well mapped, new regions sometimes appeared that demanded attention. (It was my impression that the full extent of this area, call it the subconscious, probably cannot be completely charted by contemporary psychic cartography.) However, one characteristic of the Inscape was dramatically familiar.

Gerda's inner world showed a split in the structure and evolution of the self that appeared to illustrate Kleinian psychology. The Inscape was divided between the Perpetrators and the Protectors, who established separate domains and vied over influence on the multiple system. In the course of the treatment, the creation of the "Safe Place" helped to establish a base for the "Safe People" that supported the building of more adaptive ways of being. As the good side of the split strengthened, the bad side—the "Tunnel Folk"—could gradually be acknowledged and educated. Translated into object relations terms, Gerda's sense of herself as good became coherent enough to begin to allow her acknowledgment of herself as bad—to integrate memories so ugly that only a mature sense of self, ready to manage ambivalence, could maintain her.

In this strange work, where one literally talks with the subordinate elements of the self, it has become clear to me that psychotherapy provides critical interpersonal elements necessary for psychic growth. The negative part self, monolithically based on a past of consistent, ongoing abuse, needs the modification offered by a concerned other, while the positive part self needs a dyadic presence therapeutically supportive enough to help build and reinforce inner structure that can facilitate the balancing and eventual integration of the negative.

The Safe People occupied the good side of the split, in a stone tower surrounded by picturesque, but carefully guarded grounds. They formed a sort of executive committee, a Front, that seemed analogous to the adaptive ego on the dissociative level. They were Protectors who supported functioning, managed feeling states, helped Victim Children to come to the Safe Nursery to release their stories to consciousness, and were vigilant against intrusions from the Tunnel Folk. The Safe People represented a part of the ego that had survived abuse and indoctrination, and believed in the possibility of a life of individual worth and choice. Over the course of the therapy, this group became more interoperative, flexible and receptive, and even learned to assist the evolution of the Tunnel Folk.

The Tunnel Folk occupied the bad side of the split in a labyrinthine, multileveled structure. There were many rooms representative of locations where the traumatic events of Gerda's life had happened; for instance, the bedroom with the father's reflection in the window was there. The Perpetrators—introjections of and identifications with Gerda's actual abusers, or with times when she, herself, had been forced to abuse—lived in the tunnels, endlessly repeating their hurtful activities. The Perpetrators sought out Victim Children, to return them to the replicated scenes of their victimization. The frozen, redundant nature of the Tunnel region, and the preoccupation of its inhabitants with power (either wielding it or obeying it), demonstrated the fixated and pathological nature of that part of the Inscape.

Only the ISH was able to travel throughout the entire system with some degree of safety (although with anonymity and caution in the tunnels). She seemed most at home in an area of bright fields that she said provided a region of spiritual protection for the system. In Gerda's schematic maps of her Inscape, these fields maintained a buffer zone between Safe and Tunnel territory, and steadily decreased in size as the Safe, conscious territory increased, and elements of the Tunnel territory were gradually made safe or neutralized.

Integration

Although the term "integration" is generally used to describe the merging of inner alters, it probably should more accurately refer to the inclusive therapeutic process that culminates in the emergence of the real self. Braun (1986, pp. xiv–xv) and Kluft (1988, p. 35) make this distinction, referring to the merging of alters into one as unification, and the postunification working through as integration of the no-longer multiple personality).

Gerda's psychotherapy involved this ecology of therapies. The emergence of the self—of containment, insight, and psychic transformation—was held in a progressive balance. Confrontation (ego-oriented intervention) was used primarily in the first stage of character work. As the working-through phase began, interpretation was used more, until the surfacing of the dissociative level called for the use of hypnotic techniques. Although hypnotic techniques were especially helpful in the dissociative phase, interpretation of the working through continued, and return to confrontation was often necessary as the patient regressed under the stress of increasing abandonment depression and decreasing recourse to dissociation to manage it.

Another kind of balancing act was required of the therapist in the shift from the essentially linear, cause-and-effect progress of ego work to the nonlinear processes of classic analytic working through (free association, evenly hovering attention) to the dramatically spatial and systemic development of the dissociative work. In the last, equilibrium had to be maintained between the Host and the inner alters, and between the system (outer, inner, and as a whole) and the therapist. Even in the inner world, the acknowledgment of Victims, of Protectors, of Perpetrators, and of the Helper demanded equal weight.

Character work with the Host personality created the container for the working through, which, in turn, included therapy with the defensive dissociative level of alters. Gerda said many times that this first adaptive structuring of the conscious self was critical to her ability to handle, and perhaps to survive, the pain and complexity of the working through. (The alters, however, readily reminded me that I had missed their early attempts to leave me clues as to their existence. I might have begun contact with them sooner.)

The working-through stage, for Gerda, held a struggle with abandonment depression filled by extreme rage, guilt, terror, despair, and emptiness ("Everything is ashes. My life is nothing but ashes"). Despite an essentially supportive relationship with the mother in the present time, the longing for the inner, historical mother seemed inconsolable and endless. Suicide was a frequent concern, although she telephoned me infrequently, and only under great duress. Despite her suffering, she continued to be self-supporting and socially active throughout almost the entire process.

The pain of the working through was directly related to the progress of the dissociative work. As the alters, in turn, released the portion of dissociated trauma each contained, the Host (and often other alters), who had not previously shared consciousness of the event, was shaken by this "new" knowledge, and struggled to handle it. In this way, the whole system, but the Host in particular, gradually absorbed perceptions and feelings that became part of the conscious life history. Since the dissociative defense was no longer required for a particular event, the alter who had held that experience no longer needed to be divided from the remainder of the system. As a result, a lost part of the self, split off to defend the greater self, returned as a flexible part of the whole. Although the greater self was shaken by the impact on consciousness of once-dissociated trauma, it also gained from more completeness. Protectors, who had guarded adaptive skills; Perpetrators, who had hoarded aggressive energy; Victim Children, who were loving and playful; the Helper, who was wise and giving—all brought their attributes to the continuing integration of the self.

Something should be said about the complexities of the transference on the dissociative level. Each alter brings a separate issue of trust, mistrust, allegiance, opposition, or even total incomprehension to the therapist's acknowledgment of the alter's existence. Even the ISH, who intuitively understands the therapist from the beginning, learns about the complex unfolding of interrelationship over time. Other alters, however, see the therapist as an abuser or as a mother (or both, and sometimes to the point where the transference is hallucinatory). Most intense transference issues are worked through with separate alters, and then worked through once more on the level of the Host, who now carries the (now consciously manageable) transference issue of the integrated alter.

An ongoing issue for the therapist and patient relates to a shift in relationship that, with the process of therapy, is accentuated in MPD. *Each unification of alters into the system changes the nature of the self, and, therefore, the nature of the transference and the therapeutic alliance.* Even the character work must be redone somewhat, because *the person who is in therapy is not quite the same person as was there before the last integration.*

Something also needs to be said on the issue of countertransference, which parallels the diversity and intensity of transference. Briefly, the impact of both subjective countertransference (related solely to the therapist's own history) and patient-induced countertransference (the effect of the patient's projections on the therapist) is so formidable as to be almost diagnostic (at the very least, such reactions are probably indicators of significant abuse of the patient in the developmental years). The work evokes physical as well as mental states in the therapist, and has a tendency to spill over into the therapist's social environment. The therapist experiences fascination, apprehension, exhilaration, and despair. The therapist may develop one physical symptom or a kaleidoscope of discomfort. Preexisting states may be exacerbated, or new physical problems may emerge that elude a satisfactory diagnosis and treatment. The therapist, overloaded with the data provided by the patient's alters and the technical challenge of work that is so frequently in crisis, may enter a state of stress that communicates itself to those around the therapist, verbally or nonverbally.

Until recently, the therapist's tendency to countertransference reactions has been exacerbated by a professional isolation parallel to the patient's personal isolation. There have been few professionals to turn to for guidance and support, and current pertinent literature only dates significantly from the 1980s. But the situation is changing rapidly, with the establishment of annual conferences on a high professional level, the journal *Dissociation*, and networking and additional conferences and publications on the local, national, and international levels.

INTEGRATION AND THE TERMINATION
PHASE OF TREATMENT

In Gerda's system, integration followed the orderly (not necessarily easy) process that occurs when the patient is highly motivated and the therapist has acquired enough knowledge and skill to balance character work with trauma work.

The first alters who joined hands—as Gerda, (like "Sybil"; Schreiber, 1973) described it—were the three Victim Children who had been sexually abused by the father. They became one representative child, Terri, who eventually stood for all the inner children abused by the father, and who learned to play and trust. Terri became a source of joy to the system, so that her integration at first was experienced as a loss. Terri integrated into Paulina, an unlikely combination that brought Gerda to tears. Gerda had wanted Terri to integrate immediately into her. The wisdom of the system had combined Terri's spontaneity and humor with Paulina's determination and pragmatism.

Subsequent integrations followed this pattern. Groupings of similar alters would merge as their knowledge was released to consciousness, and the remaining representative would integrate with an alter who demonstrated complementary characteristics. None of these integrations was clinically forced, but occurred spontaneously as the need to keep parts of the self dissociated diminished, and the self gathered together in a balanced way.

In the final stages of unification, the multiple system had removed itself into single representatives of its primary subsystems: Child, Protector, Perpetrator, and Helper. The Host was now consciously accepting management of the self, practically and emotionally, in a more consistent way than ever before. The Child, mainly freed from the responsibility of bearing terrors no child should have to hold, was a source of pleasure and hope to the system. The Protector, a fiercely vigilant teenager, stayed around to watch over the Child and to keep the car in repair. The Perpetrator represented the role the patient would have assumed had she permanently aligned with the cult, that of a young priestess who had grown up largely ignorant of the world of consciousness, and who, in a sense, represented the "shadow side" of the self; she had struggled hard to relinquish her power, and only did so when she understood that love could exist in freely chosen, caring forms. The Helper gradually became a moral and ethical capacity and intuitive sense that permeated and guided the self.

The Inscape was fading. Gerda spoke less and less of the past, and even the representative alters ceased to appear. Her concerns were with her daily life and relationships. The Tunnel Folk had steadily crossed over to the Safe side. The parental introjects had lost their force: parts had been assimilated as positive identifications, and parts had been rejected from the system, suggesting the acquisition of a capacity for repression as an adaptive defense.

The tunnels collapsed like a house of cards. The old belief system of childhood had been replaced by a new belief in the self and the capacity for choice.

Criteria for the Achievement of Integration

Although the literature inclines to the hypothesis that integration is a larger matter than the merging of alters only, the criteria for integration tend to stress the completeness and permanence of that merging. In Gerda's case, issues connected with dissociation were of major concern, and her healing showed the following changes.

1. The absence of alternate personalities over a significant period and in pronounced times of stress.
2. The management of feeling and conflict on a conscious, consistent level.
3. The absence of Schneiderian symptoms (voices in the head, and so on).
4. Cessation of "lost time" other than normal distraction.
5. Modification or cessation of such soft signs as headaches or ringing in the ears.
6. The capacity for symbolic dreaming (where previously dreams tended to have an abreactive quality—replicating a traumatic event or doing so in a thinly veiled form).
7. The acquisition of repression rather than dissociation as a major organizing defense of the psyche.

However, true integration is an achievement of the real self as well as of the whole self. The real self, as described by Masterson (1986), emerges with the resolution of the patient's personality disorder, as well as with the healing of the dissociative division of the self. He cites the following as an adequate clinical working scheme for defining the capacities of the autonomous real self (pp. 26–27).

1. Spontaneity and aliveness of effect
2. Self-entitlement
3. Self-activation, assertion, and support
4. Acknowledgment of self-activation and maintenance of self-esteem
5. Soothing of painful affects
6. Continuity of self
7. Commitment
8. Creativity
9. Intimacy

CONCLUSION

During the past few years, Gerda has relocated from the city and established herself in a sophisticated, semirural town. She secured a small business loan and set up a successful book-and-toy store. She commuted to her sessions, a drive of over an hour, twice, and then once, a week. The focus of therapy was on relationship, especially her deepening attachment to a young teacher and her residual wish to run away from relationship as dangerous. The couple, however, searched earnestly for closeness and commitment. They held each other and themselves to an agreement to stay and talk when they felt like running. The relationship has continued for three years, through both companionship and separation, and they are now married.

For over three years, Gerda has managed her life (which has included a number of crisis situations) without dissociating. Over two years ago, during a journey to another country, an inner child popped to the surface briefly (evoked by the echo of the continual journeys of her younger years), and then was gone.

What determines the healing of multiplicity? Time, which tests all things, will bring around unfinished business, or will simply present Gerda with the sorrows and pleasures that belong to the unity of the self. For now, it is enough to say that she has found herself, and she has also found, and entered into a committed relationship with, someone she loves and who loves her.

REFERENCES

Allison, R. B., & Schwarz, T. (1980). *Minds in many pieces*. New York: Rawson, Wade.

American Psychiatric Association (1994). *Diagnostic and statistical manual of mental disorders* (4th ed.). Washington, DC: American Psychiatric Association.

Braun, B. G. (1986). *Introduction* and *Issues in psychotherapy of multiple personality disorder*. In B. G. Braun (Ed.), *Treatment of multiple personality disorder*. Washington: American Psychiatric Press.

Braun, B. G., & Sachs, R. G. (1986). The structure of the MPD's system of personalities, in *Dissociative Disorders 1986*: Proceedings of the Third International Conference on Multiple Personality Disorder/Dissociative States. Edited by B. G. Braun. Chicago: Rush University Press.

Breuer, F., & Freud, S. (1895). *Studies on hysteria* (J. Strachey, Ed. & Trans.). New York: Basic Books, 1955.

Comstock, C. M. (1991). The inner self helper and concepts of inner guidance: Historical antecedents, its role within dissociation, and clinical utilization. *Dissociation. 4*, 165–177.

Freud, S. (1915). Repression. In E. Jones (Ed.), *Collected papers*. New York: Basic Books, 1959.

Hopkins, G. M. (1918). *Poems of Gerard Manley Hopkins* (W. H. Gardner, Ed.). New York: Oxford University Press, 1948.

Kluft, R. P. (1984). The phenomenology and treatment of extremely complex multiple personality disorder. Presented at the First International Conference on Multiple Personality Disorder/Dissociative States. Chicago.

Kluft, R. P. (1988). The postunification treatment of multiple personality disorder: first findings. *American Journal of Psychotherapy, LXII,* 2, 212–228.

Loewenstein, R. (1990). Advanced topics in the treatment of MPD. Presented at the New Jersey Society for Study of Multiple Personality and Dissociation, Princeton.

Masterson, J. F. (1985). *Psychotherapy of the borderline adult.* New York: Brunner/Mazel.

Masterson, J. F. & Klein, R. (Eds). (1989). *Psychotherapy of the disorders of the self: The Masterson Approach.* New York: Brunner/Mazel.

Prince, M. (1906). *Dissociation of a personality.* New York: Longman, Green.

Putnam, F. W. (1989). *Diagnosis and treatment of multiple personality disorder.* New York: Guilford.

Ross, C. (1989). *Multiple personality disorder; diagnosis, clinical features, and treatment.* New York: Wiley.

Schreiber, F. R. (1973). *Sybil.* New York: Warner.

CHAPTER 13

Season of Light/Season of Darkness: The Effects of Burying and Remembering Traumatic Sexual Abuse on the Sense of Self*

Karla R. Clark, Ph.D.

Traumatic sexual abuse has far-reaching effects on the personality of the victim, many of which have been well documented (Schetky, 1990; Mc-Cann & Pearlman, 1990, pp. 35–56; Courtois, 1988, pp. 89–118). Less attention has been paid to the effects on the sense of self of forgetting the

*This chapter was originally presented as the keynote address on the psychoanalytic track at the Federated Societies for Clinical Social Work meeting in Chicago in September 1991. It was subsequently published in the *Clinical Social Work Journal*, vol. 21, no. 1, Spring, 1993, and is reprinted, with some revisions, with the permission of that publication. The author would like to thank Jean Sanville, editor of the *Clinical Social Work Journal*, as well as the members of the program committee of the Committee on Psychoanalysis for their invitation to present the address and for their encouragement and support.

The author would also like to thank many friends and colleagues for their help in preparing this work, in particular, Dr. James Masterson, Dr. Eleanor Grayer, Andrea Stone, Dr. Shelly Nagel, Dr. Stephen Reed, and Stewart Clark. All of them took the time and trouble to make many helpful comments. In addition, I would like, in particular, to thank Dr. Candace Orcutt, whose thinking about trauma and dissociative states has had a profound influence upon my work.

trauma or the specific effects of remembering it. In my view, defense analysis leading to the access to and control of affects is a crucial aspect of understanding how trauma affects the sense of self and for developing strategies to treat the disturbances in it that follow (Krystal, 1988). In this chapter, I consider the defenses involved in forgetting trauma—specifically dissociation, denial, and repression—and some of their basic effects on the sense of self when they are employed consistently. A case discussion demonstrates how the analysis and control of these defenses and the resulting access to her feelings affected the sense of self of a patient who had forgotten a profoundly traumatic past.

BURIED TRAUMA AND THE SENSE OF SELF

John: Do not seek to stuff my head with more ill news, for it is full.
Falconbridge: But if you be afeared to hear the worst, then let the worst,
unheard, fall on your head.
—William Shakespeare, King John, *Act IV, Scene II*

Some years ago, one of my patients revealed a multiple personality disorder (also known as dissociative identity disorder). Another patient, Ms. A., who has a borderline personality disorder (and whose case will be discussed in detail), began to remember traumatic experiences of sexual abuse that had spanned her entire childhood. Both had forgotten the abuse, even while it was happening, and both had continued to forget this abusive history throughout their adult lives until psychotherapy stimulated recall.

In both of these cases, the origins of the patient's subsequent difficulties clearly lay in severe incestuous trauma during childhood. Was Freud correct, then, when he wrote "The Aetiology of Hysteria" (1896) but incorrect when he disavowed its ideas? I think not. Ironically enough, Freud's disavowal of his original trauma theory was a necessary precondition for the development of theories comprehensive enough to treat trauma victims. Thanks in large part to his subsequent work, here are the kinds of questions we can ask at the end of this century, questions that Freud himself could not have asked at the end of the last. When the child "forgets" that he or she is being assaulted, even while it is happening, does this further personality development in some way? Was the self protected by forgetting the things that were happening? At what cost? What defense mechanisms are involved in forgetting?

Obviously, not all childhood sexual activity is traumatic. When it is not, the child's development does not seem to suffer because of the experience.

It is when it is traumatic—as when incest, and particularly parent–child incest, is involved—that the child will be affected in ways that lead to serious disruptions in functioning.

Trauma means an experience that is (1) sudden, unexpected or nonnormative; (2) exceeds the individual's perceived ability to meet its demands; and (3) disrupts the individual's frame of reference (McCann & Pearlman, 1990, p. 10). Trauma has certain specific biological, emotional, and cognitive consequences that affect the sense of self. Among these are disruptions of the sense of self owing to the employment of defenses designed to cushion emotional shock and the overwhelmingly powerful intensities of feeling that children experience as a result of the trauma.

The combination of the direct consequences of trauma and the defenses designed to protect children from its emotional impact are expressed in behaviors and symptoms that can both affect a child's developing sense of self and alter the self already in existence. These changes in the sense of self—which are, in fact, the development of a false, defensive self (Masterson, 1985)—affect all of the self's subsequent development.

The symptomatic behaviors that develop have their own effects on how children feel about themselves, and these, in turn, influence the views of themselves that they carry into adulthood. Adults often report emotional constriction or lability; self-hatred; problems in self-activation, impulse control, and self expression; clinging or avoidant relationship patterns; sexual difficulties; problems in attachment; and other intimacy problems. They develop strong feelings of shame or worthlessness, of embarrassment, and of being different from others (Putnam, 1990, p. 116). When a person is not aware of the earlier abuse, the symptoms are all the worse for being mysterious and unaccountable. This in itself undercuts the person's sense of self-coherence and self-worth.

When the abuse is both incestuous and continues for a long time, through several developmental periods, the resultant disruption in the formation and maintenance of the sense of self will be most profound. These effects can be grouped into two classes: (1) alterations in the sense of the self owing to the nature of the interaction between the child and caretakers, and (2) alterations in the self owing to defenses against overwhelming feelings.

A sense of self, as suggested by both Mahler, Pine, and Bergman (1975) and Stern (1985), develops in the context of the child's intimate relationship with crucial caretakers, notably the mother. Disruptions in this relationship are probably at the heart of what makes incest so traumatic to the child. It is possible to think about this disruption in the context of the myriad and minute transactions through which the sense of self is formed, solidified, and maintained. According to Stern (1985, p. 132), for example, the sense of the subjective self is formed through the sharing and modification of feelings between the parent and child. The traumatically abused child may be subjected to sudden, frightening, and irrational shifts in parental availability for providing the empathic and appropriate experiences that help the child define and moderate feelings. A mother who, at one moment, may be finely attuned to the child's needs, in the next moment may be sexually overstimulating the child with no regard for the child's feelings. A father who, at one moment, is involved with his daughter in mutually pleasurable play, may, in the next, be inflicting terrible pain on her, which the child experiences the mother as being unable or unwilling to prevent. In such circumstances, a child cannot develop stable capacities for trust or for modulating feelings.

Fortunately for their survival, children are not formed simply by their transactions with their parents, but bring their own native talents and inborn capacities to each encounter. Among these are the defenses that filter, modulate, and sometimes transform experiences so that feelings are not overwhelming. Defenses, however, are a two-edged sword—at times disturbing the sense of self in order to preserve it.

For example, self-coherence, a feature of Stern's core sense of self, depends on the sense that one is physically in one place at one time and that various actions emanate from that one locus (p. 82). It is not always desirable, however, for an endangered young child to retain that sense of physical continuity. An infant or young child who is seriously hurt physically may dissociate in order to deal with the accompanying rage, fear of annihilation and abandonment, and so on, and this dissociation will, in turn, disrupt the sense of physical self-coherence. The child may thus unwittingly sacrifice the sense of self-coherence for the greater good of surviving otherwise unbearable emotions. Other sacrifices of self function may follow as the child experiences feelings as dangerous to the capacity to survive and employs defenses against them.

What is gained is survival under conditions of extreme duress. What is lost, along with the capacity to feel fully and without fear of being overwhelmed by feelings, is a sense of vitality and of being real, self-aware, spontaneous, and in tune with one's own inner workings—in short, the sense of self. This principle is dramatically illustrated in the functioning of the three defenses centrally involved in the process of forgetting traumatic abuse. Unlike the "forgetting" of neurotic or normal people, which is accomplished primarily through repression, in trauma victims varying combinations of three defenses are usually employed in forgetting. These defenses are (1) dissociation, (2) denial, and (3) repression—all of which help the child to preserve the sense of self in whatever ways are possible by protecting him or her from overwhelming feelings at the expense of developing a viable and authentic self representation. Because disturbances to the self can be caused by the very defenses that were originally designed to protect and preserve it, the systematic undoing of these defenses is vitally important in the psychotherapy of trauma victims. Defense analysis results in access to increasing levels of tolerance for feelings, which, in turn, leads to memory recovery and resulting alterations in the self representation (Masterson, 1976, 1985, 1988; Krystal, 1988).

Before proceeding to a more detailed examination of each component of forgetting as it affects the sense of self, let us consider how the terms "dissociation" and "repression" are defined here. Throughout his writing, Freud used the two terms somewhat interchangeably, and the literature has remained confusing and contradictory on the subject ever since (Singer, 1990). I have tried to use these terms in ways that seem to me both to be the simplest and to reflect their most common clinical usages.

In dissociation, the person says, "This is not happening to *me*." There are degrees of dissociation, ranging from standing off and watching someone one knows to be oneself in traumatic circumstances (depersonalization) to its most extreme forms, as in a multiple personality disorder, where the person says, "This is happening to *somebody else*." Many examples of dissociative defenses, however, are not as dramatic. For example, Ms. A., during one phase of her treatment, "saw" incidents of severe abuse as pictures projected onto my office door, in which "a girl" (who was actually herself) was involved in various violent acts. At first, she behaved as though these "pictures" had nothing to do with herself. Gradually, she was able to acknowledge that, in fact, they were pictures of her own experiences, which she could then acknowledge as being memories of her own past.

Dissociation has very serious consequences. For example, there is always (1) an alteration in thinking, whereby archaic modes of thought predominate; (2) a disturbed time sense; (3) a sense of loss of control; (4) changes in emotional expression; (5) changes in body image; (6) perceptual distortions; (7) changes in meaning or significance; and (8) hypersuggestibility (Putnam, 1990, p. 122).

Does dissociation have an adaptive function? Franklin (1990) has suggested that young children may have an inborn ability to dissociate. She suggests that the biological basis of this ability may lie in the fact that states of consciousness, from alert waking to deep sleep, appear to be more discrete in infants and young children than in normal adults. Usually, children learn on their own and from their caretakers to modulate these states. She quotes Fraiberg, however, as having described a response of abused and neglected infants of 3 to 18 months of age, in which the children appeared to screen out perceptions of the abusive mother (p. 75). We may at least hypothesize that this talent for dissociation allows the child to preserve perceptions of good aspects of the mother by splitting off these images and associated feelings from bad perceptions and overwhelmingly bad feelings about her in order to extract from a hostile environment whatever nurturance there is (see Fairbairn, 1952; Kernberg, 1975, p. 25; Masterson, 1976, p. 58).

The second defense involved in forgetting is denial. The persons says to himself or herself, "This is not happening." This defense disrupts continuity of affect and memory. It also involves perceptual distortion, impaired reality testing, and changes in meaning or significance. For example, Ms. A. was able to recall that as a child, when the pain, rage, and terror she felt became too strong, she could block out her feelings by focusing with extreme concentration on one aspect of her physical discomfort, such as feeling cold, and, by so doing, "not notice" what was happening to her. She repeated this experience at points in her treatment when, under the extreme stress of recall, she could shut down an abreaction by concentrating on feeling cold, or hot, or thirsty. In more extreme forms, at some points in treatment, Ms. A. would announce to me that none of the things that she had remembered had actually happened. At those times, she was convinced that she had made all of it up.

Denial puts people in danger of retraumatization, which makes them feel bad about themselves, because of their failure to recognize dangers that remind them of the original trauma. For example, Ms. A. frequently became involved in sexually exploitative relationships simply because she was unable to recognize that this was what they were. What denial does not disrupt is the feeling of continuity of the physical self, which it may, in fact, preserve. "This is not happening" has the positive effect of shielding the person from the overwhelming feelings associated with trauma: feelings of terror, betrayal, abandonment, and pain, and fears of annihilation and death. The person is numbed without losing the sense of continuity of the total physical self; the suffered loss is of the continuity of *experience*.

The effect of the third defense, repression, is closely related to the effect of denial, but is less disruptive to the basic sense of continuity of the self representation. Repression is an effective way of handling data about the self: what is not remembered is put into cold storage, to be retrieved if necessary. It allows for *unconscious* continuity in the self experience, although it may interfere with *conscious* aspects of continuity. For example, the first group of traumatic memories that Ms. A. retrieved had to do with violent incestuous experiences with her father. When she remembered these, she experienced shock, grief, and rage, but never felt as though the events had happened to somebody else. She reacted on one level to her rediscovered memories with relief because the memories explained many things about herself that had puzzled her. Repression was the first defense that Freud was able to identify and discuss, and it came to represent a key feature of psychoanalytic thinking about personality development. He said, "The essence of repression lies simply in turning something away, and keeping it at a distance from the conscious" (Gay, 1989, pp. 569–570). The person says, "I *forget* that this happened to me." Such matters, when retrieved, may astonish us by their existence or nature. In that sense, they may alter our sense of the narrative self by providing us with information about ourselves that we had not "known," but in and of themselves they are not experiences of discontinuity and disorientation. "I had forgotten that" has a very different meaning than does "I never knew that."

In cases of buried trauma, the individuals are not sufficiently protected by repression alone, and need to dissociate and deny as well. As a result, impairment in the sense of self is much greater. They experience themselves as more fragmented, more mysterious. They have far less access to feelings.

These defenses, used to reinforce one another, form a powerful component of the formation of the false, defensive self. This false self, formed as a way to maintain some sort of way of relating to the child's primary object, is, as Masterson has pointed out, reactivated in the treatment and acted out with the therapist. Ms. A. initially presented herself to me as a ghostly, insubstantial creature who was obedient, pleasant, and easy to be around but in some way impossible to know. This somnambulistic behavior, which was largely both created and reinforced by the defenses she used to forget her past, had been reinforced by her primary caretakers, who rewarded her when she behaved that way. She expected a similar response from me.

In psychoanalytic psychotherapy or psychoanalysis, these three defenses, reflecting the false, defensive self, will exert a tremendous, silent influence until they become conscious and the patient controls them. But what happens when the false self is challenged, the dissociated is reclaimed, the denial undone, and the repressed recalled?

TREATMENT

It was the best of times, it was the worst of times, it was the age of wisdom, it was the age of foolishness, it was the epoch of belief, it was the epoch of incredulity, it was the season of Light, it was the season of Darkness, it was the spring of hope, it was the winter of despair. . . .
—Charles Dickens, A Tale of Two Cities

Dickens' opening paragraph in *A Tale of Two Cities* serves as a beautiful metaphor for the experience of both patient and therapist in the recall and working through of traumatic abuse. This is a long and complicated journey involving many interlocking factors: defense and character analysis, transference and countertransference, abreaction, mourning, and integration.

Part of the case of Ms. A. has been presented elsewhere (Clark, 1991). At the time of the prior presentation, the patient appeared to be coming to the end of a successful analysis. However, the subsequent act of trying to separate from me, I believe, triggered access to unsuspected levels of abandonment panic and rage. Access to those feelings undid repression, opening the door to forgotten memories. The repressed memories were denied to some degree, and to a larger degree, initially dissociated by the patient even as she remembered.

The first level of forgotten memories involved incest. There also was a second, still more deeply buried level of abuse that involved her mother and much of her extended family. As we are still working on memory recovery at this more complicated level, I cannot demonstrate the effects of integrating all of the forgotten material on the self. I will try to show, however, some of the shifts in the self representation that have occurred thus far.

Ms. A., an urban geographer, is in her 40s. She currently lives alone. She has been in psychotherapy for seven years. For the first year and half, she saw me first once and then twice a week. Eighteen months into treatment, she began to come three times a week and to use the couch. Now, when abreacting, I sometimes see her daily, and she sits, lies down, or moves about as she sees fit.

The woman who introduced herself to me that first day was rather small. Although she was a trifle overweight, it was difficult to really know what she looked like, because she huddled in dark, shapeless clothes. She was slightly disheveled. Her shoes were scuffed and run down at the heel. At the end of her first hour, and throughout the early months of treatment, she stumbled over the same chair each time she left my office. Her sense of humor was keen and her wit was sharp but, while pointed, was not malicious—however, her smile, when it came at all, was a grimace that changed her mouth but did not light her face. I liked her, mostly for certain qualities of strength and depth that I sensed rather than saw. From very early on, I had the emotional conviction that in therapy she would find the sense of self that she sought. I have never really wavered for long from that early conviction about her (even in the face of what turned out to be a very difficult analysis), although I have sometimes doubted my own ability to help her.

Presenting Complaint

Her presenting complaints were not unusual. Ms. A. asked for help with a pervasive, low-level feeling of depression, which she said she had suffered from for most of her life. Her live-in arrangement with her lover of seven years, Mr. B., was precarious. Despite the fact that he had many problems, the couple's consensus opinion was that *their* problem was mostly *her* depression. She clung to him, obeyed him, and accepted his view of their situation.

Patient's History

The patient's history, as she remembered it when therapy began, included almost no conscious knowledge of incest and none of the ritual abuse that we now know she had undergone throughout her childhood. Ms. A. told me that her early family life had been very painful. Her father was physically violent and abusive. She clung to her mother, whom she experienced both as protective of her and, simultaneously, as someone she felt she had to protect. She recalled having been sexually fondled by her father when she was seven years old, but claimed that she had fought off his later advances when she was an adolescent.

She did well in school and had both friends and a boyfriend. After a fight with her parents soon after she graduated from high school, with the help of her boyfriend, she ran away from home in the middle of the night. She put herself through college.

Her problems in self-functioning began to become manifest at that time. Problems with intimacy, self-activation, and self-assertion began to become more visible as her school years came to an end and she was faced with adult responsibilities. She turned down a scholarship to graduate school in order to marry. After her marriage, she began to have numerous affairs. She was depressed and puzzled by her behavior. Feeling suicidal, she entered treatment with a male psychologist. During the five years she saw this therapist, she got a divorce, immediately moved in with another man, left him, and had a series of affairs until she moved in with Mr. B. On the side of her strengths in self-management, she did go to graduate school during this time, although she did not perform at the intellectual level of which she is capable. She developed an artistic talent to a considerable degree. She made and kept friends, although they tended to be related to her through mutual trouble or to be exploitative of her.

The patient's moderate problems in self-activation, management, and intimacy seemed consistent with her history. Two anomalies stood out, however. One was her amnesia for childhood events and her report of having dissociative experiences as an adult when she was very upset, particularly by separation stresses or by being treated abusively. The other was her relationships with men who were extremely narcissistic, emotionally abusive, and controlling. Mr. B., for one, was also beneath her in terms of intelligence and sensibility.

Early in our work, I remember being puzzled at just how bad those relationships were. The patient, for all of her problems, was not grossly disturbed, but she also was puzzled. She sensed that her history, as she remembered it, did not seem to account for the level of depression, alienation, and self-hate she had experienced throughout most of her life. She felt bad about her difficulties in managing relationships and work-related tasks. Her serious swings between frantic overactivity and disorganization troubled her. Intense feelings of anxiety and panic that she experienced at, for her, inexplicable times also frightened her and made her feel bad about herself. Consequently, the defenses involved in forgetting her history led her to have an ongoing, incongruent picture of herself and of her functioning, which was, in and of itself, depressing and deeply disturbing to her.

Diagnosis

As puzzling and incongruous as her behavior was to her, at least her intrapsychic structure could be clearly identified. This gave me some way of knowing how to work with her in order to help her to understand herself. Ms. A. had two split mental representations of herself in relation to two internal representations of her mother. In one, she saw herself as a helpless clinging child with a strong powerful mother who would protect her. This internal configuration evoked feelings of being safe, taken care of, and loved. Initially, she described this state of relatedness to her mother as their being symbiotically bonded. In the other representation, she saw herself, if she tried to act autonomously or to express herself, as threatened by a harsh, dangerous violent object. Initially, she projected and acted out this part unit, primarily through associating with men who were controlling and verbally abusive if she tried to assert herself with them. She would respond to their abuse by collapsing and clinging to them. If she left one, she would immediately replace him with another, similar man. Despite having had some academic and vocational success, she saw herself as helpless and unable to take care of herself. She was afraid of being or feeling alone. In short, Ms. A. was borderline.

Course of Treatment

Her tendency to cling through compliance was rapidly mobilized in the treatment in the form of being a "good" patient: she was rarely late, paid her bills on time, was always polite, was never angry at me, and apparently was eager to listen to what I had to say and to use it.

Although this compliance had its own set of problems, I was more concerned at the time, from the point of view of prognosis, about the way she sometimes detached in order to manage her feelings. While she had no apparent total amnesia for events in her adult life, she did have some striking memory lapses. She also seemed to stand outside herself and observe herself from a distance without making much, if any, effort to understand her motivations or to feel her feelings. For example, she told me that she had left a prior attempt at treatment about two years previously after five years of therapy, on the couch, at least twice a week. She said that the incident that had prompted her leaving was that her therapist had behaved in a rude and insulting way to her during a session. He had stood up abruptly in the middle of the session and left the office. When he returned, she asked what had happened. He simply said, "I had to go take a leak."

She told me that while she could remember the incident, she knew that she had felt nothing at the time, but had left his office and never returned. She still had no feelings about his behavior, nor was she clear about why she had reacted so violently to it. She could not remember his name without making a real effort at concentration, nor could she recall anything specific about what had and had not been accomplished during the years she had spent in his care. It was, she said, as though it had happened to someone else, someone she barely knew. Her detachment and vagueness about her failed therapy did not seem to surprise or concern her. In fact, I discovered, as I began to work with her, that she lived most of her life in this sort of detached state. I thought of her as a sleepwalker most of the time, wandering around the edges of life, rarely feeling or experiencing what happened to her.

Therapy began once a week. The goal at this point was ego repair. I thought that her detachment interfered with her knowledge of how she felt, which, in turn, made it impossible for her to know who she was. I thought that her clinging and compliance reinforced her lack of self-respect and feelings of helplessness. My intent was to help her to understand the destructiveness of these ways of handling her feelings, and to see if she would develop other ways of managing them that would be more self-supportive. This work, successfully accomplished, provided the patient with the increased flexibility in ego functioning that made the rest of the analysis possible.

Although the patient tried to be a "good patient," and to please me, she also was detached and she intellectualized. Here is an example of how this was handled and what it revealed about how she felt about herself. She told me that she was concentrating on relaxing as a way to deal with feelings of anxiety. I asked her why she chose to focus on relaxing rather than on trying to understand her anxiety. She replied, "I'm bringing here what I do at work. I have done it all of my life. I feel a pressure to succeed, to be liked, to be a good client. I am doing it right now, thinking of saying the right thing." I asked her how she felt and she said, crying, "I feel blocked, caged, like whatever you do is not going to be right. I feel crazy. I do. At least I limit it to here. I'm sitting here groping for things to talk about, censoring myself, trying to be a good girl without knowing the rules. Like when I was a little girl. Different things were expected—my mother—there were times when she wanted to be close to me and times she didn't. She would generate fights between me and Dad. She'd be on my side and then switch, and it was real confusing. I felt abandoned. I guess I never dealt with it. I left home. I avoided them for months."

From interchanges like this, it was possible to identify her contradictory self representations. A good girl, as my patient saw it, was obedient and ignored her own feelings. A bad girl was self-revealing. The patient traced this to her childhood, but blamed herself for not having dealt with her feelings about the parental treatment she remembered and for avoiding both her parents and her feelings.

Ms. A. was quickly able to challenge these initial self representations. Bewildered by her behavior and disliking herself for it, she said, "I see where situations which I create alienate me from other people. . . . At the same time I am scurrying around in some frantic manner trying to please a lot of people I don't trust . . . trying to please somebody I don't trust and on some bottom level, I don't care if they like me or I can please them. I think I anticipate in my mind rejection, and that's why I don't get involved. Here, I ask myself, does she like me, and I say it doesn't matter, it's her job, but that's a defense against rejection. . . . Where to be is to consider myself likable, so it doesn't matter so much."

This wise and somewhat accurate self-prescription demonstrated her capacity to face herself and work in her own behalf, but it also hinted at the complex transference that would characterize our work. On one level, she neither liked nor trusted me, but felt that, as with her mother, she had to be a good girl and follow orders. To counter this, she wanted not to care whether I liked her or not. However, on another level, in order to access terrible secrets, the patient was going to have to both like me and feel sure that I liked her, and we would have to trust each other deeply. On still another level, acknowledging her liking for and trust of me would allow her to feel the strong feelings that would stimulate memory, making positive feelings for me dangerous to her for much of the therapy. Consequently, until she began to remember her forgotten past, she compromised by subtly keeping me at arm's length (dissociating). She was very good at it, and I only sensed it because of two things. One was a vague and nagging discomfort about the way that she related to me. The other was that, in response to that way of relating, I had a persistent tendency, which I had to monitor carefully, to become drowsy during her hours.

The patient began to realize that her blatant detachment and her lack of feeling were against her best interests and tried to control them. "I am presently not in touch with anything remotely resembling a feeling," she said. "I think I should concentrate on my feelings about my mother and how she treated me. It seems real central. But it seems artificial, I guess because I don't want to look at it." However, despite her protests, she immediately began to speak with feeling about her life with her mother, whom she revealed to be both destructive and pathologically self-protective in her transactions with family members. Work of this sort alternated with periods when she cut off feeling and periods where she tried to be a good little girl and give me what she supposed that I wanted.

Simply asking her about this was enough at this time for her to stay on track. She dissociated, however, experiencing her feelings as separate from herself, as soon as they reached a dangerous level of intensity—one that could lead to memory. Standing aside from herself, as though she were outside her own experience watching someone else, she observed, "Part of me feels like feeling, and part of me says I don't wanna. I'm not gonna do it. And it is frustrating. The feeling, it disengages or something."

She tried to pay attention to her feelings, and as she felt more, she became even more aware of her dissociative qualities. In this mood, she went home for the Christmas holidays. She said, "I am torn between warring factions. The only way to do that is to act like a zombie, and who wants that for yourself? Everybody there lies. I should be honest. I should draw limits. I should get angry, I suppose." Instead, she lapsed into compliance. I pointed this out, and she said, "That eagerness to please is a buffer, a screen, so I don't have to look at what an outsider I feel like. So to go to take care of myself makes me see reality, which I don't want to see. . . . There's a big part of me that never gets involved in things at all. That eager-to-please thing is a mask, most specifically to myself. I feel like a robot. I have an image of the desert—a lot of wind and nothing there . . . I don't like this. I suppose I have to look at my feelings of loneliness, which are real scary. I don't like those feelings."

Her efforts to focus on and clarify her self experience led to feelings of depression as she internally started to separate out her own self representation from that of her mother (see Masterson, 1976). This led to her wanting to cling to me. She said, "I get in touch with what I feel. It is kind of feeling, like, abandoned. Yeah. That's how it feels. We talked about feeling in a desert, sort of like there, abandoned, not knowing what you're doing, with no sense of direction. It is because I am afraid to trust you. I'm afraid you won't point me in the right direction." Trying to help her to see that she was turning to me in a way that undercut her own capacities and undermined her sense of self, I said, "You begin to take care of yourself, trying to identify your feelings, and right then you turn around and say that you're afraid that I won't point you in the right direction, just at a point when you are systematically experiencing your own emotions. Do you see how that undercuts your own experience of yourself?" She said, "It's my laziness. You do it. I want to be adopted. Rather than give her up, I've decided I want to be a little kid and have another go at it or something like that. I guess that feeling of being alone is real scary for me."

She was years from knowing why she was so terrified and why she so much wanted a good mother to adopt her. Her own mother, while infantilizing her, had also participated in her torture. My patient longed for a good mother who would heal her and obviate the necessity to remember why and how her own mother had been so bad. Because all of this was forgotten, however, her longing for me to adopt her felt shameful to her, a sign of her own weakness. Six years later, she would understand the longing and, with that understanding, stop feeling bad about herself for having had it.

Meanwhile, Ms. A. was consistently tracking and overcoming her most obvious tendencies to detach and coming to understand that her clinging, helpless behavior was destructive and unnecessary. She was, therefore, less removed in her personal life, and for the first time, she began to bring in material that suggested the degree of disturbance in her relationship with her lover, Mr. B. Having overcome a level of dissociation, she began to overcome one level of her denial, as it applied in her present life. Undoing those defenses was accompanied by an increase in self-supportive behaviors, which began to have a positive effect on her self representation.

The conflict with Mr. B. intensified when she began to see more and more clearly his arrogant and deprecating treatment of her. She came to understand that a great deal of what she knew as depression was really a reaction to having consistently allowed Mr. B. to take advantage of her. As she stood up for herself more, the relationship deteriorated.

She found a good job at this point, and, with that financial security, left Mr. B. She felt stronger, much better about herself, and very interested in investigating her feelings. Her goals for treatment had now expanded. She was interested in knowing all about why she felt as she did and had such a hard time acting in self-supportive ways. She had increased her sessions with me to three times a week and was using the couch.

Under the separation stress of leaving Mr. B., however, the patient defended. She once again became dissociated, feeling very little anger, grief, emptiness, loss, or anything else. Within a week of leaving Mr. B., she had found someone else to cling to by beginning a relationship with Mr. C. He had been extremely helpful to her during a severe physical illness, and she ignored many warning signs about his personal problems.* The two quickly became engaged. Since Ms. A. completely stonewalled my vigorous efforts to confront the destructiveness of the leap from one relationship into another, I turned to pointing out the destructiveness of her clinging *behavior* to her feelings about herself. I hoped that, as she controlled the clinging, she would overcome her denial and see the problems in her relationship more clearly. She, however, reversed the field: she became strong and maternal, and Mr. C. began to cling to *her* rather than the other way around. She remained unable to see the destructiveness of the relationship and married Mr. C.

---

*Kluft (1990b) has discussed the frightening propensity of abused patients to be reabused. He attributes it in part to the patient's cognitive incapacity to recognize danger signs. One could also say that recognizing situations that are reminiscent of earlier abuse can trigger unwanted feelings about memories, so the patient will, defensively, unconsciously choose to ignore these signs.

With all of this acting out, I had grave doubts about the future of the patient's analysis. In the meantime, though, her behavior was reassuring. Her capacity in most areas to identify her own wishes, aims, and feelings strengthened still more, and since she no longer collapsed when depressed, her functioning improved. She was learning the all-important ways of managing strong feelings without sacrificing functioning and undermining her sense of self. She asserted herself more consistently everywhere in her life except with her husband. She also began to remake relationships with her family in a pattern that suited her better, unconsciously trying to take away the necessity to remember trauma. In therapy, she spent more and more time trying to focus on feelings and deal with her experiences of herself in the context of feelings about parental failures of support and acknowledgment. She said that this made her feel like a person. She acted more like one as well: her appearance improved, she lost weight, and she stopped tripping over chairs.

With a stronger, more adaptive defensive system and the improved ability to support herself, her self representation changed. A good girl became a person who could identify needs, tolerate feelings, and care about herself. In this mood, she had an experience in which, for the first time, she saw herself as having a self. She attended a family gathering, where she confronted her mother's lack of interest and investment in her and her needs. Crying, she said: "I became aware that they wouldn't go with me [to a beloved aunt's grave]. I knew that I had to get away by myself for a little while in order to deal with how this made me feel, so that I would not distract myself. I took a walk. The most awful feeling came over me. I can't describe it to you. It was as bad as I have ever felt. And then, the most amazing thing happened. Although I continued to feel just terrible, I looked down at the ground, and realized that I was walking through the most beautiful leaves. They had such wonderful colors. I reached down and picked them up, and as I walked, I arranged a bouquet. I touched the leaves. I knew again, you see, that my mother would never acknowledge me, not ever. No matter how many times I have told you that I know this, I think that I have never quite given up hope. This time, I think it really sunk in. As bad as I felt, I realized that, somehow, I could mother myself. It's not quite the same. I don't mean that it wouldn't be nice to have a mother and aunts who would go with me to the grave, to share those experiences. That's not what I mean. It would be. It would. But it is that, if that is not there, I know now that I have something within myself which can make it O.K. . . . I brought the leaves home on the plane. The leaves have faded now, but it doesn't matter. I can't explain it, but the leaves are inside."

She was now prepared to confront her relationship with Mr. C., whose behavior was neglectful and emotionally abusive. She and Mr. C. entered marriage counseling, where the counselor confronted her over and over again with her denial. She decided to divorce Mr. C.

There was a marked and dramatic intensification of all of her feelings, including, for the first time, severe feelings of panic associated with experiencing herself as a separate person. This led to a powerful surge of memory and emotion concerning what she already knew about her father's seductiveness and abusive behavior. At this point, she had had only one specific memory of incest.

She required my help in staying on track as the painful intensity of feelings made her, once again, want to defend against them. She said, "In the beginning, I started out with bad patterns of merging with my mother. I think that is what I thought would protect me from my dad. Whenever I start thinking about unmerging, I get frightened. It wasn't just my dad. It was my mother, too. I know how it worked. He built on, he preyed on, a preexisting condition. I already felt responsible for Mother. So it was easy for me to think I was responsible for him as well. . . ." She then became aloof and detached, with no visible access to feelings. I reminded her that she had told me that it felt worse to admit to herself that she was not responsible than it did to retain the feeling of responsibility, and with it the feeling that she counted. I said that, once again, it seemed that she was backing away from that feeling. Interpreting, I said, "The feeling is so unbearable that you do things to it . . . you cut off, or treat yourself like an object, or blame yourself, or accuse me of treating you like an object, all to protect yourself from the awfulness of these feelings."

She replied, "It's true. The feeling is that . . . the world is not there to help me out. I was wondering why I try so hard to get people's approval. . . . Because that doesn't fit with what I have been saying. It is not approval, it is some recognition that I am not an object. I wanted people to think I was a nice person. The operative word here is *person.*"

She began to feel good more often than she felt bad, and her daily life reflected the changes in her feelings about herself. She became a powerhouse as a planner. Her creative work took a turn for the better. She became more invested in it and increased her output. The nature of her friendships changed as, able to tolerate more feeling and to support herself better, her need for defensive denial decreased. She was able to recognize narcissistic and abusive people more readily and to stay away from them. She felt good about herself, was quite lively and vital, and began to make plans to take a trip abroad. I thought, at that point, that she was almost ready to stop seeing me.

Several things were troublesome to me, but not troublesome enough for me to question them seriously. One source of the trouble was that Ms. A., while she had certainly done work with early memories, somehow had seemed to work and rework things that she had always known rather than to recall (as others among my patients had) relevant forgotten events from childhood. I thought that access to her feelings should have provided her with a richer conscious narrative history of her own development.

Another source of some concern was that the patient, some two years after her divorce, was showing no interest in dating. I had regarded this time on her own, the first she had ever allowed herself, as a time of consolidating important gains in experiencing herself as an autonomous person. Consequently, my concern was not that she was not dating, but that she seemed impervious to any need for sexual or intimate contact, whether or not she chose to pursue it.

Ms. A. decided to end therapy, and the way that she did it made me begin to question my perceptions about her progress. She made the decision to end immediately. She showed no awareness that the core of her therapy had been feelings of fear of abandonment, or any interest in seeing what form those feelings would take when she left me. She was extremely brittle and manic about her decision. I managed to slow the process by confronting her with her avoidance of feeling, and she reset her termination date for four months away. In sessions, though, she still ignored the whole thing. Very tentatively, she started to date men. I wondered if she were looking for a replacement to cling to in order to avoid dealing with her feelings about leaving me. To my relief, she did not jump precipitously into another relationship.

What emerged, as she started to date, was great anxiety. This time she tried to feel the feelings rather than push them away. This weakened the repression barrier. She was puzzled about her fear. Unwittingly, since I had no idea how much trauma had been forgotten, I made the linkage for her. I reminded her that she had been dealing with her feelings about her father's abusive behavior for some months. I told her that I was puzzled that she had not made the connection to her anxiety about men. I wondered how she expected to feel when being with a man obviously reminded her of her earlier experiences. The stage was set. With my intervention, the Pandora's box of incestuous memories was opened.

She started to have new memories of ways in which her father had tried to prevent her from dating and to keep her for himself. Her rage mounted, and as she tolerated it, the repression gave way still more. She suddenly recalled specific incidents in which her mother had held her while her father fondled her sexually when she was three years old and of being fondled by him more aggressively when she was age five. This led to abreaction as she relived the experiences, remembering the exact placement of furniture and the exact words that were spoken, and living them through as a tiny child with a tiny child's voice and movements.

Her rage intensified still further. She tried, with some success, to track her defenses and to relate her present feelings to her past experience. "This morning I was going to supervise a project and I got lost. I got all confused and all of a sudden I realized that going out there I was being a good little girl, and I was so rageful that I couldn't do it anymore. . . . It feels like I am being dumped on by the world. I've had it. I don't want to do it any more." In asserting herself and acknowledging her self-supportive feelings of rage, connections between her past and her present experiences became available to her in a new way, improving her sense of self-coherence and continuity. "Something happened this morning. I had this dream and I woke up, and I couldn't get up. . . . It reminds me of the feeling of crying out, and not being listened to . . . not having anybody listen. . . . It was that awful time, like with my dad. . . . I became immobilized like when I was five."

The patient was extremely invested in remembering, hoping to root out all of the memories and be rid of them. "I remembered a whole lot on Saturday. I started to, and I decided to go for a walk. I felt better in the woods. It was amazing. The terrible tiredness went away, and I felt full of energy. Then I could look up and the sun was out, and I felt fine. It was great. Since I was six or seven, I have pushed this down to not let this stuff out, and now I don't have to push and push."

Repression was lifting, but she was still using denial and dissociation, just as she had as a child, both to remember and to disavow. Although it was becoming clearer that she had been systematically abused throughout her childhood, she held onto her idea that the abuse did not define her. She said, "When I first started coming here, I started talking about deserts and coldness, and then there was a hump where I started to have a self, and I think I needed that, to contain all of this. I think about people who go to those groups for people who are abused. It is not all of my identity. I am a person who was abused, but that's not all that I am." Still, through her protests, her murderous rage, primarily at her father, grew until, late in 1990, she recalled, in terrifying detail, a rape when she was 13 or 14 years old that had left her with a broken jaw, severe lacerations, and other injuries. (Those injuries have been independently verified, through scarring and dental records that the patient, denying and dissociating, had ignored.)

The worst part of the experience was that she recalled how, when the rape was over, she had tried to crawl to her bedroom and had encountered her mother in the hall. Her mother, silent, walked around her and down to her brothers' room, leaving her to crawl on unaided. This memory marked a puzzling turning point. The patient lost investment in remembering. Memories came out in bits and pieces. She was having tremendous difficulty in integrating her mother's reactions. She tried to contact her mother and discuss what she was remembering. Her mother's return letter was cold, self-absorbed, and martyred. Its only reference to Ms. A's experience: "Some things are best not to remember." Ms. A. responded, "It is important for me to keep working on this stuff. I cannot let her stand in my way. I had to deal with it. But I can't let it stop me."

Despite her protests, she was, if not stopped, stalled. I struggled to contain my own tendency to push her to remember in an organized way, feeling sure that she had reasons for renewed resistance, but being unsure of what they were. The best I could offer as an explanation, to her and to myself, was that she was, for some reason, trying to continue to protect her tie to her mother.

In the meantime, despite her difficulties, our relationship was changing markedly. At times, I still had to help her identify and contain defenses, but more and more often we functioned as collaborators—she to do the awesome work of remembering, and I to bear witness. Sometimes she would lie down and free-associate, as she had in the past. Sometimes she would get up and assume different positions, which triggered memories. Sometimes she would sit up to discuss what she was remembering with me, face to face. I thought of her as more spontaneous and real than I had ever seen her. An ethereal quality, which had been so marked at the beginning of our work and had become so subtle that I hardly knew that it was there, gave way to an experience of Ms. A. as being three dimensional and in technicolor.

The patient began to make collages. She observed that in these recent memories she was having a hard time getting clear visual pictures of what had happened. She developed a method for putting herself in a light trance (using her dissociative abilities constructively) and searching art magazines for appropriate symbols. Most of the time, she had no idea why she cut out the pictures she chose, but she allowed herself to place the images where, in her trance state, they seemed to go. Parenthetically, the act of making the collages has been very meaningful to the patient, who describes them as the piecing together of her forgotten and disavowed self.

Simultaneously with learning to use her dissociation to help her, she also began to see it as her worst enemy. "The trouble is," she said, "I feel safe right now. Totally safe. Like nobody can get me. I understand why I do this.

I do. It is almost a grandiose feeling. That nobody can touch me or affect me. Like I am totally above it, I am a million miles away. One thing that is different now is that I feel angry. Underneath it all is this total anger. And I didn't have this before. God, how do I get back in the world? I mean, I guess it's a little bit of reality nudging me. I keep thinking that I'm the victim. It's not anybody else. It's me. And nobody's going to take that away from me, but I am. By being like this, I am."

The patient went on to retrieve more memories. These increasingly focused on times when her mother caught her in sexual activities with her father and punished *her* rather than stop *him*. She began to get an increasing sense of her mother's overt and covert encouragement of the father's abuse and her mother's own frightening sadism toward her.

As the New Year began, Ms. A. assessed what was happening to her self representation. "In a way, it feels good. It explains so much about my life. There's been this puzzle. This missing piece? And, I think, for the first time, I felt as though I were really *here*. I didn't know that pieces were missing, but they were, and this explains a lot. See. I have never trusted my mother. . . . It has become clear to me why I have never really let myself shine. It is like because of the competition with her. I went walking. Often, when I walk, I want to be in the shade, but I wanted to be in the sunshine. The other thing is, in every picture of me, I am never standing up straight. And in this year's Christmas party pictures, I am standing up straight."

She reviewed her collages and was struck, suddenly and with terrible pain, by a reality that she had denied: the collages that seemed to her most frightening and suggestive of the most terrible memories all related to her mother. It took all of her strength to face the rage that welled up and to retain contact with herself. This further obviated the need for repression. The patient noted, without understanding it, that she had had a terrible dream. Once again, she had been in the desert, trying frantically to pick up pieces of things and stuff them in a sack labeled MOMA. She awakened in terror.

She balked. She announced that she was finished with remembering. She asserted that she had been terrified long enough. She did not want to feel bad any more. It was her life, and she was calling a halt to the work. Called to move from my recent role as witness to more therapeutic activity, I told her that, of course, it was her life, and that only she could know what she could stand, but I pointed out that, were she not to remember, she would have to continue to constrict her life for fearing of triggering unwanted memories and feelings. With an understandable lack of enthusiasm, she picked up the job of remembering again. What started to emerge in rapid succession were fragments of memories of ritualistic abuse, including many acts of sexual and physical abuse in which not only her mother, but other, previously valued relatives, had participated. The sessions built in rhythm and intensity, but both of us became frightened and despairing as we began to sense the depth and complexity of the work in which she was involved and the terrible evil to which she had been subjected.

At this time, I routinely acknowledged the effect that her memories had on me as she abreacted, not with extensive self-disclosure, but without denying their impact. She used this experience further to undo her own dissociation and denial, using my feelings as a bridge to her own experience. She became aware that she was treating the work of remembering in the same way that she had treated the abuse. She would come into sessions, abreact trauma, leave, and go back to work. She looked perfectly calm, competent, and attractive. She had been proud of the fact that she seemed untouched by the abuse and that she was trying to be "the least affected abused person who had ever lived." She realized that it was not in her best interests to act as though her discoveries were not affecting her. She began consciously to allow herself to feel the rage, terror, betrayal, and emptiness, and to let it show.

Her core self firmed. She mentioned to me that she had observed herself reciting something strange to herself: "These are my arms, these are my legs, this is my face, my hand, etc." She was startled (as was I) to learn that, until that moment in her mid-40s, she had not been aware of her body as having physical boundaries. Memories of rituals in which she had been systematically traumatized into feeling that she had no ownership of her physical or emotional self became more intense and specific. I finally knew why she fell over chairs.

Despite the new sense of body cohesion, she began to become even more frightened. She experienced herself as "bits and pieces, stitched together with compliance" and, as the compliance dropped off and she revealed secrets of her abuse (which carried the threat of death if she were to reveal them), she felt as though she were falling apart. It seemed incredible to me that she could hold together under the onslaught of the enormous feelings of rage and terror with which she now lived constantly. I began to wonder if she would dissociate further, becoming, or revealing, a multiple personality as a way to cope with the stress. However, the sensation of falling apart was really Ms. A.'s experience of the rearrangement of the organization of her self representation, as memory and feelings totally transformed her experience of her reality.

We now knew enough about the pattern of the ritual abuse she had undergone to understand that she had been systematically exposed to trauma in order gradually to remove any thought of herself as separate and to ensure her absolute allegiance to the group. In remembering those experiences, she said, "I used to think that I had to restore myself piece by piece. Now I understand that this fight goes on molecule by molecule."

She persisted in recall. She used her collages further to undo dissociation. As she began to notice that the images and themes repeated themselves throughout the work, her anxiety skyrocketed further than ever before. "At first," she said, "it seemed like there were hundreds and hundreds of things to remember, but maybe there are not." She began to weep and shake, and I asked her why it upset her so. She said, "Because it is not maybe going to be as hard as I thought. That means that I can, I *have* to remember, and that has many meanings. It means someday it will be over. It means losing a sense of importance. You see, that was the carrot in the carrot and stick. These terrible things happened, but then Mother made things for me, and I was treated as special by all of them. And I will lose that sense of importance.

"There's also something about the process. I come in here, and, there is the sense of battling the forces of evil, which is somehow extremely strengthening about how I feel about myself. It is just that it is very different to feel like I will have grappled with those forces and won. It's complicated, but, for example, our relationship will end, and I will be alone, and I won't have my demons to keep me company—not the little ones, the middle-sized ones, or even the huge ones."

We agreed that this was, in its way, a tremendous loss. I tried to communicate to her, and it seemed to me that she understood me well, that implicit in that loss was the most important gain of all: a self and, through it, membership in the human race. Although not everyone has endured the rituals that marked Ms. A's childhood, those rituals only concretized things that are present in the unconscious of all of us. That is the source of their terrible fascination and power. In discovering and using her real self, Ms. A. recovered her humanity, and her humanity includes these forces, as does my own, and all of ours. These aspects of ourselves are not lost but are transformed in their nature by knowledge of them.

She looked at me, and said, "I think something particularly important happened here today. " I agreed. Her story is not complete, but her humanity—her self—is on the ascendancy. By choosing to remember, as Falconbridge told King John, the worst, for all of her life to come, can no longer fall on her head.

REFERENCES

Clark, K. (1991). The psychotherapy of the higher level borderline adult. In J. F. Masterson, P. Sifneos, & M. Tolpin, *Comparing psychoanalytic psychotherapies*. New York: Brunner/Mazel.

Courtois, C. (1988). *Healing the incest wound*. New York: Norton.

Fairbairn, W. R. N. (1952). The repression and the return of bad objects (with special reference to the war neuroses). In P. Buckley (Ed.), *Essential papers on object relations*. New York: New York University Press, 1986.

Franklin, J. (1990). Dreamlike thought and dream mode processes in the formation of personalities in MPD. *Dissociation, 111*(2), 70–80.

Freud, S. (1896). The aetiology of hysteria. In P. Gay (Ed.), *The Freud reader*, pp. 96–111. New York: Norton, 1989.

Gay, P. (Ed.) (1989). *The Freud reader*. New York: Norton.

Kernberg, O. (1975). *Borderline conditions and pathological narcissism*. New York: Aronson.

Kluft, R. (Ed.) (1990a). *Incest related syndromes of adult psychopathology*. Washington: American Psychiatric Press.

Kluft, R. (1990b). Dissociation and subsequent vulnerability: A preliminary study. *Dissociation, III*(3), 167–173.

Krystal, H. (1988). *Integration and self-healing: Affect, trauma, alexithymia*. New York: Analytic Press.

Mahler, M., Pine, F., & Bergman, A. (1975). *The psychological birth of the human infant*. New York: Basic Books.

Masterson, J. F. (1976). *Psychotherapy of the borderline adult: A developmental approach*. New York: Brunner/Mazel.

Masterson, J. F. (1985). *The real self: A developmental, self and object relations approach*. New York: Brunner/Mazel.

Masterson, J. F. (1988). *The search for the real self*. New York: Free Press.

McCann, I., & Pearlman, L. (1990). *Psychological trauma and the adult survivor: Theory, therapy and transformation*. New York: Brunner/Mazel.

Orcutt, C. (1989). Psychotherapy with a borderline adolescent: From clinical crisis to emancipation. In J. F. Masterson & R. Klein (Eds.), *The psychotherapy of the disorders of the self*. New York: Brunner/Mazel.

Putnam, F. (1990). Disturbances of "self" in victims of childhood sexual abuse. In R. Kluft (Ed.), *Incest related syndromes of adult psychopathology*. Washington, D.C.: American Psychiatric Press.

Schetky, D. (1990). A review of the literature on the long-term effects of childhood sexual abuse. In R. Kluft (Ed.), *Incest-related syndromes of adult psychopathology*. Washington, D.C.: American Psychiatric Press.

Singer, J. (Ed.) (1990). *Repression and dissociation: Implications for personality theory, psychopathology, and health*. Chicago: University of Chicago Press.

Stern, D. (1985). *The interpersonal world of the human infant*. New York: Basic Books.

Stone, M. H. (1990). Incest in the borderline patient. In R. Kluft (Ed.), *Incest related syndromes of adult psychopathology*. Washington, D.C.: American Psychiatric Press.

PART III

Perspectives on Treating the Narcissistic Disorder of the Self

This section on the psychotherapy of narcissistic personality disorders reviews the developmental self and object relations theory and demonstrates its clinical application to the closet narcissistic personality disorder. Exquisite detail is presented to demonstrate exactly how the disorders-of-the-self triad—self-activation leads to anxiety and depression, which leads to defenses—operated in the therapy and in the patient's life. The material makes clear the initial therapeutic challenge the patient presents to the therapist and how it must be dealt with. The following points are emphasized again and again.

1. The patient attempts through transference acting out to evoke the therapist into responding in such a way as to reenact the patient's

pathological internal object relations in order to externalize and defend against the abandonment depression.

2. The therapist must control his or her own countertransference tendencies to resonate with the patient's projective identification, establish therapeutic neutrality, and make mirroring interpretations of the patient's narcissistic vulnerability and his or her defenses against it.

3. This connects transference acting out to therapeutic alliance and transference and enables the patient to gain access to the impaired, vulnerable self and to begin the slow and painful working through of the abandonment depression that leads to the emergence and consolidation of the real self.

In all the chapters, nodal points in the treatment are identified, explained, and supported by clinical evidence. The first two chapters detail the technical approach to the closet narcissistic personality disorder, while the second two focus specifically on the therapeutic management of devaluation and disappointment reactions, along with the countertransference they evoke.

J.F.M. & R.K.

CHAPTER 14

Disavowed Narcissism: Fusion and Externalizing Defenses in the Closet Narcissistic Disorder of the Self

Shirley Zuckerman Issel, M.S.W.

Ms. M. came in seeking treatment for inhibited sexual desire. She was unable to identify her own sexual longings, rhythm, or style. Instead, she found herself responding to her husband's initiatives with unpleasant feelings of obligation. Her treatment is now in its fourth year, and, from this vantage point, it is clear how pervasive her presenting problem was in her life. Many of her relationships were characterized by inhibition, with self-expression stifled to the point of severe impairment in her ability to manage herself in the presence of others. Her work took on similar overtones, leaving her feeling depleted and used up. Seeing herself as ill equipped to succeed in the mainstream business world, Ms. M. had gone into business for herself, yet she did not enjoy her work, often concluding her four-hour day feeling exhausted and inadequate. Encounters with clients were anticipated with distaste and conducted with discomfort. Referrals declined; income dwindled.

Not surprisingly, Ms. M.'s attitude toward psychotherapy and her stance vis-à-vis me took on a quality and tone consistent with the rest of her life.

Just as she began her own business to create a safer environment for herself, she sought treatment in the hope of being understood and accepted by a safe and nurturing therapist. Ms. M. came for reasons consistent with her diagnosis. She came in not to know herself or to understand her need to feel known, but to elicit the feeling of being understood. She came for acceptance from significant others, not to understand her difficulty in accepting herself. She was looking for a safe place to express herself, not a neutral place where she could explore her feelings of danger when she said what was on her mind. She sought soothing, not psychotherapy. She feared that genuine self-expression would result in harshness and insensitivity from me, the same response she expected from the business world.

Operating under the pressure of this fear, Ms. M. had great difficulty with her psychotherapy hour. She reported a reluctance to come to her sessions and longings to retreat to her bedroom and hide. During sessions, she was unable to focus her thoughts and would ramble on in a disorganized and fragmented manner. I found this behavior irritating. Rather than identifying my discomfort, discovering its origins in her productions and calling this to her attention, I acted out with various attempts to organize and focus her. I would make such statements as: "It seems to me that what you're really concerned about today is X." The problem with this type of intervention is not that it lacks accuracy, but that it reinforces the fusion defense and increases resistance. The patient remains unaware of painful feelings of narcissistic vulnerability associated with genuine self-expression, because the therapist, by choosing the topic of discussion, offers the patient opportunities to shield the real self with defensive fusion operations. The phrase "narcissistic vulnerability" refers to difficulties in regulating esteem. By this I mean fragmenting fluctuations in one's sense of self as physically, cognitively, emotionally, and socially adequate, sufficient, or acceptable. Relatively minor external stressors (disappointments, disagreements, misunderstandings, or errors) and internal events (dysphoric affects) become occasions for fragmenting self-doubt. In the case of Ms. M., she came to rely heavily on fusing with significant objects as a way to protect herself from her sensitivity to their approval. This fusion behavior set into motion the chain of events that I outline here. My purpose in doing so is to illustrate and elaborate on the function and consequences of engaging in fusion interactions.

What persons with closet narcissistic personality disorder (CNPD) and with exhibitionistic narcissistic disorders have in common is their vulnerability to narcissistic wounds. Both have constructed elaborate defensive structures (the false grandiose self) to protect themselves from injury, but their designs differ, with differing consequences for the self. (The fusion behavior of the person with a closet narcissistic disorder of the self stands in marked contrast to the exhibiting behavior of the person with an exhibitionistic narcissistic personality disorder, whose behavior compels fusion from others.) While it is tempting to think of the closet narcissistic disorder as less grandiose, I think the perception is misleading. It seems to me that the differences in grandiosity have less to do with visibility or volume, and more to do with the perceived origin of feelings of entitlement. For instance, the grandiosity of the exhibitionistic narcissistic disorder has its origins in a belief in the person's inherent superiority, or "correctness." It is from this belief that the sense of entitlement flows. In contrast, the entitlement of the person with closet narcissistic personality disorder is not experienced as a birthright, but rather is felt to be earned, or covertly garnered by association with or superior service to idealized objects. The grandiosity of the person with CNPD flows from the belief that by perfectly mirroring the object, the person can soothe, control, and secure the well-being and gratitude of the idealized object. Successful fusion services engender feelings of self-satisfaction and entitlement. Such persons have the sense that the object is in their debt, so when they have needs, they do not have to bear painful feelings of vulnerability and humiliation associated with direct requests. Instead, they can simply call in their chips. Trouble arises in this arrangement if the idealized object refuses or objects. Either event can expose the person with CNPD to intolerable, and thus fragmenting, feelings of injury and disappointment. The person can defend with self-righteous anger or withdrawal, but has great difficulty sustaining this position. This is so because the person's sense of well-being flows from the fusion with the idealized object. Absent a feeling of like-mindedness, in time he or she will fragment. To restore himself or herself and the fusion with the idealized object, he or she employs a strategy that is an anathema to someone with exhibitionistic narcissistic personality disorder: he or she will attack and undermine himself or herself, his or her own thoughts, perceptions and feelings. This behavior stands in marked contrast to the person with exhibitionistic narcissistic personality disorder, who deals with injury by a highly effective, sustained attack or indifference aimed at others. The result is that in closet narcissistic personality disorder, one tends to deny the self and mirror others, whereas in exhibitionistic narcissistic personality disorder, one denies others and exhibits the false grandiose self.

The fusion strategy in CNPD results in multiple negative consequences for the self. Because attention is so focused on the object, the person is unpracticed at focusing on and activating (that is, acknowledging, defending, supporting, soothing, exploring, understanding, or expressing) the real or authentic self. In Ms. M.'s day-to-day life, this translated into difficulty in advocating for herself when she came into conflict with others. In her psychotherapy session, it translated into difficulty with sorting through events of the week, identifying themes that seemed important, and exploring them in therapy. To do so, in her mind, would expose her to the possibility of narcissistic injury by harsh, attacking, derisive, devaluing objects. With almost constant projections of negative internal object images, she defended with depleting mirroring activities in the endless labor of maintaining fusion. It is only through the therapist's effective management of these events in the session that these ego-syntonic operations can be made ego dystonic and available to the patient's observing ego for control and analysis.

TREATMENT

Establishing a Therapeutic Alliance

Ms. M. managed her extreme feelings of vulnerability when she was required to start the session either by producing her idea of what a good patient "ought" to produce, or by rambling in a disorganized and fragmented fashion. These symptoms contributed heavily to her sense of herself as unable to think clearly. Vulnerable to countertransference acting out, I reacted with attempts to focus and organize her thinking. This taking over only served to provide her with an object that she could continue to idealize and mirror and, therefore, to experience fusion. When I was able to recognize this as transference acting out and countertransference acting out, I brought it to her attention with mirroring interpretations of narcissistic vulnerability. I told the patient that is seemed to me that when she was required to focus on her self (her thoughts, actions, dreams, wishes, feelings) and choose something to explore in session, she seemed to have uncomfortable feelings of vulnerability to judgment or attack, which she managed by telling me what she thought I wanted to hear. These kinds of interpretations, repeated frequently and empathically, over many months and in varying circumstances, led to the patient's ability to acknowledge her extreme feelings of vulnerability by focusing on and exploring her self.

As Ms. M. focused on her relationship with her husband, she became painfully aware of her feelings of vulnerability and her great fear of narcissistic injury. She managed this sensitivity either through subservience and inhibition of self-expression or with attempts to be perfect. Ms. M. began to elaborate on her strategy and its origins.

When we go on a hike, it's either my way or his. If it's my way, it has to be perfect. I'm terrified of making a mistake. I have to be right so I have a defense. If he's in charge, then I have to do it his way, but then he has to take care of me, appreciate my company, be glad I'm along, go at my pace, feed me, not act like I'm in the way, a burden or an obligation. I seem to have confused ingratiate with initiate.

This description of her fusion strategy lays out the basis for her grandiosity and feelings of entitlement. Her fusion (achieved through perfect mirroring) entitles her to narcissistic supplies, and protects her from the vulnerability to which a direct request would expose her. When this strategy works, she feels powerful and in control. "You know," she acknowledged some months later, "I have a deeply held belief that I run the universe. I have the power, I have to do it right and take care of everyone else." Somewhat later, she pinpointed exactly what it is that she wants from her running of the universe. "I want the parental lap—positive attention, approval, and interest. It's what I want, and I get enraged when I can't get it."

With her increased ability to focus on herself, Ms. M. came to see more clearly the substantial price she paid for her ingratiating behavior. Her commitment to controlling the acting out of her false defensive self solidified following a dream of masochistic sexual submission that was as debasing as it was vivid. The affects of shame and worthlessness that were linked to this dream were the leading edge of the abandonment depression against which she had been defending.

Before the affects and events of the abandonment depression can surface in a sustained way, there are two defensive structures that must be identified, analyzed, and contained. Not only must the self and object representations of the defensive fused part unit (false grandiose self/idealized object) be understood, but also the self and object representations of the aggressive fused part unit (harsh attacking object/fragmented self). As Dr. Masterson (1981) observes, "This perception of the abandonment depression, if not immediately defended against by the defensive unit, . . . is dramatically externalized with a projection of its object representation as causing the depression . . . the patient proceeds to avoid, deny and/or devalue the offending stimulus of perception, thereby restoring the balance of his narcissistic equilibrium . . ." (p. 16). As Ms. M. was now able to recognize and contain the acting out of her false defensive self, the perception of her abandonment depression began to emerge into consciousness and thus externalizing operation came onto center stage.

Externalization for the closet narcissistic personality disorder can function as an all-purpose defense because it focuses attention outside of the self, thus ridding the self of all need for change and for the ability to change. A successful externalization relies on the projection of internalized self and object representations onto the outside object world. The patient can then more comfortably proceed with attempts to manage the self through others. It is, in part, the complexity of this defense that makes it so effective and resistant to therapeutic effects. However, it becomes more difficult to recognize and deal with when there is a close match between internal and external objects. For example, the therapist can find it confusing when the patient's partner is the arrogant, devaluing person she describes him to be, or when her adult son is the fragmented, inadequate, and needy object she fears him to be.

Ms. M. had great difficulty in managing her husband's scathing, haughty devaluations of her and her son from her first marriage. These attacks occurred whenever the patient and her son failed to live up to his expectations. In the third year of this patient's treatment, her son returned home after his graduation from college. His plan was to live with his mother and stepfather while looking for work. In her therapy hour, Ms. M. observed that she was having difficulty in receiving her son with joy and taking pleasure in his return home. She reported feeling "anxious and off balance. He's come home broke, and I'm afraid he'll suck me dry. I don't know my own boundaries and limits. I just want to crawl into a box and hide."

She was aware that her attitude toward her son was suspect. When she told her friends that he was home, their responses were positive. She observed with concern her own negativity and aversion: "My interactions with him revolve around fending him off or trying to get him going." She felt caught between her son's need for help and her husband's demands that she set limits on the young man he characterized as a malingering user.

Torn between her husband and her son, Ms. M. had her intrapsychic difficulties nicely externalized. Her focus was entirely off her self. She had projected her fragmented, depleted, inadequate part self representation onto her son, while projecting the harsh, attacking, devaluing internalized part object representation onto her husband. Her ideas about how she wanted to receive her son were unavailable to her.

The intervention I made was an attempt to align myself with her observing ego. I stated that I found her observation that her friends had reacted differently compelling, and I wondered if she had closed herself off to similar authentic feelings because to experience them directly would expose her to painful feelings of vulnerability. Ms. M.'s response to this in-

terpretation was immediate and deep. She began to cry as she acknowledged her desire to joyfully embrace, welcome, and indulge her son. She
went on to acknowledge with horror her awareness that she had taken on
her husband's view of her son, even though his ideas and her own were
vastly different. In fact, the problem was not her husband's harsh and opinionated arrogance, but that, by focusing on his reactions, and fusing with
him by mirroring and maintaining her idealization of him, she had thereby
ignored and dismissed herself, her genuine longings for reunion, and her
natural wish to nurture her son and provide him with help during this time
of transition. Further questioning revealed that she viewed such needs as
illegitimate, and was contemptuous of them. (In other words, such needs
triggered the aggressive fused unit.) "I'm so ashamed of my longing to be
taken care of because my longing makes me vulnerable. If I express myself, I expose myself to sarcasm, ridicule, judgment, and rejection. I make
myself a target." So, she abandoned herself. Unable to advocate for herself, she was unable to advocate for her son. This view of herself as dis-
abled, too weak to support herself in the face of challenges from others,
unable to soothe or reassure herself when injured, contributed to her belief that she could only manage her son's needs or her husband's devaluations through negative distancing maneuvers (rejection, withholding, withdrawal). Understanding these issues led Ms. M. to conclude, "I don't want
either of us to be harsh with him or throw him out. I know he can mobilize himself to get a job." Because the patient's shift in self state was so sudden, and her tendency to fuse (that is, to join objects through mirroring
and idealizing) so reflexive, I followed the patient closely to determine if
her statements were an expression of her real self or if she were now fusing with me.

The next session provided an answer. She began the hour by reporting
that she was now able to find pleasure in her son's visit, giving examples of
activities they had shared. She also reported that when her husband ad-
vised her to throw him out, characterizing the young man as a malingerer
and his wife a fool for letting herself be used, she neither withdrew, mirrored, rebelled against, confronted, nor provoked him. Instead, she simply
and firmly told him that she saw it differently. "I'm not going to send him
away," she told him, "I'm enjoying his company." With this, her husband
quieted. Later, he shared with her memories of his own return home after
graduation and the hostile, rejecting reception that he had encountered.
Her actions with her son were equally self-supportive, showing signs of integration and genuine self-activation. When her son fell asleep on the couch
(instead of preparing his resumé as he had announced he was going to do),

she became concerned. Old feelings of being taken advantage of and desires to withdraw and be alone resurfaced. This time the patient contained them.

> Life requires a response! I had to wake myself up and then wake him up. I shook him and asked him if his going to sleep had to do with his resumé. He acknowledged that it did. So I sat down with him and gave him a few pointers. He finished it that day. Meanwhile, he's gotten a part-time job to bring in a bit of money while he looks for more permanent work.

For the time being, Ms. M. had emerged from the "twilight zone" of her externalization. Not only had she activated her real self, but also more realistic pictures of her husband, her son, and her self were beginning to emerge.

By relinquishing her defensive posture (refusal to mirror interrupts defensive fusion) and activating herself with her husband, Ms. M. had left herself vulnerable to injury and affects of the abandonment depression, which again triggered the return to her aggressive fused unit.

In the next session, Ms. M. reported that while she and her husband were on a hike, he had given her a look of "complete rejection." She reacted with "tremendous anger," which she attempted to manage by withdrawal when they returned home. As she described it:

> I immersed myself in my book and didn't want to be intruded upon. My attitude was, "What do I need this for?" My husband's been talking about his life for the first time, revealing stuff about himself. I'm seeing his flaws. I'm irritated with his habits. It came along with a sense of "I don't need this relationship."

By acting out her identification with the harsh attacking object, Ms. M.'s narcissistic defenses came more fully out of the closet. She defended against the hurt and anger she felt when he gave her that "look" by blaming and devaluing him. When she was able to shift her focus back to herself, she observed, "There is no support. There is tremendous rage around that. The rage around that lack of support has gone to sneering." Although detached (she was talking from the third-person point of view), she was nonetheless accurate.

> If he's vulnerable, I feel like getting revenge; belittle, make fun of, put down, and hate. I'm either a victim of contempt or I'm

dishing it out. It's unacceptable to experience it. This week has been about my contempt. I'm in a rage about a lack of unconditional love. I want my husband to support me, not be tight and chintzy. I'm enraged that he won't take care of me.

Unable to stay with her rage, (because this authentic expression of feeling made her vulnerable to attack), she squelched herself and observed in a self-critical tone, "My marriage is about having someone take care of me." It was clear to me that her negative attitude toward her dependency needs was getting in the way of her understanding herself (in fact, she was acting out an identification with the harsh attacking object, this time turning on herself instead of her husband). Rather than interpreting this (as it was not so clear to me at the time), I asked a question: "How are you thinking about your wish to be taken care of?" She responded emphatically, "Contemptuous! As a child I didn't have a right to be cared for. I couldn't ask for things from my father. He would be contemptuous." Her eyes filling with tears, she described a young and vulnerable self: "Not asking, not intruding, waiting for him to notice me and to want to be with me. My dad didn't like my sister's demands. He characterized her as fat, greedy, and intrusive. I'd do anything not to see that look in his eye. When I was *happy*, he'd give me that look. It felt *so* awful."

Humiliated for her childish displays and frustrated in her attempts to obtain legitimate narcissistic supplies, Ms. M. described a childhood memory that illustrated her fusion defense and its purpose: the creation of a false self to protect the authentic self from injury by and disappointment in significant others. She continued to elaborate on the operational techniques of mirroring and idealizing. "With Dad, my highest pleasure was to give him pleasure by performing well and looking good, but his approval was very conditional. My father looked at people in terms of their use." Acknowledging her identification with her father, she concluded: "And I've done that with my husband. Doing it makes you an object among other objects." "Why," I asked her, "do you think you've done that?" After careful consideration, she replied, "To say what I want means confronting him with my disagreement and risking his contempt. If I were to say, 'I want you to have compassion', I am vulnerable to contempt." Demonstrating the depth of her integration, she went on to identify her splitting operations: "At least I know enough not to act out that contempt. I've had a problem with putting people on pedestals, but I don't want them on a dung heap either."

I think it is important to review what has occurred in this patient's treatment that has allowed for this progress. There has been put into place a clear therapeutic alliance, an agreement between patient and therapist to control the acting out of the false defensive self through self-suppression and fusion. It is also understood by both parties that the purpose of this defensive structure is to manage the patient's narcissistic vulnerability and sensitivity. By asserting herself with her husband on behalf of her son, Ms. M. had relinquished her defensive stance, interrupted her fusion defense, and activated her real, separate self. I think this turn of events can best be understood in terms of the disorders-of-the-self triad. Self-activation (asserting her desire to have her son stay) or injury (her husband's look of rejection) stimulates feelings of narcissistic vulnerability and affects of the abandonment depression (in this case, rage), which leads to defense, contemptuous devaluation. Instead of fusion, the patient had identified with and acted out the contemptuous object, thus ridding the self of, or externalizing, bad feelings. (In other words, it is not that she is sensitive to injury, but that others are mistreating her.) Once this was out on the table, the patient could control two major defensive operations of the aggressive unit—namely, externalization and acting out an identification with the harsh attacking object (that is, attacking those who threatened her). Now another operation took center stage: the internalization of the harsh attacking object, and the ways in which she silenced, neglected, devalued, and injured herself.

In the next session, Ms. M. brought up the fact that she had become uncomfortable with the way in which she had limited herself in her career. She observed, "I'm not really making a living. My business is a gesture at work." Standing up for herself with her husband meant a lot to her; it was ego strengthening and served to contradict her sense of self as inadequate, insufficient, and unable to support herself were she to be disagreed with, to assert herself if infringed on, and to soothe herself if injured. She began to consider the possibility that she had the strength to take on a larger world. As she put it, "My boundary has enlarged." This awareness was followed by action, which she reported in the next session.

She began the next session with the following announcement: "I've been confronting the idea of working for someone else, and my reactions to others' opinions." Ms. M. had lunched with her former mentor. They had met at his place of business. "It triggered a lot," she explained.

> My feelings were triggered when he happened to refer to one programmer as 'one of my best employees.' I felt a huge desire to be what he wants and work myself into the ground to please him. It was revealing and uncomfortable. [What she was de-

scribing was her impulse to present a perfect false self in order to ward off painful affects.] I have a desire to work in a business setting, but it is combined with fear and anxiety. I'm at the mercy of the approval of those in authority, those I need or want something from. It's clear I've been unwilling to confront it for the last 30 years. It's the key to my lack of career involvement. This anxiety about wanting approval, wanting to be the best. It's what I wanted from Dad. I wanted approval. It's hard to look at. In college, I wasn't the best and I was *terrified*. In fact, I had a breakdown. It was inconceivable to me to present myself to my parents as less than perfect, or perfectly happy. My mother called me twice a day for the perfect report. I wonder if other consultants are *terrified* each day before they begin, and whether they ever talk about it. I'm so *ashamed*. It's like a big secret.

What is of note in this instance is that the patient used the session to identify and contain defenses so that she could explore and analyze (that is, work through) affects and experiences of the abandonment depression. The shame Ms. M. had identified as associated with her terror, her wish to keep it secret, and her longing for safety became subjects for exploration over the next several months. However, before this work could deepen and hold, Ms. M. had to become aware of the ways in which she attacked herself when she discovered undesirable thoughts, wishes, or feelings. This self-attack undermined her ability to trust her own perceptions and ideas. Just as she could not present an authentic self to her parents, she had great difficulty accepting her own spontaneous affects, strivings, and ideas. This process came to her attention in a vivid dream that followed the session just described.

I was surrounded by figures in black robes, higher beings. I was trying to please them. There was a Buddha-like figurine, dark green. It was a treasure. I locked it in a cabinet like your desk. Everything was beautiful. The other beings directed me. I put the treasure into a safe. I knew I was disconnected from the truth about what the treasure really was. The "safe" wasn't safe or right. It wasn't a treasure. It was an object. Its real value and beauty were locked away. And the robed beings—they were fear and control. It was a complete lie.

In her next session, she continued to identify and explore her difficulty reporting the truth about her thoughts and feelings. She reviewed her memory of her mother's calling twice a day and the requirement she felt to issue a positive report, to please her mother, to make her feel good, and to show her only the inert and beautiful figurine.

> The report has to be wonderful. You can't be vulnerable. You only report triumphs. That makes me furious. I want to tell her to stop manipulating me. Accept me like I am. Quit meddling. I feel like I must stop meddling with myself, and develop a way to look at my reactions without judgments. I crush a part of myself, the part she wanted to crush.

Next she told me a story about her father, as told to her by her sister, a story that she had told me many times before. It was a story revealing her father as harsh and attacking, a story that she knew to be true but could not accept as true, that she did not want to accept as true because it meant giving up on her idealized object and the comforting belief that she was safe in the hands of robed and higher beings. Her pain was obvious as she struggled to relinquish her denial. "How," she asked, "could this man I worshiped do something wrong?" It has become clear to me again in writing this how difficult it is to face the raw and unadorned truth of a child's powerlessness and vulnerability in the face of harshness and insensitivity from those the child needs and loves. As she stated, a few weeks later, "It's hard for me to see it, taking in what my family was. I'm reluctant to say my mother didn't meet my needs, was controlling, life killing. I've looked at it that there is something wrong with my reactions, which are from the past. I can't accept that someone would treat me that way. It must be my fault."

Having gained observing distance from her tendencies to attack and squelch herself, Ms. M. experienced a painful identity crisis. As she explained, "What I assumed was the right thing to do; isn't." Crying, she admitted, "I feel like I'm suppressing myself. It's put my view of acting naturally in a new light. I feel awkward. Like I'm giving up some liveliness to examine this." Committed to self-expression, she began to speak up for herself at home, at work, and with her friends. Often this yielded positive results with her husband. At other times, her speaking up resulted in disappointment or injury. When that occurred, she was able to contain and explore her feelings. Her outside life straightened out, but her emotional world was in turmoil. Because she was both activating herself and containing defenses, there was no place for her to go but deeper into an exploration of her fragmented self and a working through of the affects of the abandonment depression.

Working Through

Upon returning from vacation, she reported that she had lost herself. "Just being with people was scary. I couldn't define myself, say what my limits were." Crying, she recalled her fear. "There were no boundaries, no rules, no way to protect myself. I felt out of control. There is no way to be; no way you are supposed to be. It feels dangerous to me to just be." Affects of the abandonment depression surfaced. Rather than attacking herself, she was able to identify and pursue them in session. "I noticed my irritability with my husband." (Instead of focusing on what her husband did to make her angry, the patient used her irritation as a springboard into herself and her associations.)

> All I wanted to do was get away from him. It reminds me of wanting to get away from my mother. That's what my father and I did. We were cohorts escaping from her. It was freeing, full of pleasure, the two of us, going off together. To be with my mother was like being in a viselike grip. I couldn't live; I couldn't breathe. To be with her was the end of pleasure.

Here the patient stopped, reflected, and reported:

> Suddenly my view of him has shifted from seeing him as an all-powerful, perfect person who would take care of me, to a weak man. I was resentful of his weakness. I'm remembering a scene with my mother turning on the two of us, complaining that we were ganging up on her, making her wrong. We did. We looked down on her together. We got back at her.

Shifting back to the present, she observed, "I also have a desire to get back at my husband, but I'm not supposed to break out with my anger. I judge myself, I feel guilty about my reactions." Tracking the origin of her guilt, she turned back again to the past, "There was no exit. I couldn't feel angry, or bad, or that I was wrong. My mom was the one who got to be angry. I endured it. It was wounding. Waiting for it to be over. I want my mother to say 'Yes! I was a terrible mother.'" This expression of aggression toward her mother caused guilt, and the patient defended with self-attack. Now, however, she tracked herself, labeled the attack, and investigated its origins.

> A tape just kicked in. "This is stupid and unimportant. It's not
> such a big deal. Enough of this superficial wallowing!" To pay at-
> tention to this part of myself is more than I can handle. I should
> be silent, obedient, fearful. It's 1984. I'm a cog. I've agreed. The
> habits of that agreement are powerful. It takes all the strength I
> have to speak up for myself.

This very powerful session was followed by physical breakdown. The patient developed a skin infection on her torso. Her back pain increased and
she reported feelings of exhaustion and panic. Her physical complaints mirrored her internal work, the horrifying realization that "the bubble of safety
Dad and I created was a myth." She tracked her fear and panic back to her
childhood experience of being with her mother.

> There is something I want to remember about her yelling and
> screaming. I was four or six. We were in the breakfast room. There
> was no one to protect me. I'm backed into the corner and she's
> screaming. He came home. I see the door opening. He comes in
> and tells my mom that he could hear her screaming down the
> block. Then he smiled. I was terrified. He wasn't going to pro-
> tect me. He wasn't going to stop her. Only his being there would
> make it stop. What did I do? I can't remember what I did that
> was so bad.

She then began to freely associate: to a parent of her student and that
mother's harshness; to her own daughter, L., and how, at the age of four or
five L. had stood up for herself when Ms. M. had become angry; to a woman
in the grocery store who stopped her when she lost her temper with L.
"That woman stopped me. Nobody stopped Mom. I was terrified into a
corner. No matter what you do, she won't shut up. I'm cowering in a corner. When the pain stops, I'm doing it right, except not really. I don't know
how to do it right. The pain comes when I don't expect it. I have no sense
that my actions have any consequences. I'm powerless in an evil, torturing
environment where some insane being torments me. Really, really, really."
She cries, and holds up her hands, "Go away, go away."

There were two more sessions to follow, and I found them particularly
important as they demonstrated the meaning of the phrase "self-soothing,"
and the place it has in this work. The ability to turn inward to manage
painful affects is a prerequisite for sustaining working through, as illustrated
in these two sessions.

For the third time in the course of her treatment, following the session just reviewed, Ms. M. reported that she had awakened from a nightmare in a panic, unable to breathe, feeling as though there were someone who did not want her to live. She was terrified and concluded that she must face this or she could not be with people. While this last statement sounded as if it were the expression of her reality ego, in fact, it was an expression of her grandiose false defensive self. Her idea about "facing this," she went on to explain, was to "fix it, rid myself of this sensitivity, this fragility, this terror, and get back to sleep." But instead of trying to squelch herself, in the dark of the night she discovered another option. She found her way to self-acceptance and compassion:

> I told myself, yes, I am tense, intense, sensitive, easily triggered. O.K., I can accept that. I don't have to push it away and be perfect. At my core is terror and fear. I'd like it to be otherwise. I've tried to change it, but now I'm just in it. I can't remember exactly what happened, a specific incident or event to make me feel this way, but when I sit with clients and listen to my thoughts about their judgments of me I know what was done to me.

She paused and then went on with her report of the night before.

> I felt this big wave of relaxation and then I realized that I could get some tea, do some meditation, and then go back to bed. I did this and I had a wonderful experience of rest. So different from every noise-making, every nerve-ending scream. There was a sense of floating rest and relaxation. I have it so little. Never before have I had a sense of my creating it.

Retrospectively, it seems to me that this represented a defining moment in her recovery. By locating resources within herself, Ms. M. had recognized that she possessed a capacity for self-soothing. Knowing that she could turn within, permitted her further to relinquish the false defensive self. Moreover, the ability to self-soothe contradicted her fragmented self representation and fortified the ego's capacity for containment and the working through of the painful memories that were to come.

In the next session, she picked up where she had left off. "In my face since last night is sadness. I'm not going to fit the pictures anyone has of competence, happiness that in the past I've enacted. Every enlightenment course has added to the pile of how I should be. I thought it would protect me, change me, keep me from having to go back to the beginning to say, 'I'm scared and I can't handle things.' I want to defend my perfect picture of my family with: 'I'm too sensitive; it's my fault.' " Instead of silencing herself, Ms. M. supported herself and spoke out. "Mom, I'm sorry I have to do this to you, I know I'm disappointing and betraying you." Here she stopped to gather up her courage. "I can't believe how much the petty, impatient putdowns and manipulation really hurt me." She stopped and identified a critical voice. "You did it to yourself. You shouldn't blame others. Take responsibility." Answering that voice, she stated her case; "Yes I gave up, succumbed, cowered, but I'm tired of seeing myself as a victim of that environment. It's helpful to know when someone looks at me wrong, where my sensitivity comes from. You damaged me. I can't prove it, but it happened. You scared the shit out of me. You ground me down. You hurt me. I'm standing up to her. I've never said it. I've danced around it. For the first time I'm saying it from a place that doesn't require her agreement. You damaged me. You were abusive and I was hurt. I've bent over backwards, giving others the benefit of the doubt. I've misunderstood self-defense as resentful attack back. I have no right to say, 'You hurt me,' but I'm clear she did."

This last piece of work represents the beginnings of a full sense of self. Ms. M. makes a beautiful distinction when she delineates "resentful attack back" from "self-defense." To truly defend her self required her to own and expose the content and passion of her beliefs: her reality, her perceptions, her feelings, her unique experience of her childhood "without," as she states, "requiring agreement."

CONCLUSION

Ms. M. had come to treatment in search of some missing parts of herself. Like Dorothy in *The Wizard of Oz*, she wanted to find her way home. Like Dorothy, she was certain that her solution lay outside herself. She undertook a dangerous journey to the Great Wizard of Oz, believing he possessed the power and the knowledge that she lacked. Along the way she encountered and embraced missing parts of herself: a Cowardly Lion who could not stand up for himself; a dithering Scarecrow without a brain; a Tin Man with no heart. During the journey, she faced many challenges: intense fear, drugged sleep, and finally, after reaching Oz, an impossible assignment—to kill the Wicked Witch and take her broom to the Wizard. The child Dorothy gave up. The impaired adults were required to take over. The Tin

Man hadn't the heart to abandon this child in her hour of need. Hopelessness yielded to resolve. Scarecrow made the plan. When fear threatened to swamp the venture, the Cowardly Lion found his courage and faced down the screaming monkeys. Ultimately, of course, it was Dorothy who picked up the bucket of water and in her anger threw it on the Witch, melting her. And the Wizard really was no wizard at all, just another traveler trying to make a living until he could find a way home. And so he did, leaving poor Dorothy behind. Poor Dorothy? No, indeed. The Good Witch Glinda arrived to inform her that she had the power that she had needed all along. "Close your eyes . . . click your heels together three times . . . and think to yourself . . . there's no place like . . ." Well, why didn't she say so in the first place?!

REFERENCE

Masterson, J. F. (1981). *The narcissistic and borderline disorders*. New York: Brunner/Mazel.

CHAPTER 15

Mirrors of Rage: The Devaluing Narcissistic Patient

Judith Pearson, Ph.D.

Nothing impresses us more strongly in connection with the
resistance encountered in analysis than the feeling that there is a force at
work which is defending itself by all possible means against recovery
and is clinging tenaciously to illness and suffering.

Sigmund Freud

. . . which way shall I fly
Infinite wrath, and infinite despair?
Which way I fly is hell; myself am hell . . .
Milton, Paradise Lost

In his 1937 paper "Analysis, Terminable and Interminable," Freud's lexicon of therapeutic resistances expanded to include the "negative therapeutic reaction"—a term used to delineate the destructive treatment implications of a patient's intractable attachment to his or her neurotic symptoms. Freud theorized that this psychoanalytic phenomenon was a result of two factors: moral masochism, defined as the patient's unconscious sense of guilt and concomitant need for punishment; and the primacy of the death instinct as exhibited in the repetition compulsion.

Psychotherapy based on a developmental self and object relations approach rests on principles different from those stated by Freud's instinct theory; nonetheless, a patient's unwillingness to relinquish repetitive acting out of maladaptive patterns presents the therapist with a challenge as daunting as that which Freud confronted half a century ago.

This chapter explores the negative therapeutic impasse posed by a patient's reliance on devaluation as a central narcissistic defense. In order, however, to clarify more fully the dynamic underpinnings of the devaluing defense, it is useful to review some general principles applicable to the psychopathology and treatment of the narcissistic disorder of the self.

As explicated by Masterson (1981), the intrapsychic structure of the narcissistic disorder consists of two fused object relations part units that are held separate by the defense of splitting: the grandiose self/omnipotent object part unit, which contains all power and perfection and maintains the sense of being special, unique, and adored; and the empty self/aggressive-object part unit, consisting of an object representation that is attacking, unloving, and punitive, and a self representation that is small, empty, and humiliated. The empty/aggressive unit is characterized by the affect of the abandonment depression (pp. 14–16).

The etiology of the narcissistic disorder lies in a parent–child interaction whereby the child becomes burdened with the bargain of performing idealizing or mirroring functions for the parent in return for being seen as lovable or special. Real-self goals are sacrificed to the parents' narcissistic needs, while false-self grandiosity, hungry for constant mirroring and idealizing supplies, provides defensive restitution for the painful injuries of the attacked and empty self. In the interpersonal sphere, the parents' continuous reinforcement of the child's unmodulated grandiosity supports the fantasy of fusion, which gets carried into all future relationships.

The disparity between the narcissistic patient's grandiose false self and impaired real self is well illustrated by a dream presented by a young male patient whose financial successes were as indisputable as his relational failures. In the dream, he was having some renovation done on his yacht (a prized possession imbued with great narcissistic investment). As a part of this project, the beautiful hardwood floors, with their mirrorlike polished surfaces, were lifted, revealing a rotting, dirty, unsupported infrastructure. The patient was discomfited by the dream. "That's me." He said. "That's what I'm afraid is inside. And truthfully, I never want to find that place, because even if I could get to it, which I doubt, I'm not sure I could ever recover."

That commentary serves to point out the narcissistic patient's powerful drive to preserve the defenses that guard against the painful affects associated with the impaired self. Success in the endeavor necessarily requires the warding off of any circumstance that interrupts the continuous global activation of the false-self grandiose unit. In general, such ruptures are occasioned by attempts to pursue realistic as opposed to narcissistic goals, or by perceived empathic failures on the part of objects in the patient's world. When these circumstances arise, harsh aggression is often unleashed onto the offending object in the form of rage and devaluation. For example, one patient, an exhibitionist narcissist, came in for her third or fourth session and said chummily: "Well, now that we've gotten to know each other a little better, what do people call you?" When I replied, "Dr. Pearson," she looked startled, then angry, and then responded, "Well, you can call me Mary, Queen of Scots."

A second patient, a closet narcissist fairly far along in the course of treatment, gave equal, if gentler, testimony to the use of narcissistic devaluation as a defense by musing with surprise: "You know, I think I deny the power of other people by dismissing them. Sometimes my so-called superiority is just a way of covering my vulnerability. Underneath, I feel like a piece of crystal that could be shattered into all those little fragments."

As can be seen, the psychotherapeutic arena shows most narcissistic patients primarily demonstrating transference acting out of early idealizing or mirroring patterns. Projection of the empty/aggressive unit takes a secondary role, appearing only on occasions of perceived empathic failure by the therapist. The patient's defensive responses can then be interpreted by linking them to the impaired self's exquisite sensitivity to and fear of attack. This therapeutic strategy, appropriately designated a mirroring interpretation of narcissistic vulnerability (Masterson, 1993, pp. 76–79), serves the dual purposes of supporting the real self by acknowledging the pain and disappointment that it has suffered, while addressing the destructive defenses employed by the patient each time a narcissistic injury is encountered. Thus a normally obliging and reasonable patient began to discuss an incident in a restaurant where he was well known, but where a new rule forbade the acceptance of personal checks in payment of the bill. The patient flew into a rage at the waiter's refusal to accept his check. In reviewing the event, the patient acknowledged the source of his anger, noting how the waiter's refusal threatened the terms of his internal "bargain" with his parents: "I guess somewhere I felt I had a right to expect a particular kind of treatment. I was special. Because I was a good customer, the rules should not have applied to me, so I felt his refusal as a rejection." The patient's discussion of this incident led him to recall his anger at me when I charged him for a session that he had had to cancel because of an unavoidable out-of-town business meeting. At that time, his feeling was one of "being punished" for something that was not his fault. He truculently agreed to pay, but indicated that my behavior was unduly rigid. Predictably, when the time came to pay, he "forgot" his check. In reviewing these events, the patient summarized: "I guess when someone treats me as ordinary it makes me feel small and unrecognized—annihilated, the way my mother's coldness made me feel."

As treatment progresses, the constant working through of such nontraumatic disappointments will allow for the creation of new internalized structures. Reliance on early maladaptive defenses gradually diminishes to be replaced by real-self activation as the abandonment depression is worked through. An adolescent girl facing the loss of her internal idealized father illustrates this process when she comments tearfully: "I guess I just made him up as supportive. He was never really involved at all. Now I not only have to deal with my conflicts, but I also feel like my father inside is dying."

Despite differences in overall therapeutic capacity, all of these patients were sufficiently intact to more or less consistently demonstrate the transference acting out of idealizing or mirroring patterns of attachment based on the projection of the grandiose-self/omnipotent-object unit.

In some patients, however, both core self structure and ego defenses are so primitive and fragile as to preclude the therapeutic mobilization of idealizing or mirroring patterns. The pervasive need to defend against internalized persecutory objects leads to reliance on rigid, pathological defenses that serve the purpose of projecting and denying intolerable feelings. The ability to sustain activity in the external world, which ensures the more successful narcissist some measure of supplies is, in these less capable patients, limited or damaged, as observing ego and tolerance for delay or disappointment are easily breached, replaced by poor impulse control and a failure to tolerate and master anxiety.

In treatment, the patient demonstrates a predominance of paranoid trends, which infiltrate the therapy and create massive obstacles to the patient's capacity to form a working alliance. Internalized representations of parental intrusion, abuse, and devaluation lend strength to these projections. Further, all objects become imbued with shades of the patient's own unresolved oral aggression, as shown by one patient, who uneasily stated: "I hate the light in here; sometimes it makes you look like a vampire."

In the fight to ward off these dangerous and engulfing imagos, splitting remains a major weapon, as the patient clings tenaciously to the fantasy of fusion with the magic "all good" object, while avoiding any real dependency that could result in annihilating humiliation or persecution. Thus the therapist, or any object, is held to the measure of the internalized ideal, who is seen to contain all elements of beauty and power, while being totally dedicated to meeting the patient's narcisstic needs. Even small failures to meet this fusion fantasy will precipitate fears of persecution and attack, triggering concomitant rage. In relationships, and in the patient's transference acting out, these internalized patterns become manifest in ruthless infantile needs to possess and dominate the object while destroying or devaluing any evidence of its independent existence.

More simply put, these patients, who experience virtually continuous rupture of the grandiose defense, must rely instead on defensive projection of the aggressive part unit. As Yeats declared, "The center cannot hold, and . . . anarchy is loosed upon the world."

CASE ILLUSTRATIONS

Case of Mr. D.

The dynamics addressed are exemplified by the case of Mr. D., a 31-year-old man referred to the Masterson Institute following his involvement in a street fight. Mr. D.'s initial presentation was one of intense, fragmented anxiety and emotional lability covered by a veneer of superficial charm and glib intellectual formulations. He was thin, unshaven, and scruffy, and looked more than a little wild.

Mr. D.'s early history was stormy and chaotic. His memories included instances of abuse by his narcissistic, temper-ridden father; neglect by his sometimes Valium-addicted mother; and a clear recollection of bearing witness to a favorite aunt's suicide attempt. Mr. D. also spoke of his earliest memory, seemingly less traumatic, but equally telling. At about the age of two, he recalled needing his mother to help him toilet himself. Unable to find her, he deposited his feces in a plastic bag, which he then proudly saved for her to see and admire. She instead became angry and shaming, and gave Mr. D. a hard spanking. This memory is one I hold onto in the treatment, often thinking as he comes in flaunting some piece of entitled and irrational grandiosity, "It's that stuff in a bag again!"

Despite his history of neglect and abuse, Mr. D. early on was given the feeling that he was special. Bright, attractive, and the oldest boy, he was designated as the child destined to succeed. Unable to hold his own in a school or work setting, Mr. D. defended against his feelings of depression and humiliation by judging himself superior to those mundane contexts. He saw himself as unique, a martyred, Christ-like figure, gifted with rare sensitivity and great artistic talent. His mission, he believed, was to give the gift of his wisdom to the world through his art.

Mr. D.'s vision of himself, however, was constantly under siege. His capacity for self-supporting work was limited, and his narcissistic sensitivity and paranoid projections left him with the task of continuously fending off feelings of being misunderstood and attacked. His response, quick-trigger rage and devaluation, led to trouble, even in his art classes, where his acting out ultimately defeated the expression of his appreciable artistic talent. Thus Mr. D.'s acute sensitivity and consequent lashing out cost him the regard of several mentors who might have been sources of healthy narcissistic supplies. In response to these ruptures, Mr. D. resorted to soothing himself with spending sprees, pornography, and drug and alcohol abuse.

Mr. D.'s course of treatment has been shaky. When he first began to see me, he was living with his parents in their cramped New York apartment. His daily activity consisted of wandering aimlessly around the city and stopping at museums or sitting in coffee shops. He was angry, depressed, and paranoid, and talked about his fury when people in the streets "jostled him on purpose" and tried to "push him around." Often these incidents were marked by verbal quarrels. Occasionally, they ended in physical fights.

In session, Mr. D. had trouble keeping his thoughts together, and would spill enormous obsessive sentences into the room, which seemed directed at keeping a watch on his crumbling self. Despairing statements that he used to have something special but now could not find it and that he was afraid that "what happened to him" had taken it away from him forever would alternate with rageful accusations against "assholes" who could not understand someone with his purity and sensitivity. Often, I was one of those assholes.

Sometimes Mr. D.'s preoccupations would center around his ambivalence toward coffee, an ambivalence I saw as indicative of his need for and fear of any self-regulating object. "Coffee takes me away from myself," he would say. "I never know what's me and what's the coffee, and it keeps me from having a through line to my center." But then he would add: "I really need that pickup. It gives me energy, and helps me feel alive."

During the initial phase of Mr. D.'s treatment, almost everything he did was as an attempt to ward off his massive experiences of emptiness and anxiety. He drank to excess, sitting in bars to late at night and talking to various women, from whom he would extract statements of admiration, while denigrating them as vain and shallow whores who only wanted to "talk about themselves" and "get laid."

As treatment progressed, it became clear that Mr. D. was masking his own sexual insecurities with a layer of holier-than-thou righteousness. "People just use sex like masturbation," he would say, "but I'm different. The

mere physical thing is not important." At the same time that he was running for the moral high ground, however, Mr. D. was masturbating excessively and expensively through the use of telephone sex.

In my initial work with Mr. D., I was faced with a dilemma. I knew therapeutic work could not proceed as long as he had no structure in his life,
and he was still dependent on his parents. It was also clear that he was engaging in enormous self-destructive acting out of a kind that ordinarily
would merit unremitting confrontation. At the same time, it was obvious
that Mr. D.'s fragile sense of self, combined with his propensity for paranoid projection, would make confrontation difficult, if not impossible. In
the final analysis, however, it seemed clear that allowing Mr. D. to continue
in his untrammeled fashion would leave me in the position of being a therapeutic eunuch, and leave him where he had always been—with an unconcerned, uninvolved parental figure who allowed his rage and grandiosity to run wild. I decided to use mirroring interpretations where I could,
and confront when I must, with the caveat that my confrontations would
also affirm his vision of himself as an artist.

Mr. D.'s initial responses to my interventions were as might be expected.
When I addressed his street fighting, he would turn vice into virtue, stating: "I don't care what you think. I stand up for myself and for what's right.
I confront people when they shit on me or on anyone. You probably would
have sat by and let the Holocaust happen." At various times, he accused
me of being shallow, of being a therapist only for the money, of trying to
convert him to my bourgeois way of living.

In my turn, I asked him if he did not think that it was a waste for someone with a genuine talent to be spilling his energy into the telephone lines
and the street. He said he was smarter than I was. I said he was smart, but
not smarter, and asked why a smart guy who wanted to communicate
through his art settled for communicating with his fists in a way that had
once before, and might again, get him into serious trouble and stop his career.

I commented on his oft-stated wish to find his center and his "real" feelings, and asked how he expected to accomplish that task when he was discharging his feelings every minute, could not keep his voice modulated,
and would not even sit in his chair. At the same time as I confronted Mr.
D., I also interpreted his extreme sensitivity, comparing his responses in
the street and in session to those of veterans who get back from the war
and start shooting when a car backfires. I stressed his vulnerability—a trait
Mr. D. integrated as part of his pure and sensitive artistic temperament.

Mr. D. slowly responded, finally coming in one day and saying "You know, it's true what you say about my feelings. I can't stand being criticized. I guess it reminds me of how my father used to put me down, and my mother would yell at me for everything." Within a year, Mr. D. had moved out of his parents' house, begun an art class, and found some rather unsteady work as a waiter.

A second year has passed since those events, and Mr. D. is far from better. Nonetheless, slow but positive outcomes are accruing from the treatment. In sessions, I still confront when Mr. D. acts out, but as his acting out has lessened, my role has increasingly shifted to one of being a mirroring object. Mr. D. comes in and talks, and I listen. He is clear that there are times when my saying *anything* distracts him from himself, and despite the fact that I find myself feeling deanimated and controlled, I know that he is right, that my presence threatens his fragile narcissistic balance and sets in motion the train of vulnerability and paranoid projection that leads to his explosions of narcissistic rage and devaluation. So when I can, I stay silent.

In accord with his internal fusion fantasy, Mr. D. receives my silence as support, but his use of me as a mirroring object now also includes requests for more direct acknowledgment, as he brings me copies of pictures he has drawn or of stories he has written. At those times, Mr. D. will comment on how vulnerable he feels showing me his productions. I, in turn, feel much like a mother of a very young child being handed a creation that demands admiration. On one such occasion, Mr. D. came in describing a successful period of painting. I listened, nodding affirmation at Mr. D.'s reports of his success. The end of the session surprised Mr. D., who looked wistful and stated: "I waited all week to tell you this, and now I don't want to leave." He paused briefly, put his jacket on, along with his defense, and said with a mischievous grin, "You don't do overnights do you?"

Mr. D.'s case clearly illustrates the way in which the shattered grandiose defense gives way to the continuous projection of the aggressive unit as a means of shielding a fragile and beleaguered self. Through it all, however, Mr. D. has clung fiercely to his narcissistic vision of himself, holding to his only, albeit shaky and distorted, source of self-esteem and self-activation. Thus far, the goal of the treatment has been to allow him to reconsolidate that vision, while doing the ego repair necessary to facilitate restructuring of his maladaptive defenses. Mr. D. has shown some capacity to utilize the treatment to help him in this work of self-repair. What has helped me in my work has been the fact that Mr. D.'s rage and devaluation were matched by his longing for an object on whom to project his mirroring and idealizing needs. This tendency was evident both in his relationships with his mentors and in his prior love affairs. It also became manifest in the treatment, where it can serve useful therapeutic aims.

Case of Ms. F.

In the case of Ms. F., different, and in some ways more difficult, facets of the devaluing defense become evident. It was her resistance that, at one point, prompted me to consider abandoning Freud's concept of "negative therapeutic reaction," to replace it with the more contemporary notion of transference acting out from hell.

Ms. F., a slim, raven-haired, perfectly groomed woman in her early 50s, carries herself with the stiff, rigid posture of someone constantly enjoined to stand up straight. Her presenting complaints included depression, intense and pervasive anxiety, and a sense of emptiness and meaninglessness in life. She came into treatment following the breakup of her 10-year marriage to a successful Wall Street financial analyst who fled across the country to a younger woman, complaining that he could no longer tolerate "living with Leona Helmsley."

Unlike Mr. D., Ms. F.'s history was one of being a pampered youngest child of wealthy doting parents who idealized their children and gave them lavish gifts and praise, but expected beauty, brilliance, and success in return. The death of an older, much admired sister caused Ms. F.'s mother to close even tighter ranks with her youngest daughter. Time, former treatments, and a succession of disappointments had taught Ms. F. that the world will not match her parents' indulgence. But the recognition has been a hard pill to swallow, and one laced with bitterness. In consequence, Ms. F. still shows a stubborn refusal to substitute realistic goals for her lost Eden. Having had her narcissistic dream shattered, she has made it her mission to reject all dreams as not worth having. Devaluation has been elevated from the status of occasional desperate defense to a way of life that not only affords her protection from future disappointments, but also grants her immense gratification through the discharge of aggression.

In Mr. D.'s case, mirroring objects, when they mirrored, stilled the pangs of narcissistic hunger. For Ms. F., burdened with the memory of a dead sister who aroused both love and envy, the situation was more complex, taking on a resemblance to Marc Antony's plight with Cleopatra, who, he claimed, "made hungry where most she satisfied." Ms. F.'s resolution of the dilemma was to attack and denigrate that which she desired, and, therefore, envied. Her transference acting out consequently reflected not only narcissistic fears, but also narcissistic entitlement, envy, and talionic rage.

As treatment progressed, the exploitive, controlling underside of Ms. F.'s doting parents became increasingly apparent. Listening to Ms. F. talk about her mother would often lead me to the thought that the mother had to have been invented by a conspiracy led by the combined forces of Woody Allen and Emily Post. Unable to relinquish her own needs for fusion with her daughter, Mom could not resist any opportunity to "help" Ms. F. "better herself" by correcting every aspect of her behavior and her physical appearance. These intrusions remain internalized in the form of constant preoccupations about her weight and minor skin flaws. At this point in her life, those concerns have been heightened by the inevitable marks of advancing age, so that Ms. F. spends a great deal of time poring over the latest magazines in search of miracle potions designed to restore fading youth.

Her father, idealized by Ms. F. as rational and powerful, could more accurately be termed demanding and domineering. Willing to buy his children out of any scrapes, he exacted the price of total control over their lives, and Ms. F. vividly remembered how Dad's attacks on a former fiancé ultimately resulted in the breakup of the engagement.

In her treatment, Ms. F.'s behavior constitutes an extension of what Masterson (1981) has called a "sitdown strike" (pp. 54–63), which in her case was manifest by disdainful repudiation of all current activities or future possibilities. I, of course, was not exempt from her contemptuous outlook. A perfect mirror of her mother's censorious attitudes, she systematically dismantled every facet of my therapeutic persona, as her defensive attempts to avoid looking at her own vulnerabilities led her to focus on mine. I remember, for example, one summer session in which she played Hannibul Lecter to my Clarice, commenting: "Your outfit's O.K., but I don't know how you can wear such ugly shoes."

As with Mr. D., I both mirrored Ms. F.'s vulnerability and confronted her acting out. When I mirrored, she would reply with such comments as: "I know everything you're saying, but so what? It's too late to do anything about it." Confrontations met with a similar fate. When, for example, I confronted her raising her voice in a session, she replied: "Obviously, if you hadn't said something ridiculous, I wouldn't have had to behave that way." At times when I smiled, she accused me of being condescending. At times when I did not smile, she said that I was cold and removed.

Driving home from sessions, I found myself feeling, at best, small, angry, humiliated, and hopeless, and, at worst, sadistically tortured and deliberately being driven crazy. Slowly, through my massive countertransference haze, the idea emerged that Ms. F.'s behavior was a way to let me know how hard and painful life had been for her. By projecting her small, flawed self onto me, while enacting the role of her unremittingly critical mother, she not only was repeating in behavior what she could neither fully remember nor verbalize (Freud, 1953, pp. 366–376.), but was also communicating feelings that some part of her wanted to be heard and understood.

I began to interpret this piece of projective identification, indicating that it seemed to me that her behavior toward me was in part a way to help me understand how she felt having to respond to the continually impossible and inconsistent standards that were set for her. She acknowledged that this was so, admitting finally that when all was said and done, the only source of power she still had faith in was the power of her denigrating talionic rage. If living well was not to be the best revenge, then revenge itself would have to do—even at the price of her self-destruction.

Ms. F. is now ending her first year of treatment. Although she denies any change in herself as a result of therapy, changes are evident. These shifts have largely taken the form of reducing acting out in Ms. F.'s external life, thereby confining it to the therapeutic arena in the form of transference acting out. And change has begun even there.

In a recent discussion, when Ms. F. once again was pointing out that I was cold and "didn't understand her," I responded by noting that her extreme sensitivity led her to fend off almost any intervention I made. "You are so attuned to attack and intrusion that it is hard for you to hear any remark as something other than that," I said. "That leaves the door where I can enter without needing to be repelled like an invader a very small one indeed." Ms. F. nodded, adding quietly, "And the few times that you do get through, *I* hate you for succeeding—it makes me feel so small that I want to slam that door in your face so you'll hurt too."

In the process of working with Ms. F., I have learned a great deal. She has taught me something about technique, and even more about countertransference. And she has many times achieved her mission, leaving me so smarting from my own feelings of impotence and defect that I lose the focus on her.

The most severe reactions I have experienced occurred, predictably, when her accusations were on target, and these times have been more than enough. Slowly, however, I am learning to manage both her reactions and my own. Primarily, I think this change has come about because I have begun to relinquish my own grandiose wish to be the special therapist who can cure this patient of her unhappiness. Wittingly or not, Ms. F.'s insistent devaluation of virtually all my therapeutic efforts has left me little choice but to accept what I have so often told her—that the ultimate success of the treatment rests in her hands, and not in mine. Despite her voluble resistance, I can only believe that underneath it all, Ms. F.'s message to me, received in the form of my countertransferential response, is that this is the only resolution she *may* accept.

IN SUMMARY

These cases were presented in an attempt to illuminate some of the dynamics underlying the devaluing narcissistic patient's attempts to protect a vulnerable impaired self by discharging and projecting aggression associated with the internalized persecutory object and the hungry envious self. A review of some of those mechanisms shows the following.

1. Projection of the internalized harsh object and the rage associated with it. For these patients, the maxim holds: "The best defense is a good offense."
2. Repudiation or coopting of any independent source of help. This process defends against the twin threats of the separate existence of the object and the oral greed and envy of the self. Mr. D., as do many narcissistic patients, demonstrated this trait by initially rejecting an interpretation, only to come in with it three weeks later as his own idea.
3. Refusal to relinquish unconscious wishes for omnipotence and entitlement associated with the internalized fused grandiose-self/ omnipotent-object part-unit. Mr. D.'s grandiose fantasies are plainly apparent. In Ms. F.'s case, this principle was demonstrated not only by her stance of entitlement, but also by her bid for specialness through being the worst of the worst if she could not be the best of the best.
4. A vengeful talionic thwarting of the internalized object's narcissistic goals, the latter representing power through Pyrrhic victory as the one sure victory. In the case of Mr. D., his continued life failures served this end. As for Ms. F., her not-so-unconscious wish to deprive me of the narcissistic pleasure of her progress undoubtedly constituted one of the more significant impediments to her improvement.
5. Persistent reliance on projective identification as a means of coercing the therapist to resonate with and act out the projections. This means of communication offers the possibility for the thera-

pist to recognize, contain, and ultimately interpret the dynamics associated with these primitive internalized self and object relations.

Freud alerted us to the difficulties entailed in doing treatment with a patient whose pathology becomes manifest in grave and persistent resistances to the therapeutic process. A note of encouragement, however, may be gleaned from the paradox that in the cases reviewed here (as in most cases), it was often precisely the negative aspect of the patient's negative therapeutic reaction that became the most telling analytic informant.

REFERENCES

Freud, S. (1963). Analysis, terminable and interminable. In *Freud: Therapy and technique*, pp. 233–273. New York: Macmillan.

Freud, S. (1953). Further recommendations in the technique of psychoanalysis: Recollection, repetition, and working through. In *Collected papers*, vol. II, pp. 366–376. London: Hogarth Press.

Kernberg, O. (1975). *Borderline conditions and pathological narcissism*. New York: Science House.

Kohut, H. (1971). *The analysis of the self: A systematic approach to the psychoanalytic treatment of narcissistic personality disorders*. New York. International Universities Press.

Kohut, H. (1977). *The restoration of the self*. New York: International Universities Press.

Masterson, J. F. (1993). *The emerging self: A developmental, self and object relations approach to the treatment of the closet narcissistic disorder of the self*. New York: Brunner/Mazel.

Masterson, J. F. (1981). *The narcissistic and borderline disorders*. New York: Brunner/Mazel.

CHAPTER 16

Neutrality Under Attack: Devaluation in the Therapeutic Relationship

Bill Robbins, Ph.D.

To devalue is to diminish the worth of something, to attack, to criticize. Criticism can be a relatively constructive, objective investigation of merits and faults, as when we use our critical faculties to point out meanings or shortcomings in order to change. The function of devaluation, however, is to hurt or to annihilate. While criticism can be constructive, devaluation always has a dual function, that of weakening, hurting, or even annihilating the object while protecting the defensive false self.

Whereas persons with borderline and schizoid disorders of the self may use devaluation to manage intrapsychic conflict, the narcissist uses devaluation commonly as a principal defense.

One of the hallmarks of the disorders of the self is the use of projective identification and splitting. The aggressive component of the split object relations units differs in distinct diagnostic categories. With the borderline disorder it is withdrawing (WORU). With the schizoid disorder, it becomes a persecutor—sadistic object/self in exile (S/O:S in E). In the narcissistic disorder, it is seen as harsh and attacking (aggressive, empty). All of the disorders of the self convey an image of an aggressive unit that is punitive and coercive.

Devaluation in the therapeutic encounter is an exceedingly active form of projective identification, in which projections are verbally forced onto the therapist. Through the defense of projective identification, the patient externalizes and reverses self and object representations. The patient exchanges his or her own identity and takes on the role of the aggressive object representation, generally a parental image, and the therapist is forced into the role of the self representation, a childlike image. The patient now acts in the role of the threatening object and the therapist is forced into the role of the victimized self, to feel the now-disavowed worthlessness and fear. The patient has emptied these feelings onto the therapist, and can regain a fleeting feeling of psychic equilibrium. The devaluation has protected the patient from painful internal feelings.

Because it carries with it a manic excitement and a feeling of power, devaluation is ideally suited to protect the false self from fragmentation. The acting out of aggression helps to promote a mania, which fuels the engine of grandiosity and invulnerability. Devaluation can also function as a form of retaliation against the harsh object, externalized onto the therapist, who is experienced as the one who has inflicted the pain. It is a weapon to punish the therapist, and helps the patient to distance himself or herself from vulnerability and disappointment.

DIAGNOSTIC DIFFERENCES

Schizoid Disorder

Devaluation can be used quite differently by different character styles. For example, Mr. L., who has a schizoid disorder of the self, has a profound inability to love himself. Safety demands that he maintain an optimal distance, not too far, but definitely not too close—the schizoid compromise.

Mr. L. recently found himself the object of a woman's affection, the realization of a lifelong desire. But this experience conflicted with his sense of himself as being a troublesome burden in relationship. The intensity of his girlfriend's interest created a degree of intrapsychic conflict that had to be acted out to be relieved.

Mr. L. projected his own devalued feelings onto his new girlfriend so as not to contain them within himself. He described his conflict of the previous weekend: "I was drowning in affection and I felt she was not for me and I pulled back. It's such a problem to allow myself to be loved. I feel a bad taste now. When people are attracted to me, I feel there is something wrong with them. The more she expresses those feelings to me, the less favorably I see her and I feel that's not what I want." Mr. L. was devaluing his girlfriend to maintain his intrapsychic equilibrium through a safe interpersonal distance.

I used the vehicle of interpretation to point out what I thought Mr. L. was doing and why he might be doing it. Because of his sensitivity to intrusion, and the potential for my intervention to reenact his experiences of victimization, I prefaced my remarks with an explicit invitation to comment on and contribute to their accuracy. In response to what he told me, I outlined my understanding of the dilemma he faced in being loved. As his girlfriend got closer to him, it opened him to the inner fear of being controlled, even taken over, and those feelings were very threatening. I then wondered if, in order to manage himself and those feelings, he was putting onto his girlfriend alternating projections of the self ("something wrong") and of the object (a harsh, controlling master) so as to justify maintaining a safer distance between them.

I also wondered if, to protect himself from the damage of closeness, he was doing to her what he knew had been done to him—to see her in an unfavorable light and force her to pull back. In effect, I was helping him understand the specific purpose of his devaluations: to create a compromise distance that was not too close, but not too far.

Borderline Disorder

Ms. F., who had a borderline disorder of the self, was continually challenged when she dealt with self-activation. Activation of thoughts, feelings, or behavior led to anxiety and depression, which she managed by giving up her endeavor. At these times, she would often experience me as a critical evaluator, and she would act out her split self representation of being helpless and inadequate. Or she would own the intrapsychic turmoil but devalue herself ruthlessly as a liar, as stupid, and as spoiled. These maneuvers served to protect her from what were felt to be dangerous impulses, especially when they were self-affirming.

At such times, I would point out, in a more confrontative style, the disorder-of-the-self triad, and that her self-activation led to a very specific anxiety about being abandoned by the object, which then had to be immediately defended against—in this case, by undoing her self-activation with devaluative self-criticism. This helped her to recognize the full impact of the strategy she used to protect herself from her anxiety and her depression.

Although I had worked with her for a number of years, a subsequent interaction took place that startled me and brought to my attention how painful devaluation can be and how significant can be its consequences.

I announced to her that I would need to change her appointment time. She responded that it was opportune for her, because in another month she would be changing jobs and would need the time change herself. My schedule contained three open hours.

I offered her one of the free hours and she declined for what seemed a legitimate reason. I offered her a second option. She said that it would impose a great hardship. I then offered her the third of the free hours. She was pleased, and accepted the time. But then she added: "What's happening? Are all your clients deserting you?" I felt wounded, but it was at the end of the session and I distanced from the feeling, mistakenly thinking I had let it pass. But I had not let it pass. I wrote down the earlier choice of time that she had told me was unsuitable.

The next day, when a new patient called, I offered him the time Mrs. F. had chosen. By chance, Mrs. F. was a few moments late for her next appointment, and I, unaware that two patients had the same hour, ushered in the new patient. When Mrs. F. arrived, she waited for about 15 minutes and then left. At the end of the hour, I found a legitimately angry message on my answering machine. I had lost my therapeutic neutrality and had made an unsettling blunder that had to be repaired. I had responded to her devaluation by withdrawal, which led to denying her her own hour. It brought home to me my own vulnerability, and led me to take another look at the issue of devaluation.

If I had not acted out and retreated from therapeutic neutrality, I might have explored with her some of the dimensions of her remark. Was it possible that she was identifying with my being abandoned by my patients and, in fear that that could happen to her, was only asking for clarification? Or was she perhaps feeling guilty and frightened at getting her own needs met, and needed to attack me to handle her own anxiety? In either case, the devaluation seemed to be used to manage the fears associated with a potentially withdrawing and abandoning object.

NARCISSISTIC DISORDER AND THERAPEUTIC NEUTRALITY

The devaluating transference acting out of patients with narcissistic disorders generally presents a more complex problem. The easy access to aggressive, manipulative, and competitive feelings exacerbates the intensity of their devaluations. This leads to a central therapeutic dilemma.

Empathy, a fundamental of therapeutic neutrality, is inordinately strained by devaluation, and often makes therapist countertransference acting out the rule rather than the exception. Additionally, because of the patient's exquisite sensitivity to criticism, confrontation becomes too injurious and risky. The person with an exhibitionistic narcissistic disorder, like the one with a closet disorder, regulates his or her sense of self from the responses of others. The demand for mirroring, coupled with a strong sense of entitlement, can fuel a cold, sometimes ruthless, rage against anyone who threatens to destroy the patient's grandiosity.

While the function of devaluation for someone with a schizoid disorder of the self is to maintain a safe distance; and for someone with a borderline disorder, it is to protect from abandonment; for the person with a narcissist disorder, its function is to maintain the grandiose self-image. Furthermore, he or she is armed and ready to fight to sustain it.

Probably no other defense demands so much from the therapist as the devaluating acting out of the narcissist disorder. The ability of the therapist to manage himself or herself and maintain a neutral therapeutic platform is put to its acid test. Even with less aggressive defenses, the therapeutic relationship between patient and therapist is a complex interpersonal dance. The patient reveals hidden, sensitive thoughts and feelings. The therapist is expected to remain neutral, not to resonate with criticism or disdain, and to stay available to the patient throughout these disclosures. But when devaluative thoughts and feelings are projected onto the therapist for the patient's protection, they can easily provoke the therapist's vulnerabilities.

When a patient devalues and attacks the therapist, the therapist's defensive responses are often reflexively enlisted in the service of protection. It becomes very difficult for the therapist to be empathic when the patient is attempting to force the therapist to experience the feelings associated with the fragmented self. If one of the goals of treatment with the narcissistic-disordered patient is to help him or her to manage aggression, therapists are, in the interest of preserving therapeutic neutrality, also required to do the same.

Additionally, the demands for perfect mirroring, exact attunement, and admiration not only are antithetical to a therapeutic alliance, but can stir envy and resentment in the therapist. Underneath the therapist's discomfort with some of the more blatant narcissistic self-entitlements can be a sadness and rage at the necessity to manage unresolved infantile grandiosity.

Thus the central danger in deserting therapeutic neutrality is that the therapist may respond to a harsh, attacking patient by attempting to ward off feelings of victimization by denial of, retreat from, or retaliation for the injury. Either way, the patient's defenses intensify.

CASE OF MR. C.

History

Mr. C. had been one of my more problematic cases, specifically because he used devaluation as a principal defense. He had been referred to me by his physician, when he sought help in coping with his stressful work situation. An attorney in a high-powered law firm, he was in line for a promotion to a partnership, but there was stiff competition. His office was rife with what he perceived to be secretive alliances, backbiting, and potential treachery.

Mr. C.'s history revealed that he had had to learn early on to protect himself from feelings of fear and anger, because any expression of such feelings endangered his relationship with his mother. She could by physically abusive, but more often she was unpredictable. She could be charming and seductive and enlist Mr. C. in fusion fantasies of her own, or she could be ruthlessly rejecting. When his mother pushed him away, Mr. C. had to manage the pain of being assaulted by the person whom he loved and whose love sustained him.

In a household with three siblings, Mr. C. soothed himself with the knowledge that he was the brightest and most favored in the family, and the one who most consistently could calm his mother's anger and frustration. This self and object fusion with his mother was the basic source of his grandiose self-image. It included a sense of superiority and of being special to her, the omnipotent object, and an illusion that he was not really part of the family, but superior to it.

There was, however, another component of this fused self and object representation—the pain and anxiety of a more dangerous and hidden fragmented self. This arose in relation to an often weak, unconfident, but very punitive caretaker, his mother, and to the sense of chaos and lack of direction that pervaded their environment. His identification with his mother's aggressive defenses was likely the origin of his defense of devaluation.

While sadness was very difficult for Mr. C. to access, fear and anger were not. When these emotions overtook him in childhood, sometimes as a result of a disagreement, especially when his mother would lose interest in him or become interested in a new lover, he would retreat to the attic of his home, where he had set up model airplanes that hung from the ceiling in combat formations.

He would discharge his rage by battling the enemy and triumphing as the victor. In this way, he could avoid facing his rage and helplessness directly. It was a metaphorical but very real struggle between victory and annihilation, which survived into adolescence and adulthood.

Mr. C. learned to protect his vulnerability to rejection and criticism in important relationships by making sure that he felt victorious whenever possible. In adulthood, he transformed the battle into the arenas of knowledge and superiority. He was, in fact, very bright and quick, but also extremely sensitive to any indication that he might be exploited or abused.

He had also mastered (for he initially saw it as a strength) a dissociative ability to distract himself reflexively when in a position of helplessness. This was a very important protection from distress, but it also deprived him of the knowledge of many of his own feelings.

Treatment

Coming into therapy presented Mr. C. with a unique problem. It required him to focus on himself, in the absence of my admiration of the exhibition of his grandiose self. Feeling and revealing his weakness in front of me made him vulnerable to attack, a painful and difficult experience for him. When I did not start the session and direct him, he handled his difficulties by a series of intense and persistent devaluations.

Upon entering the room, he would often criticize the temperature of the office or its ventilation, using a devaluating tone to reduce his fear and uncertainty on beginning the session. At other times, devaluation would be enlisted to deal with his disappointment when I did not respond to his entreaties to say something that might enable him to feel better about himself. "You're a shitty therapist," he would shout. "God damn it, say something."

He would devalue me when I could not soothe him or help him with his difficulty in becoming aware of feelings or when I did not deescalate his fears and help him deal with his stressful interpersonal difficulties at work. He would also criticize me for dust in the office, some ants on the floor, a mistake on his bill, my looking at the clock, my raising my fee, my colorful sports jacket, or my seven-year-old car, which he had seen.

Some of the devaluations were more subtle and were reflected in his body language. His facial expressions could clearly show disdain, and early in his treatment he would often display a smile of superiority when he entered the office.

Additionally, he became involved with a number of other authority figures who helped to dilute his involvement with me. Among other meanings, these relationships reflected an additional devaluation of his therapy. He was in group therapy and would consistently compare me with the other therapist. I was portrayed as inept while the other therapist seemed extraordinarily gifted and helpful. He was also in a very close relationship with a therapist uncle who meant a lot to Mr. C., as he not only had helped Mr. C. through an earlier crisis, but often responded to Mr. C.'s requests for advice. Mr. C. often discussed his therapy with the uncle, who gave Mr. C. his opinion on many issues related to treatment.

Although his uncle's advice contributed a greater intellectual understanding by Mr. C. of what was happening to him, it also diluted his emotional connection to the treatment. It allowed Mr. C. to titrate his relationship with me and to protect himself from fears of full involvement. He attempted to relegate me to relative insignificance as a way of dealing with his fears of exploitation and abuse, which he projected onto me.

Mr. C. was also using devaluation outside the office to buffer his fears and feelings about himself. He felt a chronic fear of displeasing his superiors at work, and yet a need to shine as the star of the office. He would disparage his colleagues as dullards, because he considered himself to be more cultured, better educated, and more worldly. He found it helpful to focus on the fools at work so as not to focus on himself.

Mr. C. was using the same well-crafted skills he had developed in childhood. His major weapons were devaluation and distancing. The war was primarily a defensive action to protect him against vulnerability, but it also was a way to punish me, his colleagues, and anyone who did not meet his insistent demands for mirroring.

Whenever I recognized these maneuvers, I would intervene with a variety of mirroring interpretations of narcissistic vulnerability associated with being in treatment. Beginning with a mirroring component that focused empathically on the understanding of the pain to his self, I would remind him that he had come into treatment to understand why his self-esteem fluctuated so markedly.

It seemed to me, I told him, that when he was required to turn his attention on himself, to explore and attempt to understand this situation, it was either too dangerous or too painful for him to contemplate those feelings. Then, labeling the defense, I added that I had to wonder if, by focusing on his annoyance with events outside himself (the temperature of the office, my car, my clothes), he was not managing his fears by focusing his attention on me. I also wondered if he were experiencing me as a dangerous adversary, for he seemed to be attacking me, trying to render me ineffectual, helpless, and harmless.

Mr. C.'s responses varied. He might, somewhat begrudgingly, mirror me by agreeing with my interpretations. "You may be right," he would say. But the maneuvers were still too entrenched and my interventions not forceful enough to make any enduring change.

This period of his treatment went on for many months. As a consequence of my countertransference acting out, my inability to control my own narcissistic vulnerability in the face of his devaluations made it difficult for him to control these devaluations. It weakened, even aborted, any attempt to establish an idealizing transference acting-out pattern of relating to me.

This process often develops slowly but naturally, if the therapist does not act out and retreat from neutrality. But in the earlier testing stage, I had often been taken aback by his consistent devaluations and had become somewhat immobilized; therefore, I was not able to follow through to examine and interpret his mirroring resistance to my interpretations.

While outwardly I was making accurate mirroring interpretations, more personally I was often accepting his projection onto me and experiencing myself as inept and useless. I was taking responsibility for a sense of failure, his inability to access feelings, and his strong resistance against emotional recognition of the therapeutic relationship.

In the face of his attacks, I was feeling helpless and he was feeling superior. Because Mr. C. was quite perceptive in recognizing my limitations—the shortcomings in the delivery of some of my interpretations, as well as the occasional shifts in my own self-confidence—his devaluations were wounding my narcissistic sensitivity, confirming my feelings of deficiency and imperfection. Coupled with internalizing these feelings of inadequacy, I also was defending against his attack by denial, not allowing myself to be consciously aware of many of his more subtle devaluations. Therapy at this stage almost came to a standstill. My immobility, a retreat from neutrality, was actively reinforcing a major resistance. Therapy cannot work with two scared people in the room.

As I pondered the immobility of therapy with Mr. C., I began to gain control of my own countertransference acting out. I was becoming less sensitive to his devaluations, less fearful, more able to think clearly in the face of his defenses. However, there was one more obstacle that had to be surmounted. His emotional numbness that followed most of my interventions, or any momentary attempt to focus on himself, made him almost impervious to my mirroring interpretations.

Finally, I recognized that there was no choice but to get the message across by upping the ante. I had to make an all-out assault on his devaluative defenses by confrontation. I knew there was a chance of losing him as a patient, and of his losing the opportunity to work through his difficulties, but there was no other choice.

I told him that he was using his devaluation of me for a number of purposes: to dump his frustrations at work on me; to protect himself from experiencing any vulnerability in his relationship with me; and, in general, to maintain this very familiar but fleeting feeling of superiority. I admitted that he might feel better for the moment, but asked if he were not really just digging the hole deeper and depriving himself of learning about himself.

I told him that whatever transient satisfaction he was getting out of these maneuvers, it was not therapy and I was no longer going to be the dumping ground for his ultimately self-destructive efforts to feel better about himself. I also added that I thought he was no longer an innocent bystander, and that he was now quite aware of the destructiveness of his own behavior in treatment, as well as outside. Finally, I told him that if the devaluations were to continue, they would doom the treatment to failure and he would have to find another therapist.

It was a strong confrontation, forcefully delivered, and had a very significant impact. In theoretical terms, my firmness in helping Mr. C. control his transference acting out was encouraging him to move from a mirroring into an idealizing transference. Without this new dynamic, he and I could never have reached a therapeutic alliance.

Mr. C.'s first response was fear—of me and of my abandoning him. It put him in touch with some affect, which had always been elusive. In attempting to understand his devaluations, I hypothesized that part of his testiness with me, as with others, may have been an effort to escape from an essential numbness that often characterized his internal experience. Like an addict, he needed situations of great intensity and excitement in order to feel alive and vital, and his maneuvers were attempts to generate them.

My confrontation, combined with the management of my countertransference acting out, now set the foundation for the control, as well as the understanding, of his devaluating defense, which had become such a significant part of his defensive armament and, I imagined, contributed substantially to the character he displayed to the world. Once the confrontation was on the table and it was clear that I meant business, the devaluations gradually decreased in intensity, although it was still necessary for me to keep interpreting or confronting his criticisms on the spot, every time they occurred.

Mr. C. began to exercise greater control. He would announce his devaluating thoughts, but they were one step removed from action. At this stage, I might confront or interpret unnecessarily, and he would ask me calmly and movingly not to push him as he knew what was happening. Finally, the devaluations were brought under control. He could express the feeling that at times I did not fully understand his inner workings, rather than attack me for my imperfect formulations.

As he exerted his willpower and concentrated on controlling his transference acting out, the therapeutic relationship slowly but measurably deepened. Mr. C. was learning that if he controlled his aggression, safe avenues were still available whereby he could express his pain and disappointment, both in others and in himself. I, in turn, was learning that my essential task, addressing his devaluations and their meaning from a neutral platform, necessitated the management of my own vulnerable feelings when attacked and bruised.

In the next few months, especially as Mr. C.'s treatment began to make a difference to his life and his feelings about himself, he expressed remorse for his previous behavior. He seemed honestly shocked, in hindsight, at the consequences of his devaluation. It had imperiled his relationship with me, and had led to the extra time spent avoiding the focus on himself. He began to understand how his need to protect himself by trashing others and his portrayal of an image of superiority were creating additional challenges to his survival at work, as well as to the viability of any romantic relationship.

Additionally, as a by-product of this understanding, and as a measure of the deepening of the idealizing relationship, he began spontaneously to examine the appropriateness of his use of the outside therapeutic relationships. He began to realize how his search for mirroring—from the group therapist, from his therapist uncle, with the partners in his law firm, with me, and in other relationships—had blinded him to an understanding of his real self. For the first time since the beginning of treatment, he started a serious relationship with a woman. Also, to my surprise, he began seriously to reevaluate his career goals and to contemplate life in a family and work situation in which he would not be so driven by a need to display and to be admired.

CONCLUSION

Therapy with a person with a narcissistic disorder of the self, predictably under the onslaught of devaluation, requires an ability by the therapist to tolerate his or her own narcissistic imperfections. Thus it is fundamental, in spite of their limitations, that therapists appreciate that they are good enough therapists, and that their motives are essentially in the patient's best interest. Therapy is stalled when both people in the room need to be perfect.

Additionally, it is important to depersonalize the attacks that may have been the patient's essential protection against fragmentation. Such attacks are not really directed at the therapist, but at the therapist as a stand-in, usually for parents who were unavailable or intrusive. Through the defense of identification with the aggressor, patients project their fragmented selves onto others so they may take on the role of their own parents, and thus protect themselves from feelings of victimization or from realizing their own vulnerability.

Also, on occasion, it is appropriate for therapists to respond with anger at being devalued, and they may have to permit themselves to get in touch with their own rage at being used in such a way. Although that does not give them license to be rageful, the fear of it can be immobilizing.

Although it may not be necessary to interpret every devaluation, it is important not to allow the patient to get away with a devaluating stance over time. The devaluating transference acting out needs to be converted to an idealizing transference acting out. It is only at that point that a therapeutic alliance can be established and working through can be contemplated.

This goal might be accomplished by interpretation, but it may be necessary to use confrontation. Either way, the problem must be dealt with. If the patient is permitted to destroy the therapist emotionally, he or she will be repeating the destruction of one more object who might provide some relief. It will reinforce a self representation of a dangerous, destructive, murderous self.

Patients may already feel responsible for their past fractured and broken relationships. Therapists who allow the patients to render them ineffectual are colluding in perpetuating the patients' murderous fantasies and in their equating fantasy with reality. Underneath the facade of devaluation is remorse and fear of the loss of the only methods they have had at their disposal to remain sane.

A distinction must also be made between criticism and disappointment and devaluation. They are not mutually exclusive. A patient can use devaluation to express an accurate yet troubling perception of the therapeutic relationship. Therapists must consider the expression of criticism or disappointment seriously, as well as point out and explore its devaluating nature.

Finally, as with so many of the obstacles to growth in clinical work, therapists learn more about themselves through the process of therapy, which ultimately brings meaning to both participants in the therapeutic relationship.

CHAPTER 17

Therapeutic Management of Disappointment Reactions with the Closet Narcissistic Disorder of the Self

Bill Robbins, Ph.D.

Mr. A. began treatment by telling me how confused he felt about his work and relationships. I listened attentively, but offered few comments.

Although he often had great expectations in starting a job or a relationship, he said, he could not seem to find the right match in either. He was often in more than one relationship at a time. A few weeks earlier, another in a series of lovers had left him, and he felt that things in his life were once again getting out of control. He had awakened with a hangover with little memory of where he had been or with whom he had been, and he realized that he should get some help.

He then switched to talking of his successes, in both his relationships and his work, but he also mentioned the sadness that sometimes overcame him, as well as occasional concerns about his adequacy. My assessment during the interview leaned clearly toward a closet narcissistic disorder of the self.

At the end of the session, he asked for a fee reduction. After discussing his finances, and remembering that he had told me of the high salary he received in his new job, I refused. He responded by telling me that he was in therapy only because his insurance paid for it. He just wanted what he called "pep talks and feedback" from me so that he could make his own decisions and move on with what had to be done.

This was clearly a protective response to a narcissistic injury—his disappointment at my failure to mirror him adequately. This would quickly become a critical issue for the treatment.

In his second session, Mr. A. told me that he had complained to a friend about me, but that the friend had convinced him to return for another visit. He then told me he intended to quit because I was not giving him enough feedback. It was clear that Mr. A. was very disappointed in me, so the first thing on *my* agenda was the issue of disappointment. I offered a somewhat general interpretation of how he seemed quite disappointed, but that he dealt with those feelings by getting angry at me and wanting to leave.

He readily agreed, but the interpretation was insufficient in itself. The concept of disappointment is not one that is easily grasped by the patient the first time around, when projection and transference acting out are strongly in force.

It became necessary to respond to Mr. A.'s explicit demand for me to talk and direct him more and to interpret his disguised communication, the desire to quit, as a reflection of his sensitivity to a failure in mirroring. A response at this critical juncture had to satisfy his need to be understood, as well as elicit his observing ego's interest in what I had to say.

I was addressing the expectation of and need for a positive response from others, and the disappointment that resulted when the expectation was not met. I used a number of interventions to elaborate on my first interpretation. I told Mr. A. that it seemed that when he does not get what he feels he needs and wants, either a fee reduction or more input from me, he seems to experience an unpleasant disappointment, and he protects himself from those feelings by distancing from me, by contemplating quitting. When I do not respond to him in a way that makes him feel a reflection of my special interest and caring, he is faced with managing his feelings about himself by himself.

I also suggested that the same was true of his need for feedback. When he has to provide direction and enthusiasm for himself, he is faced with focusing on himself, and that while I did not yet know what that was like for him, I presumed it felt quite uncomfortable. In order to dilute his discomfort, he reached out to me, so as not to feel the discomfort in himself. When he bridled at this interpretation, I had to use a more forceful confrontation. I added that he could likely find another therapist who would respond to his demands, but that would only drive his difficulties further underground and they would become even harder to understand.

It was not my task, in this situation, to try to find a solution to his problem, and certainly not to use myself as the solution. Rather, through the analysis of his responses to me, I was attempting to help him begin to understand the profound effect his feelings of disappointment had on how he responded to other people.

These interpretations had to be followed by a number of others. They form a paradigm that helps in understanding the polarities of the split object relations units of the narcissistic disorder of the self. They include the libidinal unit, a fantasy of an idealized and omnipotent object paired with a grandiose self that feels special, wonderful, admired, and perfect. The reverse, the aggressive unit, is composed of a harsh attacking object and the feeling of an impaired, unworthy, worthless, fragmented self. It is a relational continuum with perfect mirroring at one end and painful disappointment at the other. Both are of consequence in treating the narcissistic disorder of the self.

Disappointments invariably occur and are defended against as early as the first session, and ultimately can become chronic impediments to treatment. They can create crises in the treatment, resulting in the patient's terminating, or, more often, they may become a source of continuous challenge. The patient is demanding that the therapist respond in a particular way to maintain an illusion of fusion and quickly repair the injury of disappointment.

It is precisely in the analysis of the consequences of the lack of mirroring that working through will become possible. The concept is simple, but the challenge lies in recognizing the injury, and then understanding its meaning for the patient.

As far as Mr. A. was concerned, whenever possible and appropriate, I tried to express myself with what Masterson calls mirroring interpretations. They began with a mirroring component, focusing on the self, describing the patient's pain and attempting to ally empathically with the patient's sensitivity to pain. The mirroring would help Mr. A. feel understood and, in particular, more receptive to the final component of the intervention, which is the interpretation of his protective operations, the defense. It is this final component that has the potential to elicit resistance, and thus must be preceded (at the beginning of treatment, if at all possible) by the mirroring.

Subsequently, I summed up his situation by suggesting (with mirroring and a focus on the self) that the distress he felt when he had to manage his feelings about himself by himself (and then labeling the defense) led him to insist on perfect reflection from me, as well as from others (employers and the women in his life). I went on to point out that the aim of these demands was to keep hidden from himself and others the confusion, sadness, and feelings of inadequacy that he had named, but had only touched on during his first visit. Mr. A. said he felt understood and was interested enough to continue treatment.

Occasionally, due to countertransference acting out, I have resonated with a patient's defense against disappointment. This occurred initially with Ms. B., who came into treatment in a state of great distress. Twenty-three years old, a recent immigrant from South America, she had married a considerably older man whom she described as "a dream come true." It was her first intimate relationship. But three months into the marriage, she was beginning to realize how different they were.

She spent most of her first session telling me about the supportive and nurturing environment of her childhood home and its contrast with her present situation. Her husband seemed to be extremely insensitive and demanding of her. She told how he went out late at night, was not home when she came home, never called her to tell where he was or when he would be returning, rarely complimented her for tasks well done, discouraged her from making individual decisions, and engaged her in bitter and humiliating arguments. Perhaps most painful, she now found him critical of her physical appearance and he was withdrawing sexually. As an unwelcome, added stress, her much-esteemed father would soon arrive from South America for a visit.

I left the session feeling really sorry for her. She seemed to be a nice young woman, and I felt confused, sad, and protective of her. I felt that I wanted to shield her from this unhappy state of affairs. With a blurring of boundaries, and my identification with her projections, I began to feel a fatherly concern more appropriate to that of a parent for a child.

By her next visit, I had realized that I had strayed away from therapeutic neutrality. Knowing that my Achilles' heel is often a tendency to resonate with a patient's externalization defense helped me regain a more objective stance. I had been taken in by her externalization of her problems onto her husband. This does not mean that her husband was not the source of much of her discomfort, but I realized that there was an even greater discomfort that was causing her agitation.

At the second appointment, when she continued to describe her unhappy situation, I rather quickly made an interpretation of her disappointment, but now within the context of her focusing on herself rather than on her husband. I began by recalling that she had been so enthusiastic about both coming to the United States and marrying someone whom she considered "a dream come true." Now she was finding that her judgment and her understanding of reality left a lot to be desired.

I thought that what was most disturbing to her was a profound disappointment, not only in her husband, but also in herself. I added that she seemed to be suffering from very distressing and painful feelings about *herself*, but it was so difficult to tolerate those feelings that she focused most of her anger on her husband, and on wanting to leave him, so as not to have to experience them.

This interpretation had an immediate effect; it opened the floodgates of her feelings. She immediately confirmed my interpretation, and told me that she had come to the United States primarily to gain the admiration of her family. After she arrived, she decided to get married, mostly to escape from the intolerable and overly critical relative with whom she was living.

She realized now how disappointed she was in herself. In tears, she went on to relate how much energy she spent on making sure that others admired her and thought of her as special, and how she devoted herself tirelessly to others to elicit that kind of support.

We were now on firm therapeutic ground, with room for further interpretations of how her need for mirroring and feeling special made her so vulnerable to meeting others' needs rather than her own. At that moment, a transferential reenactment was not evident enough, so the interpretation had to be made with regard to an outside relationship. The next step would be to bring her sensitivity into the relationship with me, to analyze in her relationship with me her acute sensitivity to disappointment and her protection against it, so as not to feel painful feelings about herself.

Mr. C., who also came to see me in distress, illustrates a very common theme in couple relationships that is seen when obviously mismatched partners seem unable to separate. Mr. C. began by telling me of his tumultuous relationship with his girlfriend. He was attracted to her and wanted her desperately, and yet he and she could not seem to maintain any harmony when they were together.

He described how, when things went well and they felt close, it was like nirvana. However, usually something would happen between them, and the situations would become so mercurial that they often ended up in violent, sometimes physical, arguments. Mr. C. could not live with her and he could not live without her. "Should I send her flowers?" he asked. Could I suggest something that he could do to win her back? Mr. C. was protecting himself from the feelings that would arise if he were to contemplate the reality of his situation. Disappointment was being warded off by "help me fix it."

Understanding the polarized intrapsychic structure and the mechanism of splitting would enable me to concentrate not on how to solve the problem, but on interpreting, in a way he could understand, the internalized self and object relation that I saw being reenacted. This might lead Mr. C. to understand himself better and allow him to make decisions based on that new knowledge.

My interpretation to him was that there must be something very appealing about his girlfriend, but that he and she did not seem compatible in other ways. It seemed too painful for him to face the problems that existed—in him, in her, and in both together—and to face the realization that the relationship did not seem to work at all.

I suggested that this disappointment must arouse such uncomfortable feelings in him that he seemed determined, in spite of all he reported, to ignore the facts of the relationship. I was again pushing back the externalization, based on my understanding of object relations and the consequences of the failures of mirroring. My therapeutic agenda disregarded, at least for the moment, any amelioration of the couple's situation.

In response to my intervention, Mr. C. opened up somewhat and talked about his defeats in relationships. He told how he often found women who were initially compliant and supportive of him, but then would turn on him and want everything from him in return. Obviously, my interpretation had touched a resonant chord. Sadly, however, Mr. C. called me before the next appointment and terminated the treatment. I inferred that it was more important for him to fix the situation than to understand it more fully from the vantage point of his self.

These are all examples of the pervasiveness of the role of disappointment in the treatment of the narcissistic disorder of the self and of the ways in which patients deal with the effect that those experiences have on themselves.

In discussing the part self and part object representations that are ascribed to the narcissistic disorder, we are describing the polarities of fused representations of relationships. The fusion of a satisfied, often grandiose self with an idealized, admired, and admiring omnipotent object is contrasted with the fusion of a harsh, attacking object and a devalued image of self.

Because of the fixation on splitting, such patients seem to vacillate between these poles. If they are not feeling good, they are feeling bad. If they are not feeling great, they are feeling awful. If they are not feeling supported and attended to, they are feeling alone, unworthy, and rejected. These are the theoretical concepts that must be turned into clinical usefulness.

The patient requires perfect attunement, two minds thinking and feeling as one. This is not something that will readily be admitted, but one may hear such things as, "I want a relationship that is like my pulse, always there and unconditional, or I will be pulverized." This statement clearly delineates the fused libidinal unit, "like my pulse, always there and unconditional," from the fused aggressive unit, "or I will be pulverized."

The therapist thus has to walk a tightrope between allowing an idealizing transference to develop and not responding countertransferentially to the patient's need and desire for a fused relationship.

In general, the experience of disappointment often seems to arise as a result of the failure of an external source of encouragement, admiration or specialness, attention, praise, or perfect understanding. The loss of these supplies results in the varied symptoms of narcissistic injury—the loss of a sense of completeness, identity, and stability of one's self-perception and one's expectations for oneself.

Stabilizing reflections from important symbols of authority, whether individuals or institutions, are often fundamental to the maintenance of a satisfying sense of self. Without these reflections, disquieting feelings of disappointment and loss create substantial discomfort and depression.

In the therapeutic situation, if the therapist is being himself or herself, at times imperfect and limited, the patient may feel the need to devalue—or, conversely, to idealize—the therapist's behavior and habits, so as to push aside the patient's own experience of disappointment in his or her own limitations. Again, the disappointment is in his or her self when connected to what is perceived as a less than perfect object. Although the dynamic may be initiated by external sources, the source of feelings is within the self.

Ms. D., a clinical social worker, came into the office and rearranged the pillows on the couch. She was annoyed. "You know, it would be nice if you put the pillows in a consistent place before I came in. I always have to re-arrange them after your last patient. My God, who would sit this far away anyway?" "In fact," she went on, "according to formal analytic technique, the pillows should be in the same place each time a patient arrives." Ms. D. was disappointed in me. As the guardian of her thoughts, wishes, and needs, I have failed to provide for her. It is a small but significant narcissistic injury.

Ms. D. continued: "But I wonder if you are doing that purposely, so as to help me understand my feelings about your having other patients." She had protected herself from feelings of disappointment by rationalizing and idealizing my behavior, which I then reflected to her with a mirroring interpretation of her pain on perceiving me as less than perfect, which had an immediate effect on her feelings about herself. She diluted those feelings by rationalizing my behavior so as not to concentrate on herself.

Sometime later, Ms. D. was talking with feeling about something quite important to her. We could both hear the audible click of the answering machine as a message was being received. Once again, she was quite annoyed. "Why can't you do something about that?"

She and I had had this conversation many times before, and I have made many interpretations of her sensitivity to things not being the way she wants them to be and her expectation that I should provide a trouble-free environment for her.

She went on: "I'm quite sensitive to my clients. Why can't you be to me?" Then she changed the subject and tried to go back to what she was talking about previously. Ms. D. did not want to deal with the significance of the disruption. She had protected herself from feelings of disappointment by distancing from me, which again had to be interpreted.

Ms. D. had grown up with a serious speech impediment. Up until her early teens, her stuttering was humiliating and painful. She experienced her defect as one in which, in spite of her very high intelligence, she could not communicate to others, and never would. When she finally overcame her problem, she took up public speaking and oration and became an accomplished speaker, a source of great pride to her.

In the treatment situation, she kept herself unaware of many of her imperfections through a forceful denial system. The ones to which she could admit became sources of self-admiration. She was pleased that she could be so open to others about her limitations.

Through a process that exposed an idiosyncrasy on my part, as well as a forceful projective identification on her part, I would often find myself, especially during mirroring interpretations, slowly groping for the right word or a clearer way to communicate a concept to her. She could become critical or hostile in her response.

Sometimes she would offer me rather good advice. "Why don't you take a deep breath?" she suggested. She assured me that she would be happy to wait. She also suggested: "What if you thought your idea over between sessions and presented it to me the next time we meet?"

When she was clearly "driven up the wall" by what she considered my ineptness, she would cover her eyes while I spoke, so as not to have to witness such a horrifying event as her therapist's perceived limitations.

I often interpreted her discomfort at her disappointment in seeing her own limitations in me and her difficulty in refocusing on her own feelings. These interpretations were only minimally received. In addition, her constant criticisms challenged me to experience my own limitations as acceptable and not as narcissistic wounds.

Following one particular dream, she began to integrate the understanding of my interpretations. In the dream, three people were present: her mother, herself, and another person, who seemed retarded and spastic. Her mother was scolding the retarded person as the patient looked on. She was mystified by the dream and could offer no associations.

I interpreted that she was put into a situation in which either she had to deny painful feelings, especially those that arose around her early childhood limitations, or she had to accept herself, with the consequence of being subject to the memory of so many years of feeling anxious and inept, and of risking humiliation by her parents.

She took in my interpretation, became teary, and then talked of her dilemma. "I'm not good at treating you as a human being, and I don't know if I can get through that—even when I try not to be critical and judgmental, and try to be empathic. The residue of judgmentalism, which is so destructive to the relationship, has to do with my not being able to accept defects in others that I refuse to acknowledge I have in myself. I don't stutter anymore, yet I still have it in my history. I got in the habit of not remembering. It still is too painful when you lose your train of thought. Why don't I accept my own imperfections?"

Ms. D. could now begin to investigate and understand her strong response to her disappointment in me. Additionally, it was yet another example of other disappointments she faced in people who were close to her. To find so many of these people imperfect and disappointing necessitated her need to distance from them.

In summary, these clinical examples emphasize that when working with the narcissistic disorder of the self, the experience of disappointment and the defenses against it can be a distinct challenge for the therapist. However, it can also be a rich source of information about the patient's character structure and a path toward working through. In understanding these responses to disappointment, both the therapist and the patient have a fundamental key to personality growth and change.

PART IV

Other Treatment
Strategies

In this section, the horizons are extended beyond the boundary of individual psychotherapy for disorders of the self. Dr. Fischer, in Chapter 18, combines the Masterson Approach with that of W. Bion to present an innovative approach to group psychotherapy. Dr. Seider and Dr. Orcutt, in Chapters 19 and 20, apply it to couples therapy. In the last two chapters, Dr. Grubb applies the approach to the use of antidepressants and to the understanding of comorbid conditions. He makes the important point that an understanding of psychodynamics is crucial to appropriate drug therapy.

J.F.M. & R.K.

CHAPTER 18

Group Psychotherapy and Disorders of the Self

Richard E. Fischer, Ph.D.

The literature on the disorders of the self is quite clear in consistently recommending an individual psychoanalytic psychotherapy that is tailored to the needs of the patient (Masterson, 1976, 1981, 1985, 1988a, 1988b). The role of alternative treatments, such as family and group psychotherapy, has been unjustly relegated to a position of relative unimportance.

Throughout the years, group psychotherapy has been a devalued form of psychotherapy. It has been seen as a potential treatment for economically deprived patients and for those who have not been responsive to individual treatment. This dismissal of the benefits of group psychotherapy has been unfortunate, since most patients with disorders of the self suffer from serious problems in interpersonal relationships and intimacy conflicts. Group psychotherapy, with its identification and clarification of interpersonal distortions, can be an extraordinarily useful approach to help many of these patients identify their defenses, maladaptive patterns, and difficulties in relationships. It can be an extremely useful secondary adjunctive treatment synergistic with individual psychotherapy for many disorders of the self.

This chapter describes a group treatment that is compatible with and reinforces the individual psychotherapy of these patients. It is an integration of the work of Wilfred Bion on the interpsychic structure of groups with the work of James Masterson on the intrapsychic structure of the individual's personality.

GROUP STRUCTURE AND PROCESS

The manifest task of a therapeutic group, or the work function as defined by Bion (1961), is designed to identify, clarify, manage, and resolve interpersonal conflict. This is analogous to what has been defined by Masterson (1976) as the therapeutic alliance and the reality ego in individual psychotherapy. The group relates on a rational level with an adaptive approach to problem solving.

When the group is in a work mode, there is a belief in adaptive coping with conflict and negotiation, and a dismissal of magical solutions to interpersonal problems. There is a demand that cooperation takes place and that primitive need and fantasy consciously be renounced.

In the pregroup interview, this manifest task of the group will be explained to group members. Most people coming into a group will describe their interpersonal problems. The purpose for most members is to identify maladaptive interpersonal problems and defensive distortions that take place in interpersonal relationships, and to use the group as an in vivo laboratory to explore these maladaptive behaviors and to develop new and better forms of relating.

The therapist, during the initial interview, will help the patient to identify these maladaptive patterns, and may point out the nature of these defenses, how the group can be useful in identifying them, and how the group can be used to help resolve and develop new forms of behavior. While the initial presentation of all of the patients in the group is one of work and cooperation, as soon as these eight or so members gather in the same room, anxiety, conflicts, depression, and fears begin to develop that propel the group to move from a position of problem solving to one of fear and ultimately to defense.

GROUP FEARS AND CONFLICTS

The first fear that arises in a therapeutic group is the dread of ambivalence and conflictual relationships. It is as if the group has an unconscious motivation to keep all goodness within the group and to extrude all badness from the group. The group seems to move through an introjective–projective cycle. Good interpersonal experience is introjected, and the group attempts to contain it within the group, while bad conflictual experience is extruded and expelled from the group. There is an analogous situation that takes place with the individual patient. Masterson (1976) has described the oscillating cycle of the borderline patient, where good experience is held onto in the form of the rewarding object relations unit, and bad negative aspects of experience are projected in the form of the withdrawing object relations unit.

The group has a similar split-oscillating cycle. However, when the group members decide to extrude negative experience, they literally eject or evict a particular member. It is important to understand that on the level of group experience, one's part object representation is an individual group member. This dread of ambivalence and fear of conflictual relationships, combined with the introjective–projective cycle, makes a group structurally very similar to a person with a low-level borderline personality disorder who seems perpetually unable to tolerate ambivalence.

The second group conflict is the ongoing difficulty in integrating the wish for contact and the wish for separateness. The underlying fundamental need is a longing for interpersonal contact without surrendering the individual self. However, most group members are caught between the two poles on this continuum. At one end of the continuum is the fear of schizoid withdrawal, of isolation, and of banishment from the community, and on the other end is the fear of the group absorption of the individual self. Patients would often describe this situation as a fear of not being accepted by the group and of becoming a group "moonie" or robot. This conflict is the classic one between the individual identity and the group identity. Of course, the healthy individual recognizes the need for group affiliation and the need to maintain an individual sense of self, and these two identities are not in conflict. However, very early on in the group development, these two needs come into conflict.

The next group fear is the dread of integration of disparate and separate identities and the simultaneous fear of splitting and disavowal of identities. One sees this classic conflict in race relationships that seem to oscillate back and forth between the wish for integration and the fear of integration—the wish for separatism and the disavowal of other races and cultures. In its extreme forms, there can be a loss of individual cultural identities, such as all cultures falling under a communist umbrella, and in another extreme form, there can be violent ethnic uprisings and scapegoating of other cultural or ethnic groups.

The next group conflict is the wish for and fear of integrating the basic assumptions of group life with the work function of the group. The basic assumptions are basic illogical defenses used by the group to maintain a sense of cohesion. The work function operates on a manifest conscious task, and moves according to rational principles. As with the borderline patient, who has a reality ego, there is an increased need to bring the irrational defenses under the direction of the reality ego. Similarly, there is an opposing resistance to this domination by the reality ego, as the individual or the group will have to relinquish pathological fantasy gratification.

The last conflict is the need to maintain a sense of self and to resist the boundary pressure that is put on the individual identity by the group. Very often the group therapist will hear different patients complain that they are not good in groups, or they are not able to resist the group pressure, or they seem unable to conform to the group needs. Such patients, rather than declaring themselves as not suitable for the group, are identifying a particular type of interpersonal problem of theirs that can be worked on in the group context. It is my premise that all people discover an individual sense of self within the context of multiple groups, and very often the individual sense of self is reinforced and affirmed when asserting itself against the antagonistic forces of the group. While an individual patient may feel that he or she has to conform with the group in order to grow, very often such a patient has to be successful in resisting the underlying group pressure and group needs.

DEFENSES AGAINST THE GROUP TASK AND GROUP FEARS: THE BASIC ASSUMPTIONS

All individual therapists using the Masterson Approach are aware of the difficulties that a borderline patient has when faced with the task of individuation. This task, along with separation stress, exposes the patient to the threat of abandonment panic or depression, which mobilizes the pathological defenses of the ego. A similar process takes place within the group. The manifest task of the group is similar to the reality ego and the therapeutic alliance of the individual patient. However, when those eight group members get together, and it mobilizes group fears and group conflicts, the reality of the ego of the group is given up, along with the work function of the group, which produces magical, irrational defenses to preserve and maintain the continuity of the group. It is as if the fears and conflicts that are operating in the group trigger a terrifying anxiety of group disintegration, and the group as a unit mobilizes these defenses in order to preserve the continuity of the group, and to ward off frightening feelings of group disintegration.

Masterson (1985) spoke about the therapist's need to be the guardian of the individual's real self. An important axiom of group life is that the group therapist must realize that the sum is truly greater than the parts. It is essential that the group therapist continuously monitor the collective anxiety, fear, defense, and resolution at that particular moment.

This is a very difficult concept for many individual therapists to integrate, as the primacy of the individual has always been a hallmark in individual psychoanalytic psychotherapy. It is also very difficult to conceptualize a group self, as it is not physically visible, nor is it always apparent. The task, nonetheless, of the group therapist is to keep a watchful eye on this conceptual unit, and to clarify the manifest task of the moment, the group fears and anxieties, the reactive defenses, and the group resolution. This does not mean that the group therapist never focuses on an individual patient, but sees the patient's role as that of spokesperson for the covert unconscious group needs. The individual patient in the group can be considered as being a spokesperson at a particular moment, as a representative of a crucial conflict.

For example, if the group has been struggling with frightening feelings of anger and competition, it would not be unusual for a schizoid patient to become a focus of the group, as the group needs to disengage from conflict and to withdraw from contact. The model is as follows: each individual member is a humble servant of the group's needs or a soldier in the group's army. Masterson (1981) has emphasized the borderline triad and the need for the therapist's cognizance of this dynamic relationship. The borderline triad emphasizes the role of separation–individuation mobilizing depression, which activates defense. It is well known at this point that the borderline patient moves through a continuous cycle of this triadic relationship. The group has a similar sort of triad. Interpersonal conflict mobilizes group fear, which, in turn, mobilizes group defense, and this, in turn, produces group resolution. The nature of the resolution, however, is not always in accord with the reality principle.

BION'S ASSUMPTIONS ABOUT GROUPS

Bion (1961) highlighted three basic assumptions of group life. The first basic assumption is one that he called dependence (BAD). In a basic dependent group, one notices the group searching for an oracle or a deity, from which all security, nourishment, and direction come. This is similar to the rewarding object relations unit that has been described by Masterson (1976) in the individual borderline patient. In a basic dependent group, there is no evidence of spontaneity or individuation. The group seems to conduct itself like a fundamentalist bible class in which there are both believers and atheists. The group generally runs like a theocracy.

If the group leader rejects the role of the omnipotent and omniscient guiding force, then the group becomes angry and looks for another theocratic leader. This angry dismissal of the group leader who does not resonate with the dependent needs of the group is similar to the withdrawing object relations unit that has been described by Masterson. A basic dependent group denies group responsibility to self-activate. The leader can feel like Moses leading infantile children of Israel out of the desert.

It seems that all the individual patients in the group want an individual relationship with the therapist, and only the therapist is respected as a source of guidance or advice. Much advice giving goes on in the group, and there is little expression of feeling or belief in the merit of exploring feeling and fantasy. According to Bion, the dependent group brings up feelings of greed and envy, and there is a fear of being cheated or starved in such a group.

The external object, or leader, exists for one reason—to provide security and a magical feeling of protection. The group leader is often referred to as Buddha, Christ, or God, and there is an excessive devotion to the leader and a belief in his or her magical abilities. An example of an institution that exploits this basic assumption is the church. Another is the 12-step programs in which participants are given a book that, they are told, will lead to mental health, recovery, or salvation. A dependent group is not run like a democracy nor does it respect logical approaches toward problem solving. Instead, it operates like a religious sect or cult, and has a need to stifle individuality. It is very rule ridden and dogmatic, and differences are not tolerated. Very often, a confessional phenomenon takes place whereby the group tries to rid itself of badness or sin.

Bion (1961) often emphasized the group's unconscious fear and dread and its resistance to learning from experience. There seems to be a basic need in group life to believe in the omnipotence and omniscience of one particular leader, and a general avoidance of learning to resolve interpersonal conflicts. If the therapist resists resonating with the projections of the dependent group, the group will turn to someone else to resonate with the group need. According to Bion, the group will choose the sickest member of the group to take on the leadership position, a dynamic that he calls the holiness of idiots or the genius of madness. It is not unusual for the replacement group leader to be psychotic, paranoid, or psychopathic. While the group in a basic dependent assumption has a wish for a deity, there is also a dread of relinquishing control and a fear of dictatorship, as all defenses were designed to cope with group anxiety. It also creates fear and tension, and as this anxiety develops in the group, there is a need to move on to the next mechanism of defense, which will help to, at least initially, reduce the anxiety that has been mobilized.

The next basic assumption described by Bion is the fight–flight group. A fight–flight group is characterized as seeking security through the search for a hated enemy that the group fears and flees from, or hates and fights. One notices in such a group a tremendous level of fear and anxiety, which is most similar to the Kleinian paranoid–schizoid position or the withdrawing object relations unit described by Masterson (1976) in his discussion of lower-level borderline patients. This is the most primitive of basic assumptions, and there is the greatest loss of tolerance, delay, and even language as a vehicle to resolve interpersonal conflict. It is not unusual to see people shouting at each other and engaging in verbally abusive behavior, while the leader tries unsuccessfully to clarify the dynamics through verbal interpretation. The basic assumption fight–flight group can often lead to the scapegoating of particular members or the banishment or condemnation of, or aggressive discrimination against, various members. This group dynamic on a societal level is responsible for racism and the persecution and genocide of various subgroups. It is as if the group searches for security by evacuating "bad elements"—a process that exists on family, corporate, national, and international levels. The leader must be firm, interpret the process, and at times be confrontative to protect various members from the potential violence of a fight–flight group.

Whereas most people are aware of the possible hazardous effects of this fight–flight dynamic, one can speculate that positive results can ensue from such a group process. For instance, I would speculate that the individuation process naturally activates and mobilizes an enormous amount of aggression that needs a group or an object to serve as a container. During the initial individuation process, this aggression is securely bound through the relation to the hated object.

Another need for fight–flight dynamics seems to develop when ego boundaries or interpersonal borders are vague and poorly defined so that the relationship between the self and the other becomes tenuous, often resulting in the need to highlight oneself against the bad other. The examples of fight–flight dynamics on an international level are clear. The Middle East has been caught in such a group dynamic for hundreds of years. The civil war in the Balkans, with the tragedy of ethnic cleansing, is another example of a fight–flight dynamic that has developed to murderous proportions. One can look at this as the result of a larger group process that has evolved on the European continent. Although the previous relationship between the Communist world and the free world resulted in many tensions, there was also a clear demarcation of boundaries between the self and the other, between one group and another. As the Communist world collapsed, Europeans were once again left with a vague sense of their borders and the mobilization of traditional ethnic rivalries developed to help clarify boundaries. In our society, we tend to search for victims and victimizers, and feel quite comfortable with a model that focuses on the abused and the abuser.

If we take group dynamics seriously, however, then a new model of collective collusion in a group process has to develop. For instance, the situation in the Balkans is taking place with a simultaneous awareness of genocide and a denial of its existence. As the world remembers the Holocaust, the group process seems to be unfolding once again in order to gain a collective sense of security and to redefine boundaries. This model maintains that all participants in the group process are responsible and are collectively colluding in an interactive system to create a new sense of group definition and to mobilize covert unconscious needs.

The ramifications of this model can be generalized to help in developing new perspectives on the interactions between therapists and their patients. The old model of a neutral, somewhat detached, therapist who observes the intrapsychic structure of a patient while being removed from the process no longer seems viable. A model that places the therapist in an ongoing introjective–projective interaction with a patient, in which the therapist both shapes the intrapsychic structure of the patient and is affected by the patient's projections, seems more on target conceptually.

The relationship between a group leader and the group is also complex (Bion, 1961). While the therapist does have a unique position in observing group process and in commenting on these interactions through the interpretive approach, the therapist is also affected and modified by the covert unconscious needs of the group. While not always conscious of his or her relationship to the group process, the therapist must always be aware of the fact that he or she is as much a part of this process as are the patients. In fact, to gain insight into the process, the group leader must first be caught by these unconscious processes, struggle with the dilemma, and then through his or her understanding begin to communicate interpretively to the group in order to have an effect on the resultant process.

This model of collective collusion will also develop new conceptualizations of countertransference, if therapists are seen as continuously interacting with patients, modifying their structures, and, at times, being shaped by their projections. Therapists have one distinct advantage in that they are trained and aware of the unconscious forces with which they struggle and which they try to understand. If they are open and receptive to these forces, and at the same time try to become aware of them and to communicate that awareness, then an effective psychotherapeutic interaction can take place.

This model will also draw new conclusions for the relationship of the group and the individual. At times, the individuals in a group are shaped by the covert unconscious needs of the group. Similarly, the individual, with his or her unique character structure, will shape the group process and modify its development. It would be naive to assume that each group will produce the same group process. A better explanation would focus on the unique contributions of the individuals affecting the group process, and would also be open to the possibility of the group's affecting the individuals.

This release of hatred and a search for a common enemy as part of a group process must be accepted as part of group life in order to identify the process when it happens and contain its destructive impact. The societal institution that exploits this fundamental group process is the military, and the results of the process are not always negative. It is my opinion that fight–flight dynamics are typically used in the early stages of group identity to firm up boundaries and borders, and to defend against a more diffuse and tenuous sense of self. For instance, the United States, in declaring its independence from England, did so against the English enemy. Israel, in declaring itself, did so in defense against European anti-Semitism. Finally, the Palestinians, in their search for a national identity, are doing it in an adversarial relationship with the Israelis. It seems that most national identities form and evolve against a hated adversarial other.

Malcolm X, the movie directed by Spike Lee, is a fascinating study of the relationship between an individual personality and the groups that were operating during that period. The study of Malcolm X shows a personality during early adulthood that was quite diffuse and unable to adopt a working, functioning identity other than to be a con man and a pseudo-antisocial personality.

One can say that Malcolm X suffered from an identity diffusion or a poorly defined sense of self. However, an alternative explanation may search for an understanding of the group process during that period. It is important to understand this identity diffusion in the black male population as resulting from the unconscious communication of group racism in which the black and white populations collectively colluded in the scapegoating of black men, leaving them with a nonworkable, economically disenfranchised sense of themselves. While in prison, Malcolm X began to discover a sense of himself under the leadership of a Black Muslim inmate. He developed a sense of who he was in opposition to the "white devil."

As his identity became more secure, he began to flourish as a participant in the Black Muslim community. However, Malcolm, a strongly individuated personality, began to search for new, alternative expressions of himself that came into conflict with two hostile group containers of that period—the Black Muslims and white racist America. If the individual grows past the tolerance of the group container, then there seems to be a collision between the individual self and the group self.

This raises a number of interesting questions. Can a child individuate beyond the capacity of the parental objects? Can a patient improve beyond the disorder of the therapist?

As Malcolm's individuating self moved beyond the capacity of the two groups of that period, a major tragedy was in the offing. In my opinion, when the individuating self moves beyond the capacity of the group container, then a position of interpersonal catastrophe is reached that can only be resolved by one of two methods—revolution or the slaughter of the individuated self, which I am calling martyrdom.

It is as if the conflict between the individuating self and the rigid group container cannot be maintained, and a revolution takes place when the self overthrows the existing group and builds a new group that is more consistent with the needs of the individual. The other possibility is the group murder of the individuating self, where that individual becomes a martyr.

In a revolutionary group, the old structure is not lost, but is reabsorbed into the new group structure and kept in the memory of the group. For instance, after the Communists overthrew the leadership of czarist Russia, the memory of the old order was still retained in a modified form 70 years later. Similarly, if the group destroys the individuating self, it retains a memory trace of the individual that is reintegrated into the group at a later period, as the group evolves, matures, and is able to absorb the ideas of the slaughtered leader in a more integrated form.

This process clearly took place in the case of Malcolm X. Twenty-five years after his death, the groups of that period have evolved, moving from their basic fight–flight dynamics, and are now able to reabsorb the ideas of Malcolm X in a more metabolizable manner.

This process is clearly seen in group psychotherapy. If a particular personality is unable to be integrated into the group, the position of interpersonal catastrophe is reached, which is resolved by the group's extruding that particular group member. However, that group member is retained in the memory of the group, and is often brought up at particular points in the group process as a lost spokesperson.

The final basic assumption described by Bion is called pairing (BAP). During a pairing group, there is an alliance or a union between two or more group members, which is interpreted by the group as a sexual union to create the new unborn messianic leader. According to Bion, the purpose of this group is to create a new sense of hope in the unborn messianic leader, but it is hope that is based on religious magic and not on the work of conflict resolution and interpersonal management. Examples of pairing assumptions are seen on an international level every Christmas season, when a spirit of messianic hope dominates, but then abates when the holidays end.

This phenomenon is very similar to the type of transcendent invulnerable sense of self that has been described by Masterson (1981) as resulting from the fusion of self and object images in the narcissistic personality disorder. It also helps describe the sense of hope that people feel in romantic love and in the institution of marriage.

The basic assumption and its false sense of messianic hope must be differentiated from the real hope that is involved in the work function group through the management, clarification, and resolution of interpersonal conflicts. Bion cites several examples that exploit this basic pairing assumption. The aristocracy, with its emphasis on breeding to create an elite offspring, was an example of pairing fantasies that were operating on a national group level. Communists, with their emphasis on a union of workers to create a new person, is another example of such an assumption. A more nefarious example of this pairing assumption was that of the Nazis, who tried to create a new race by encouraging the breeding of Aryan individuals and exterminating non-Aryans.

All three of Bion's basic assumptions must be understood as irrational, magical fantasies that are mobilized by the group in order to defend against unconscious fears of disintegration. They can be seen as attempts to preserve the continuity, survival, and perpetuation of the group, when the group is most concerned about disintegration, death, and extinction. According to this position, the basic assumptions of group life are most analogous to the primitive defense mechanisms of disorders of the self that have been described by Masterson (1976).

While the study of group process, the work function group, group conflicts, and basic assumptions is the model that is being used by this author, other theorists (Yalom, 1969) have criticized Bion and the group process model as a form of psychotherapeutic treatment. According to Yalom, the basic assumptions described by Bion are interesting but incomplete, and he speculates that there may be many other basic assumptions that are operating in groups at various times. While this criticism may be correct, I feel it does nothing to diminish the valid contributions of Bion in at least highlighting and describing several key dynamics that are operating to deal with group anxiety and conflict.

Yalom further criticizes Bion's work when concluding that the interpretation of group process does not effectively use the most important ingredients to mobilize change in group therapy. He speculates that the individual may be lost in such an interpretive approach while too much emphasis is being placed on the group dynamics. He emphasizes an approach that focuses more on the individual dynamics in the group, and utilizes the process of interpersonal learning and new social role development that can develop in the group.

I have two objections to Yalom's criticism. First, if the group therapist ignores group process, then it will be pushed underground and acted out in more covert forms, eventually resulting in the disintegration of the group. This is very similar to Masterson's (1976) view that if the structural entity of the individual is ignored, it will lead to a mobilization of acting out and a breakdown of the therapeutic alliance. My second concern is that Yalom's emphasis on interpersonal role learning and modeling relies on the avoidance of intrapsychic structure and its manifestations in group life and on a more superficial social learning approach that borders on a reparenting model of change.

My firm conviction is that intrapsychic structure that is ignored can only express itself in alternative routes (most notably, acting out), and that new interpersonal learning that is superimposed on such a system of denial can only result in superficial compliant behavioral change that is less durable. However, I do agree with Yalom's concern that the individual can get lost in the massive, routinized, somewhat stereotyped interpretations of group process.

The group psychotherapeutic model that is being recommended here employs two primary interventions: interpretation of group process and focus on the individual dynamics, particularly on how that person is used as a spokesperson for the covert unconscious needs of the group at that moment. This heightened awareness of the individual's behavior in groups can focus on the person's vulnerabilities, and how his or her particular characterlogical structure is exploited in groups.

The model of treatment that I am recommending (as opposed to Yalom's) also views group psychotherapy as a secondary adjunctive treatment to individual psychotherapy. All participants can engage in group interaction and get a further working through of intrapsychic structure in their individual therapies. While I agree that Yalom's criticisms have merit regarding the psychotherapeutic intention of group psychotherapy for the individual, I must disagree with his belief that the therapist should avoid the clarification and interpretation of group process.

GROUP MATURATION AND DEVELOPMENT

As a group matures, a number of developments take place. First, the basic assumptions of the group not only become less harsh, but they shift from opposing the work of the group and being extremely disruptive to advancing the work of the group.

This is similar to the initial projections of the rewarding object relations unit of a borderline patient. At first, such projections are radically opposed to the psychotherapeutic work and the development of a therapeutic alliance. As the treatment progresses and the reality ego of the patient becomes stronger, such projections are utilized in the service of work to gain further understanding, insight, and development.

While the initial assumptions of group life are attempts to preserve the group and to deal with the disintegrating fears and anxieties, the later work of the group becomes manifest by showing an integration of basic assumptions with the work function. Thus the group with a stronger reality ego and commitment to the work of the interpersonal resolution begins to examine its own basic assumptions, resulting in further growth and development. In other words, there develops an integration of the two primary modes of group functioning—the work function and the basic assumptions come together in order to service the purpose of group insight and maturation. There is an integration of the rational logical needs of the group and the magical, illusory, and transcendent fantasies.

A second development that takes place as the group matures is the relative ease with which new members can be introduced and the diminished upset that results from the loss of old members. It is as if the group structure has become sturdier and is able to handle the evolutionary process.

A third change is the increased capacity of the observing ego of the group, which results in the improved identification of group conflict, basic assumptions, and the improved skill in conflict management, interpersonal functioning, and containment of maladaptive personality distortions.

Through the continuous interpretation of group process, the basic assumptions become less harsh and anxiety provoking, and the group will rid itself of excessively disturbing members through more democratic procedures that emphasize discussion, clarification, and the joint recognition that some members are more appropriate for the group than are others. The violent exclusion of members during the early phase of the group begins to transform itself into the somewhat mournful recognition that not all individuals are appropriate for the group.

GROUP PSYCHOTHERAPIC TECHNIQUE

Masterson (1986) has rightfully declared the position of the individual therapist as the guardian of the real self. A similar position must be maintained for the group therapist. However, the focus of the group therapist has to be the collective self of the group, and in order to preserve such an awareness, the therapist must assiduously avoid the focus on individual dynamics and structure. The group therapist must maintain a heightened awareness of the group self—its dynamics, structure, defenses, and covert unconscious needs. The therapist must continuously search for the dynamics of this larger structure, and view it as an entity that needs to be understood, clarified, and targeted as an object of intervention.

The primary intervention in group psychotherapeutic work for disorders of the self is the interpretation of group process. The interpretation must include a focus on the task of the group, the conflicts and fears that are operating in the group, and the basic assumptions, and on how various individuals are being used by the group to preserve its structure and to express its covert unconscious needs.

This model of group psychotherapy views the individual participant as a soldier in the group's army. For example, a paranoid patient may be used to mobilize a fight–flight dynamic, or if the group is trying to disengage from excessive anxiety caused by a particular conflict, it may call on the schizoid patient to help with the process of disengagement. It is as if the group takes a very accurate characterological X-ray of each group participant, scanning the psyche of each member upon introduction into the group, and exploits and recruits that person to service the particular need of the group. The group, according to Bion, is always concerned with the integrity of the group, and in order to maintain itself, it has a tendency to ignore the needs of the individual. The group therapist, however, by focusing on the individual as an exploited participant, can help the individual take a stand in opposition to the fear that the individual is being submerged in the group process.

Masterson (1981) has described some of the countertransference paradigms that operate if the therapist resonates and identifies with any of the structural projections of the patient. The group therapist has a similar task—

to maintain a position of technical neutrality by resolutely avoiding resonance with any basic assumption projections, and stay clear of providing group gratification through identification with those projections. The group therapist who does maintain a position of neutrality, and does not resonate with any of the three basic assumptions, will produce the same irritation, anger, or devaluation of his or her role that the individual therapist will observe from maintaining a position of technical neutrality. The benefit of maintaining such a position will be the improved reality ego of the group, clarification of interpersonal conflict, and the development of the structure and cohesiveness of the group as a work modality for the study of interpersonal conflict.

Masterson (1976) has described the movement from a testing phase of psychotherapy to the working-through phase. The patient seems to be more able to contain defenses and projections, modify behavior, and become increasingly aware, observant, and understanding of thoughts, affects, and fantasies. On a group level, a similar process can be noticed, as maturation and cohesion of the group lead to a greater ability by the group members to observe group process, gain insight, modify interpersonal behavior, and be less reliant on the activity of the group therapist. The leader of the group can take a less active position as the structure of the group and the abilities of the group members become stronger.

The interpretation of individual dynamics should be ignored by the group leader as it may be unconsciously colluding with the group's need to rid itself of a bad member, and may reflect the therapist's need to resonate with this group dynamic. Instead, the group therapist can focus on the individual's relationship to the collective group need, and on how the group has called on that particular personality to express its conflict. The intrapsychic working through for the individual must be addressed with the individual therapist. As the interpretations of group process strengthen the reality ego of the group, there is a shift away from magical defensive resolutions and a move toward the clarification and negotiation of interpersonal conflict. While some therapists have focused on the leader's need to police the group and to avoid a scapegoating process, this author suspects that severe scapegoating is the result of the therapist's failure to interpret group process (in particular, fight–flight dynamics) and does not necessarily evolve as a natural process.

It seems to be difficult for the individual therapist to let go of the notion of the primacy of the individual self and to focus on the group as an entity. It is as if the fantasy of individuation taking place in a vacuum is maintained by most therapists, as opposed to the more realistic position emphasized here that considers the constant interplay between the individual and the group.

Individuation takes place in a group context. For example, can a black person, no matter how highly individuated his or her self is, truly develop in South African society? Similarly, can any theorist fully develop ideas in isolation? Psychoanalytic theory has always evolved in the context of groups. Freud developed his ideas in the context of the psychoanalytic movement. Kohut similarly developed a group of self psychologists to promote his ideas. Finally, Masterson, in order to develop his theories, established the Masterson Group and Institute.

The truly individuated adaptive self recognizes, consciously or unconsciously, his or her need for groups as a container of individuation rather than taking a negativistic or oppositional stance toward those groups. Therefore, when the interpretation of group process is recommended as the primary tool in group psychotherapy that cannot be confused with relegating the individual to an inferior status, but must be seen as emphasizing the importance of the interplay between the individual and the group. Finally, this model of treatment maintains a clear focus on the combination of individual psychotherapy and group psychotherapy, in order to gain maximal benefit from group involvement.

PATIENT SELECTION FOR GROUP PSYCHOTHERAPY

Therapists often ask which disorders of the self are appropriate for group psychotherapy. It is my opinion that the intrapsychic structure of the particular patient is not extremely important in the selection of patients for group treatment. Most intrapsychic structures are appropriate for group selection, with the exception of the psychopathic disorder of the self, since this patient has a conscious intent to exploit the group or to destroy its effectiveness.

Similarly, there are contraindications to each of the disorders of the self, making patient selection a task that must be carried out with discrimination and accuracy. Each individual participant can be seen as a characterological spokesperson for the group needs at a particular moment. For example, a clinging borderline patient may be used to represent the thwarted attachment needs of the group, while a detached schizoid can be used by the group members to disengage and withdraw from one another. In a similar way, a narcissistic patient may be used to reinforce cohesion, as he or she unconsciously speaks for the fusion needs of the group.

A group therapist becomes very cognizant of the idle and superficial conversation that takes place prior to the group's convening. He or she must also take note of the initial conversation, or who the spokesperson is, and the content of the talk, as this sets the tone for the theme of the group. The individual patient is not consciously concerned with the group and its evolutionary development, but is there to identify maladaptive defensive interpersonal styles, to develop better management of these conflicts, and to try on new ways of communicating and relating to others.

The group, as an interpersonal laboratory, acts as a potential for acting out, but soon becomes a container if the group process is clarified through the use of interpretation. It is a very useful conceptualization to see the group as an experimental laboratory where the participants identify interpersonal distortions and defenses and use the conflictual patterns that emerge to gain containment and mastery. This model, however, emphasizes the need for a conjoint individual psychotherapy to work through the anxiety and conflict that become exacerbated during the group process. Working through is not possible through the utilization of group therapy without the addition of individual psychotherapy.

While the intrapsychic structure of the patient may not be that important for group selection, the ego strengths of the participants are extremely potent variables. Group cohesion and development depend on the homogeneity of ego strength in outpatient groups. In other words, participants in an outpatient psychotherapy group for the disorders of the self seem to require a minimal level of moderate ego strength, and lower-level patients with severe ego deficits will produce a severe regressive pull on a higher-level group exhibiting group anxiety about integration, which will lead to the mobilization of primitive defenses of group extrusion and scapegoating. I have found that this kind of group psychotherapy is contraindicated for those patients who have acute symptomatic stress, an underlying addictive process, a psychotic disorder, or a serious mood disorder. Furthermore, persons with low-level disorders of the self with serious ego deficits and reality distortions usually should not be admitted since they threaten the cohesion and continuity of the group. When such patients are brought into the group, a collusive relationship seems to arise between the subject and the group to extricate the group from the presence of that individual in order to maintain a sense of survival.

Individual patients seem to have different perceptions of the group according to their intrapsychic structures. For instance, patients with a psychotic organization often view group interaction as a threatening loss of self and a major stress on already tenuous ego boundaries, resulting in psychotic distortions that heighten group anxiety. The antisocial personality senses opportunity in the group experience, and mobilizes group revolt, and utilizes the process to exploit group anxiety for personal manipulative reasons. The person with an exhibitionistic narcissistic disorder perceives the group as a source of admiration and acknowledgment and a gratification of fusion needs by positioning himself or herself as a subject of authority. The person with a closet narcissistic disorder, on the other hand, views the group as a potential source of shameful exposure and anxiety and uses other members as a façade to hide behind. This patient may also use other group members to express frightening aspects of the self. The borderline patient views the group as a potential for being loved and cared for but at times sees it as a frightening, attacking, scapegoating entity. The schizoid patient tends to see the group as a place in which to map out a safe interpersonal space—somewhere between connection and disengagement.

While most of the disorders of the self can benefit from outpatient group psychotherapy, a mid-level to upper-level ego-functioning patient is most responsive to this modality of treatment, as the participants need enough free energy to observe their interpersonal patterns and identify their distortions. Although this requirement is essential for outpatient treatment of disorders of the self, it is not necessary for the inpatient treatment of such disorders since the hospital milieu serves as a secondary container to prevent severe regressive acting out.

In summary, group psychotherapy provides an exceptional opportunity for many persons with disorders of the self to master the inherent conflict between the self and the object. The conflictual relationships that take place in group provide a natural boundary pressure on the self that provokes two primary defenses. The first defense is schizoid withdrawal or isolation as a protective moving of the self away from the group. The second defense is group fusion and attachment, which is a defensive absorption of the self by the group. Both of these defenses work against the developmental need to maintain a sense of self within the context of group pressure. The group acts as an in vivo laboratory, moving the participants toward the goal of relatedness with a maintenance of the self. In the initial phases of group development, members will often complain and devalue the group or the therapist. The therapist will hear complaints about the group's being cold and nonsupportive, and a collective need will be expressed to flee dangerous interactions or to transform the group into a warmer and more loving environment. If the group members are simultaneously participating in individual psychotherapy, they will soon identify these perceptions as external manifestations of their internal world and will use the group to contain the perceptions rather than act on them. Furthermore, the participants will learn that they can only strengthen a sense of self within the context of conflictual interpersonal relationships, and the group's acting as a vehicle for conflict provides each participant with the opportunity for mastery.

In summary, group psychotherapy can be a useful adjunctive treatment to individual psychotherapy.

COUNTERTRANSFERENCE IN GROUPS

If the therapist does not maintain a neutral interpretive stance toward the basic assumptions, then a position of countertransference and potential group arrest has developed. The following are several classic countertransference positions that can take place in a group psychotherapy situation. The first position is called "the loving leader." This group leader identifies with the basic assumption of dependence and becomes an oracle giving guidance and advice to the group members. An infantalization process takes place as such a leader encourages regressive dependent behavior, and group members, rather than identifying interpersonal distortions and defenses, feel cared for and use it as a stress reducer for real external conflictual relationships.

The second countertransference position can be called "the appeaser or the false prophet." This therapist projects all bad interpersonal relationships outside of the group and identifies group members as good, concerned, caring, and available people. It is not unusual in this group to hear complaints about the spouses and intimate partners of the various group members. The group begins to feel like an alliance against the external world, and the interpersonal conflicts in the group are ignored.

The next group therapist who falls into a countertransference trap will be called "the ally." This therapist is seen as favoring some patients over others, and unconsciously is viewed by the group members as a seductive or hostile threat. The therapist is viewed as potentially splitting the group, exacerbating unconscious fears of disintegration and scapegoating.

The final countertransference position is carried out by the group leader who can be called "the demonic leader." The demonic leader usually has a paranoid or psychopathic personality, and exploits the fight–flight dynamics of group life by maintaining leadership through the persecution of various participants. In its extreme form, it can result in group murder of one or several participants, but more typically involves the persecution or ostracism of various group members. Modern history is replete with demonic leaders ranging from Hitler to today's cult leaders.

The final countertransference position has to do with the conflict between individual therapists and group psychotherapists. When an individual therapist refers a patient to group, that mobilizes the therapist's anxiety about exposing his or her work to another therapist and to a group of patients. It is essential that both therapists operate from positions of theoretical compatibility, be able to discuss various fears and apprehensions about working together, and be willing to explore mutual countertransference problems. If the two therapists coordinate their efforts, any splitting mechanisms that are being used by the patient will be confronted and contained. If the therapists are not compatible, then the patient's splitting mechanisms will be utilized to act out and destroy both treatments simultaneously.

Most patients with disorders of the self, when presented with the threat of group anxiety, will immediately mobilize themselves to take a position of divide and conquer. This usually, but not always, takes the form of devaluing the group and idealizing the individual therapist. Individual therapists can identify with this idealization by some patients, while referring difficult patients to the group. It is important to emphasize, however, that the group cannot be seen as a wastebasket to hold difficult or intractable patients. The outpatient group experience affords the opportunity for persons with middle-level disorders of the self to identify interpersonal distortions and should not be used by individual therapists as a way to remove difficult patients from their practices.

CLINICAL PROCESS

The Opening Phase of an Outpatient Psychotherapy Group

The group begins with the members sitting in anxious silence. Some question how to begin and others ask if there are rules of order. Ted turns to me and asks, in a sarcastic manner, "What's up, Doc?" The group laughs. One person says, "I hope this is not a stereotyped group with a bunch of hostile patients and a therapist who sits there like Buddha." Another member asks me if I could give some advice on beginning.

I tell the group that there seems to be considerable anxiety about beginning, which the group handles by turning to me for direction. Ted, in his usual way, says, "I guess we are stuck with a paper tiger for a leader." Jeff speaks up, "Unless, of course, you want to be the leader." Another member interjects that a problem in the group may be that they are looking for complete direction. There is a prolonged period of silence. Jean, a passive-aggressive borderline, begins by saying, "Why don't we introduce ourselves?" Everyone decides that first names are friendlier. This is followed by another prolonged silence. I note that although the group has settled on first names, the issue seems to be trusting each other enough to reveal themselves to each other. First names were chosen because the people were not ready to be known by each other. Ted quickly concludes that my interpretation is "bullshit." He says, "Outside of here, I have great friendships." Jeff responds, "Then why are we all sitting in a group of personality disorders?"

Jean says she would like to begin. The group calls it the hot seat. She talks about the intimate details of her sex life with her husband. Some group members give advice. Ted flirts with her, and says that she should leave her husband. Jeff said, "You come on as a nice guy, but I don't trust your motives." The group is quite harsh with Jean and very critical of her. I tell the group that they seem to be trying to deal with the frightening task of opening up to each other but the attempt to reveal intimate matters so quickly only reinforces the fear that this is a dangerous place and process. Ted quickly responds by saying that he has been in much more supportive groups than this one. Other members conclude that the group feels unsafe.

The next several sessions focus on turning to me for advice, devaluing my leadership, and the hot-seat phenomenon, where members give superficial presentations and receive superficial advice. Ted continues to devalue the group and names the hot seat the electric chair. Jeff seems to be the guardian of the group, and Kate complains that her depression has become worse since she joined the group. The group seems to focus on external relationships and concludes that all outsiders, spouses included, are bad.

I interpret the fear of presenting problems in the group, and the need to walk away with the safe conclusion that the problem is out there. Ted continues to ridicule me and Jeff promptly protects my role as the leader of the group. The group continues to focus on outside people, and interactions in the group are primarily giving advice. The group process becomes more devalued and labeled as a "cold place." My interpretations continually focus on the tremendous fear of revealing oneself to strangers that has caused the participants to blame the group or the environment.

By the seventh session, Kate comes in late and turns her back to the group. She says that her therapist has called it a "nonnurturing environment" and told her to terminate her membership in the group. She continues by telling the group that she can call her individual therapist at any hour of the night and that he hugs her and tells her that she is a wonderful person. She goes on to describe a dream in which she is at a funeral and no one can comfort one another. The priest is unable to provide support. Ted then says that Kate's problem is the therapist. He says, "I'll run this group in my office and charge less money." Jeff says, "We have problems, but do you think we are crazy?" Another member says she has to leave the group for financial reasons. Someone else turns to me and says, "Do something. This family is falling apart."

I interpret the enormous anxiety about being locked into a process like this and that there seem to be two group wishes: one is to preserve the group as a container to deal with feelings and the other is to destroy the dreaded container. I then add that the group has called on two spokespersons for this conflict. Jeff seems to be the guardian of the group, and Ted seems to be the hit man. I then express confidence in the group's wisdom in resolving the conflict. Ted waves his hand at me in a diminishing manner. Kate terminates the group during that session.

Tom unsuccessfully tries to recruit the members and does not show up for the next group session. Another member leaves for financial reasons. The group is badly fragmented at this point, but is stronger and more committed to the therapeutic process.

A number of lessons can be learned from this initial period of group development. First, there was a continuous interplay of the basic assumptions of dependence and fight–flight. The initial threat of group cohesion and containment provoked the defenses of externalization and devaluation, and a search for a magical oracle to relieve the group of the interpersonal conflicts of trusting and communication. The hostility to developing this group container for interpersonal communication came from several sources, such as an outside individual therapist, Ted; the group; and, finally, myself as part of the group process of ambivalence. It is important to understand that every participant, including the therapist, is a reflective mirror of the internal fears of the group, and since this group was ambivalent about building a group container, all voices became spokespersons for that fear, including mine. My ambivalence clearly expressed itself by refusing to take a more confrontative and firmer stance toward the destructive attitude that Ted was communicating in the group. Furthermore, I was not careful in my screening of patients from other therapists who did not work in a style compatible with the Masterson Approach, which set into motion the dangerous process of splitting between the individual therapist and group therapist.

This opening phase of the group also clearly illustrates how group process can be used as a natural screening device for disorders of the self, as the process will gradually eliminate psychopathic individuals, low-level personality disorders, and outside therapists who threaten the cohesion and integrity of the group's development. Finally, a statement must be made about the passive or ambivalent leader. There seems to be little room for passivity or ambivalence on the part of the therapist, particularly in the early phase of group development, as such a stance will only become part of the group's unconscious need to destroy an interpersonal container that must be maintained for further clarification and understanding of interpersonal distortions.

The Middle-Phase

Three years later, there is a relatively cohesive group dealing with ingroup interactions, and defending by focusing on outside group issues. The group deals with unbearable conflict through the search for magical alliances. Some members talk about being friendlier with other members. There seems to be an affiliative search within the group. The women and men seem to be sitting on opposite sides of the room. At times, someone verbalizes having a brief sexual feeling for another participant in the group. The women begin to talk about the insensitivity of the men.

I interpret the frightening aspect of sexual tension and the group way of dealing with it by sitting on opposite sides of the room. The group members spend several sessions disengaged from one another and begin to focus on Karen, a schizoid member, becoming angry at her silence and her attempt to "deaden the group." I point out that the group is still not ready to face certain tensions and has chosen withdrawal and disengagement as a way of dealing with this. The consequence is feelings of deadness, which they prefer to blame on Karen.

Kathy, an upper-level borderline patient, talks about wanting to get together with the others after the group. Steve complains that the group has trouble getting together in the office. Kathy presents a dream about having an anxiety attack on the subway and being saved by holding onto Steve's hand. The group becomes scattered at that point and begins to focus on Alice, as she becomes tangential and difficult to understand. Steve calls her crazy and recommends that she leave the group. The women begin to shout at him for being insensitive.

I point out that the recognition of certain feelings for each other is so threatening that the group wants to either direct interaction outside of the room or throw disturbing people out of the group. Kathy spends many sessions discussing her attempts to become pregnant. Group members talk about yearning for her pregnancy. They call it the magical baby. Steve complains that he is not getting enough attention and asks why Jane, the Ice Princess, never talks to him. She says that she is shy, but would like to communicate with him. I point out that the group members are very tentative about direct contact with one another and seem to be playing a game of hide-and-seek. Kathy says that she finally has become pregnant. There is a sense of joy in the room, and one member calls it magical. For the next several sessions, interactions are superficial and fleeting. Kathy's pregnancy becomes the focus of all group discussion.

I interpret the underlying conflicts about direct feeling, particularly between men and women, and focus on the effort of the group to move away from this through the discussion of the magical child. Steve begins to attack Alice, saying that she does not belong in this group. I point out that dealing with disturbing feelings belongs in this group—magical solutions do not.

Several sessions later, Kathy calls and cancels her attendance in the group. She has had a miscarriage. The group descends into a feeling of depressive despair. Members talk about getting nowhere in solving their problems. They feel that their efforts are futile. I interpret their fears of lost hope and wonder why all their hopes were based on Kathy's pregnancy rather than working on their interactions. Steve says, "I guess life goes on." Other participants agree with him, but all conclude that a piece of them has died.

A number of conclusions can be stated about the middle phase of this group's development. First, there seems to be a greater ability to face interpersonal conflict, but there is still a reliance on the basic assumption of pairing and fight–flight to defend against heightened anxiety. There also seems to be a growing tension about intimate feelings, particularly sexual ones that threaten interpersonal contacts within the group. Finally, there seems to be a combination of work that takes place in the group, and periodic flight into basic assumptions to defend against heightened anxiety, fear, and conflict. In general, the group is more cohesive, with a greater integrity, purpose, and durability to deal with emerging group conflict.

Recent Group

The group begins with a tense awareness that nobody in the group is happily married. Dave complains about his ex-wife. The women become angry at his arrogance. Susan says that he acts like a Nazi with women. There is silence. She says that she feels great tension between the men and the women in the group. She adds that she feels embarrassed at that moment. She goes on to say that she has been feeling a sexual attraction to

Dave and that she becomes hostile whenever she feels that way. The group begins to focus on Susan's problem with men. I say that the group members would prefer to talk about Susan's problem with men rather than face certain feelings that are taking place in the group.

Dave changes the subject and begins to talk about a new love relationship. The group focuses on the problems in that relationship and begins to dismantle it. One member says that the group does not allow love to be experienced. One male patient maintains that he feels left out of the loop. Susan says that her feelings toward Dave are really quite minimal.

I wonder aloud if the group feels that loving feelings will bring out intolerable competition and envy, which would result in the group's dismissal of loving feelings inside and outside the group.

Steve says that the room is hot and asks about opening a window. Susan says she hopes the group will end soon so that she can leave. Several members comment on the tension in the room.

At the next session, all the men are late. The discussion is superficial and disconnected. The group's focus is on a schizoid member's distance.

I point out that this focus and the men's lateness suggest that the group still does not want to face problems with intimate feelings and needs. A low-level borderline patient begins to attack various group members and the group calls her crazy. There is shouting in the room. I just say that this group has a much easier time fighting than it does dealing with loving feelings.

Dave says that he would like to get back to Susan's feelings toward him. He says, "I like you, but I really have a mad crush on Jane, the Ice Princess." Susan looks shocked, as do most of the group members. Jane says that she is flattered but annoyed because people always love her as an exotic fantasy. She talks about how her father made her the object of his adoration rather than deal with his problems with her mother. Dave says he thinks that he and Jane could make a perfect baby. Steve says that he may be envious of all that is going on, but that Dave should consider knowing a woman before making a baby.

I point out that the group is still threatened by the direct expression of intimate feelings, but magical avoidance solutions do not seem to be working anymore. Everyone feels that this is a very tough issue that needs to continue to be considered, and they ask me not to bring in any more nutty patients who distract the group work.

Several conclusions can be drawn from this phase of the group's development. First, there is a much stronger reality ego in the group, which enables the participants to make a greater identification of conflicts and defenses that are operating during the process. There seems to be more direct work taking place within the group as higher-level issues of sexuality competition and envy are being addressed. There seems to be a greater commitment to the work and identification of interpersonal conflict, and there seems to be a legitimate request to avoid the introduction of group members who might distract the group from continuing with the work.

Perhaps the group was giving a signal to the group therapist to avoid any unconscious collusion with group resistance. If the therapist were to introduce persons with low-level disorders of the self at this point, it would only steer the group away from the crucial process that needs to take place.

CONCLUSION

Group work can be of great value as a secondary adjunctive treatment for many disorders of the self. While it is true that only individual psychoanalytic therapy can work through the intrapsychic structure of disorders of the self, group psychotherapy can be used to identify interpersonal distortions and maladaptive behavioral patterns, and to help contain defenses that interfere with positive interactions. It is also important to understand that reaching the goal of individuation and emancipation of the self does not take place in a vacuum, but always operates in a group context.

In the future, it will be appropriate for most individual therapists to ask what combinations of treatment will be most effective in helping their patients to identify maladaptive defenses, improve containment, and facilitate more positive communication and interaction on a personal level. Group psychotherapy is certainly not appropriate for all disorders of the self, but is extremely useful with interpersonal problems.

All disorders of the self suffer from an impairment in interpersonal relationships. The group process and the identification of interactions within the group provide a marvelous experimental laboratory in which many persons can be helpful to identify these patterns, modify them, and develop new and more adaptive interpersonal styles.

GROUP PROCESS: THE MEMBERS

Initial Group

Ted: Psychopathic disorder of the self—self-proclaimed therapist. His therapist initially saw him as having a low-level narcissistic personality disorder.

Jeff: Closet narcissistic personality disorder. Family history includes taking care of family after his father abandoned them. Feels overly responsible in relationships.

Kate: Low-level borderline personality disorder with mood disorder. Has a history of a harsh, depriving, and passive father. Present therapist resonates with RORU and reparents her.

Other group members include an assortment of disorders of the self.

Middle-Phase Group

Steve: Exhibitionistic narcissistic personality disorder (50 years old). Tries to monopolize the group and direct the interaction. Currently struggling with a bitter divorce and business failure.

Kathy: Upper-level borderline personality disorder (35 years old). Comes from a large family and experienced maternal neglect. Responsible for keeping family interactions intact.

Karen: Schizoid disorder (35 years old). A silent group member. Views relationships as controlling and persecutory.

Jane: Closet narcissistic personality disorder (25 years old). Foreign-born, quiet member, but is seen as exotic and seductively alluring. Known as the Ice Princess.

Alice: Borderline psychotic (35 years old) with reality-testing problems when under stress.

Recent Group

Dave: Forty-eight-year-old schizoid who complains about feeling alienated in relationships; recently divorced.

Susan: Closet narcissistic personality disorder (35 years old) with conflicts around gender identity. Provocative interactions followed by withdrawal.

Steve: Same patient from the middle-phase group.

Jane: Same patient from the middle-phase group.

Sarah: Thirty-year-old borderline psychotic who views relationships as dangerous and hateful.

REFERENCES

Bion, W. R. (1961). *Experiences in groups and other papers*. New York: Basic Books.

Masterson, J. F. (1976). *Psychotherapy of the borderline adult: A developmental approach*. New York: Brunner/Mazel.

Masterson, J. F. (1981). *The narcissistic and borderline disorders: An integrated and developmental approach.* New York: Brunner/Mazel.

Masterson, J. F. (1985). *The real self: A developmental self and object relations approach.* New York: Brunner/Mazel.

Masterson, J. F. (1988a). *The search for the real self: Unmasking the personality disorder of our age.* New York: Free Press.

Masterson, J. F. (1988b). *Psychotherapy of the disorders of the self: The Masterson approach.* (R. Klein & J. F. Masterson, Eds.). New York: Brunner/Mazel.

Yalom, T. (1969). *The theory and practice of group psychotherapy.* New York: Basic Books.

CHAPTER 19

Couples Therapy of Patients with Disorders of the Self

Ken Seider, Ph.D.

The study and treatment of patients with a disorder of the self has largely been carried out within the confines of individual psychoanalytic psychotherapy or psychoanalysis. Although the initial pioneers in family and couples therapy were trained in psychoanalytic theory (Nichols, 1984), with few exceptions, there has been little cross-fertilization between those clinicians who can be characterized as systemic and family focused and those who are intrapsychic and individually oriented.

In this chapter, I will provide a rough outline of an integrated approach to couples therapy that utilizes the developmental self and object relations theory of the Masterson Approach. My intention is to describe clinical theory and techniques, as well as some of the signposts that indicate the transitions through the phases of treatment. Borrowing from Freud's famous chess analogy (Freud, 1913), I intend to provide a rough outline of the opening, middle, and closing moves.

DISORDERS OF THE SELF

Patients with a disorder of the self have pathological false-self organizations, whose defensive function is to avoid dysphoric affects, often at the expense of reality considerations and the expression of the real self. The false-self organization arises as a compromise formation, whose function is to maintain an attachment to the outside world. The false-self organization results in individuals' having impairments in their real-self capacities. They will have difficulties in intimacy, commitment, sharing, and empathy, as well as in the acknowledgment of others. They will report problems with self-soothing, self-acknowledgment, self-activation, creativity, and spontaneity, as well as not having a feeling of aliveness.

In general, the patient exhibits a disorder-of-the-self "triadic" defensive operation—separation and individuation, which activates dysphoric affect, which then is defended against, until appropriate therapeutic interventions are made. Knowledge of the triadic nature of defenses is useful, but a detailed and precise appreciation for the specific intrapsychic structure is necessary in order to engage the patient in a psychoanalytic process of treatment. The Masterson Approach offers an integrated developmental self and object relations theory that provides such a differential approach to diagnosis and treatment.

A thorough review of the Masterson Approach to differential diagnosis and treatment is not within the scope of this chapter, but has been treated extensively in the literature (Masterson, 1976, 1981, 1993; Klein, 1989, 1993). A brief overview is warranted.

The four diagnostic categories are the borderline, the narcissistic, the schizoid, and the antisocial disorders of the self. One can think of these disorders as modes of relating to oneself and others. For the borderline, it is reward for regression and withdrawal for separation and individuation. With the narcissistic disorder, of which there are two subtypes (exhibitionistic and closet), it is regulation of self-esteem by maintaining a sense of omnipotent grandiosity in order to avoid being harshly attacked for having flaws. For the schizoid, it is a sense of the interpersonal world as being unsafe, where to be attached is to become appropriated, but to be unattached is to risk being cut off from all personal relationships, to feel isolated and cosmically alienated. With the antisocial disorder, the self is totally detached and emotionally uninvolved with the object.

DIAGNOSIS

When conducting couples therapy from the Masterson perspective, the focus throughout all phases of treatment is on the couple's intrapsychic structures. With few exceptions, all of the therapist's responses to the couple are fed through a diagnostic understanding of each partner and are directed at modifying the defensive operations that are at the root of the couple's problems.

Case of Mr. and Mrs. A.

A couple came to me for their initial consultation with the presenting concern of how long therapy would take and how expensive it would be. From the outset of our first meeting, there was a push on me to respond to these concerns about the length and cost of treatment.

In the course of the first hour, the husband, in a somewhat distant and devaluing fashion, indicated that he expected little from couples therapy. The wife, in a complementary way, related her anticipation that she would be forced to endure her husband's mistreatment and dismissal of her, and that she would be made to have sex with him. The separation–individuation challenge of beginning couples therapy had activated, within each of them, defensive operations that were reflective of their intrapsychic structures. The problem in that initial meeting with the couple was to arrive at a differential diagnosis.

Differential diagnosis in couples therapy is arrived at in the same fashion as it is with individuals (Klein, 1989), with the added source of information that is culled from the partners' interactions with each other. Often couples at the outset of treatment will evidence interlocking projections and projective identifications that represent an acting out and activation of the negative internalized self and object relational part units. It has been my experience that the identification of these destructive interactional sequences aids in arriving at a differential diagnosis.

With Mr. & Mrs. A., I responded toward the end of the hour with a mirroring interpretation (Masterson, 1981, 1993) to the husband. I said, "One thing that I think is going on for you is that the prospect of investing yourself in this couples therapy and reinvesting yourself in your marriage makes you get in touch with feelings of hurt and rejection and you respond to those feelings in yourself with thoughts of leaving and stopping as a way of protecting yourself from those painful feelings." This was responded to by the husband with a strong "Yes" and an elaboration of how he also used the same distancing defense at home.

With the wife, I interpreted her schizoid dilemma. I stated to her, "I think investing here stimulates in you the fear that I and your husband will take you over and you will be forced into things, and that your own interests will be disregarded. I think you respond to this by taking a step back and removing yourself to what feels like a safer distance." Her response was affirmative and elaborative too.

In this vignette, I have differentially responded to each partner, based on a working hypothesis of his or her intrapsychic organization. I responded to this couple's concern about fees and length of treatment only when I could determine what their concerns meant to them. With the husband, I utilized a mirroring interpretation that was in keeping with my initial hypothesis of his having a narcissistic intrapsychic structure. With the wife, my interpretation was of her experience of interpersonal space in terms of her schizoid structure. It would not have been helpful at the opening of this couple's treatment to respond to the content level of their concerns, laying out the fees and approximate length of time treatment might take. What was called for was maintaining an intrapsychic focus.

The initial meetings with couples are primarily diagnostic. I will meet with a couple for one to three sessions, at the end of which I will provide the couple with my assessment and recommendation. In addition to the standard evaluations that make up the Masterson Approach to the disorders of the self (that is, self and ego functioning, developmental history, intrapsychic structure, and the nature of the individual's relationship to the therapist, or transference acting out), one must also assess the severity and tenacity of the negative and positive projections within the couple.

Most often, couples with disorders of the self come to treatment as a result of the activation of negative projections. The tenacity of these negative projections and projective identifications is often a prognostic indicator. Mr. & Mrs. A. responded readily and positively to my interventions, exhibiting good therapeutic potential.

Case of Mr. and Mrs. B.

Mr. and Mrs. B. had been through a number of couples treatments that failed. They began, though, with a clear picture of what their problems were. For each of them, it was obvious that the *other* needed to change. The wife described her husband as arrogant, demanding, devaluing, highly offensive, and insecure, and as expecting sex "no matter what." All that was needed was for her husband to change and she no longer would be "reactive." A mirror sketch was drawn by the husband of a highly seductive, vicious, biting, withholding, insensitive, and grossly unreasonable woman. All that was needed was for the wife to change. They did not have much capacity, at the outset, to reflect and focus on themselves, to identify what needs and feelings within themselves contributed to their difficulties.

These partners with exhibitionistic narcissistic disorders of the self failed to recognize what was at the base of their difficulties. For each of them, when they focused on themselves and made genuine moves toward intimacy, very painful feelings about themselves would become stimulated. For the wife, it was the feeling of being totally worthless and being stomped on, which, she reported, was the way she had been chronically treated in her family of origin. For the husband, it was the feeling of being nonexistent and suddenly abandoned—which was how he had often felt in his alcoholic family where his mother would suddenly leave the family for extended periods with little more than a note of farewell.

What each had very little capacity for, at the outset of treatment, was containing the painful affects that were stimulated by moves toward intimacy. My initial interpretations to this couple rolled off like water off a duck's back. Although each would briefly reflect on my comments, experience a sense of being understood, and then touch on his or her painful feelings, it would be only a matter of seconds before each would be off in the same direction of blaming the other. These painful affects were chronically projected and dumped onto the other, where the battle then became interpersonal rather than intrapsychic. They responded to me like a closed unit, unwilling to let me in, evidencing little therapeutic potential.

The strength and persistence of behavioral discharge of intrapsychic conflict need to be evaluated at the outset of treatment. The less persistent and intractable the interlocking projections are, the better is the prognosis.

At the end of the diagnostic evaluation, one should have a clear idea of each person's differential diagnosis, of how each person's intrapsychic organization is contributing to the couple's difficulties, of how these difficulties interlock, and if the modality of couples therapy is an appropriate one. After arriving at an initial understanding of the couple's problems, this is shared with the couple in plain language and a course of treatment is agreed upon.

INITIATION OF TREATMENT

Frame

Treatment is initiated against the backdrop of the therapeutic frame. The frame for couples therapy is the same as that for individual therapy with regard to responsibility for sessions, time, fees, and so on (Greenson, 1967; Langs, 1974; Masterson, 1976). In the literature, though, there has tended to be confusion about the role of the couples therapist. For example, the Scharffs, in their groundbreaking work *Object Relations Family Therapy* (1987), advocated that one can conduct an individual psychoanalysis with one of the members of the couple while also seeing that patient in couples therapy. In my opinion, this is neither possible nor desirable, for a variety of reasons.

Several years ago, a therapist came to me for a consultation that speaks to this very issue. She had begun seeing a couple, whom she had thought of as being neurotic, for difficulties in communication. Several months into their couples therapy, their difficulties had improved significantly, at which point each asked to see her individually, and the therapist agreed. After having seen them each individually for a couple of years, the man decided to leave the relationship. This was a gradual and unfolding decision for the man, but the therapist was bound by confidentiality not to reveal anything to his partner. Predictably, when the woman, who turned out to have a narcissistic disorder, learned of her partner's plans to leave, she felt betrayed by her therapist. Her injury and rage were so intense that it led her to file charges with the Board of Medical Examiners and to initiate legal action. At the outset of treatment, it needs to be made clear that a couples therapist can only wear that hat, and must refer patients elsewhere if a course of individual treatment is indicated.

Neutrality

The stance of analytic neutrality is of central importance in the conduct of couples therapy. The therapist limits his or her activities to clarifications, confrontations, and interpretations; educational or counseling-like suggestions are avoided. Although the therapist is an authentic, interested, and empathic human being, his or her job is to assist the couple in reflection and not to react in a directive fashion.

In addition to providing a reality screen upon which the patient's projections can be viewed, tested, and integrated, it serves the added function of demonstrating to the couple the possibility of a different kind of object relationship with each other. Over the course of time, the couple will internalize the therapist's stance toward them and begin to approach themselves and each other in a more realistic and less distorted fashion.

The couples therapist's neutrality serves as the starting point from which the couple can begin to align their observing egos with, and begin to develop a working relationship (Greenson, 1965) with, each other and the therapist. The stance of neutrality adopted by the couples therapist enables the therapist to piece together a coherent picture of the couple's problems. The picture arrived at is systemic and not a linear one (Watzlawick, Beavin,

Jackson, 1967; Hoffman, 1981; Keeney & Ross, 1985). The therapist who maintains a stance of neutrality will not 'blame' one partner more than the other for the couple's difficulties, but will arrive at a balanced view of how each person contributes to the couple's problems.

Systematic Triangulation

Often when couples first present themselves for treatment, they are in a very high state of distress. Sometimes, in the first session, they are on their best behavior, and act civilly toward each other. But at some point, the difficulties for which they sought therapy become manifest; that is, there is an activation of the negative interlocking projections, and they begin to act out in treatment. This phenomenon is one of the reasons that the beginning of couples therapy can be easier on the therapist than initiating an individual therapy. The partner is the object of the transference acting out, rather than the therapist. Although these data are useful diagnostically, if the destructive interactions are allowed to continue too long without being addressed successfully by the therapist, the therapeutic space will become filled with acting out, and what goes on in the consulting room will be no different from what goes on outside of sessions.

As Freud laid out in his paper "Remembering, Repeating and Working Through" (1914), the objective of treatment is to get patients to stop discharging their conflicts in behavior and to get them to remember and work through their problems intrapsychically. This tendency to externalize conflict is especially great in patients with disorders of the self, and is further exacerbated when patients are seen cojointly.

To interrupt the transference acting out sufficiently so that a therapeutic process can begin, I systematically triangle myself into the couple's conflict. Bowen was the first to outline how two-person systems engage a third party in their interactions when tension and anxiety exceed certain limits, which he called triangulation (Bowen, 1976; Kerr & Bowen, 1988). This principle of regulating tension within two-person systems is utilized by the therapist (Sluzkie, 1975). The partners' direct communication with each other is blocked, and each partner is then sequentially engaged with the therapist. The objectives are to assist the couple in detoxifying their communications and to encourage reflection and exploration of what lies beneath manifest problems. Strategic therapists, focusing on the interactional dimension of the therapist's activity, have referred to this as interdicting interactional sequences (Watzlawick, Weakland, & Fisch, 1974). On an intrapsychic level, what the therapist is trying to do is to stop the transference acting out, so that the intrapsychic conflict is no longer discharged in behavior and is accessible for self-reflection and analysis.

To illustrate, again consider couple A. When Mr. A. raised the issue about my fee and the length of therapy, this activated in Mrs. A. the feeling of being controlled, and she quickly shot back, "You are always so controlling." He responded, "I don't want couples therapy added to your list of things I'm doing wrong. Furthermore, all you are interested in is getting me to do things. And besides, what's the point to it all? We haven't had sex in a year." Very quickly, Mr. and Mrs. A. were at each other.

I responded by first engaging Mr. A. Through the use of clarification, I focused him on his experience of himself, and what feeling was beneath his concern about the length of treatment. When he identified feeling hopeless about ever changing things, he was able to articulate that he felt like giving up before starting. I then turned to Mrs. A. to clarify what lay behind her statements. She was able to express her concern that she was very fearful of couples therapy, and was deeply worried that she would end up being controlled and forced to do things that she did not want to do.

By interrupting their interactions with each other, and through the use of clarification, I was able to begin to tease out the subjective feelings in each of them that were activating the projections. For Mrs. A., it was the fear of being controlled, and for Mr. A., it was the fear of being criticized. The effect of the therapist's systematically becoming triangled in the relationship in this way results in calming things down and in making it possible for each member of the couple to focus on the subjective sense of self, and to begin to identify and express needs in a real and constructive fashion.

ACTING OUT OUTSIDE OF TREATMENT

While the therapist's activity in this initial phase of therapy is to calm things down in the sessions, simultaneous attention is given to reducing destructive interactions outside of sessions. The goal is to have the couple use the therapy sessions as an arena in which they can work things out. By creating a context in which each person feels listened to and understood, the couple is enticed into expressing and demonstrating their difficulties within the session, while containing their acting out outside of sessions. What results as this is gradually accomplished is an intensification of conflict in the sessions where they are subject to therapeutic intervention. Once this has been accomplished, the couple enters the working phase of treatment.

Case of Mr. and Mrs. C.

Mrs. C. called to set up an appointment for herself and her husband shortly after their honeymoon. Mrs. C., a successful professional, was extremely upset with her husband. She had discovered after their wedding that her husband had been involved in a number of business dealings with an unethical business partner. Mrs. C. had determined that Mr. C. was not aware of his partner's problems at the time he did business with him, but she found the fact that he had hid this from her deeply troubling. What was even more troubling was that she was unable to talk to him about it.

Mr. C. was very upset, as well. He felt that his wife was constantly criticizing him, and he could not understand why she became so hysterical. He would try to convey to her that it was not a "big deal," but when he did this, Mrs. C. would blow up and threaten divorce. After the initial diagnostic sessions, the outline and the intrapsychic meaning of this destructive interactional sequence were clear.

Mrs. C.'s diagnosis was difficult to ascertain. Initially, she presented as having a closet narcissistic disorder, attempting to bask in the glow of her husband's achievements and becoming narcissistically wounded when he disappointed her. What emerged upon closer scrutiny was a theme of wanting to be taken care of. As I switched from mirroring interpretations to confrontation, the borderline triad emerged. When she activated herself in the marriage, it would set in motion a predictable sequence. She would first thoughtfully express herself to her husband. She would then begin to experience herself as becoming emotional and would start crying. Very quickly, the tears would lead her to reach out in an almost helpless fashion. When she was not responded to, she experienced intense feelings of hopelessness. This then would activate in her the withdrawing object relations unit (Masterson, 1976), which she would, through projective identification, put onto her husband. She would now feel powerful—exploding, threatening divorce, and calling him names.

Mr. C. had a narcissistic disorder and was extremely sensitive to criticism. When his wife would engage him and he would begin to respond, that set in motion an increasing subjective awareness of feeling bad about himself, which he would deal with by pushing Mrs. C. away and by attempting to get the two of them onto the "real" business of purchasing expensive homes and constructing an exotic lifestyle. This interlocking sequence was repeatedly played out, resulting in many sleepless nights in separate bedrooms.

After I brought this sequence to the couple's attention, they were able to limit their destructive interactions outside of the sessions. Both agreed to deal with those issues for a time only in the sessions. They had also taken some constructive steps in structuring their time together, reporting that for the first time since they were married they had spent several enjoyable days together.

Predictably, there was an intensification of their conflict in sessions. This culminated in one session in which Mrs. C. became hysterical, took off her wedding ring, and said, "It's hopeless. We're never going to make progress." Mr. C., wanting to leave the office, said, "I've got to get out of here. I can't take this." They were now faced with a situation in which they were functioning better in their marriage but were feeling worse. It was at this critical juncture that I was able to interpret to them the interlocking nature of their difficulties, how steps toward intimacy had set in motion a sequence of internal responses that led to the present blowup.

I commented to Mrs. C. that it seemed that whenever she attempted to express herself deeply and intimately to her husband, this stimulated feelings of hopelessness, and then all of her awareness of the real improvements in their marriage went out the window. I added that if she were in a vacuum, this process would be hard enough to contain, but that her husband's withdrawal fueled her fears and made it an even greater challenge to regain her perspective. To Mr. C., I commented that when he made genuine attempts to become engaged with Mrs. C., this made him aware of feeling inadequate and so he would withdraw to protect himself from feeling bad. Furthermore, his wife's behavior reinforced the sense that the problem was out there, rather than in his own feelings about himself. I focused on this interlocking aspect of their negative projections with the intention of underlining the intrapsychic origins of their conflicts.

Following the intervention, both Mr. C. and Mrs. C. calmed down significantly. Mrs. C. responded by saying that she knew she ended up feeling that it was hopeless and that she did not really know why the improvements in their relationship did nothing to alter the feeling. Mr. C. responded that he loved his wife, that he did want to talk with her, and that he did not really understand why it was so hard to do so at times. In essence, Mr. C. and Mrs. C. were beginning to examine themselves and trying to understand their joint difficulties. The focus had gone from the other to the self. They had begun to reflect on the damage that was being done to their relationship by this pattern. This shift in focus marked for them, as it does for all couples, the beginning of the working phase of treatment. They were now in a position in which they both could recognize that steps toward intimacy stimulated in them feelings that they dealt with by projecting conflict into the relationship.

THE WORKING PHASE

In the working phase of treatment, the couple has begun to establish a working alliance (Greenson, 1965). I use Greenson's term to differentiate it from the therapeutic alliance (Zetzel, 1956). Essentially, the partners ally their observing reality egos in a collaborative fashion. Rather than projecting their conflicts into the relationship, they work together to understand what lies beneath their problems. This alliance serves as the foundation upon which each can identify his or her own needs and the needs of the other and overcome the obstacles to intimacy. At this point in treatment, many of the difficulties that the couple first presented have receded into the background. What now comes into center stage is the couple's examination of their own defensive operations and how these contribute to relationship difficulties.

At this stage, the isomorphic (Levenson, 1983) nature of therapy becomes more apparent; that is, the content of sessions often mirrors the process of interaction. The partners begin to collaborate with each other in identifying and overcoming difficulties. The climate of interaction has changed. There has been a shift from blaming the other to helping the other, from hiding one's problems to examining them. Often at this point in treatment, the couple will collaboratively embark on new projects, have a baby, do work around the house, buy a new home, or one of the partners will return to school. While these separation–individuation acts of the couple are the result of real self-activation, they will also set into motion defensive false self-mechanisms, but now these defenses can be subjected to mutual self-examination.

The work of the therapist at this stage is focused primarily on tracking and interpreting the couple's interlocking defensive operations. This includes stringing together for the couple defensive sequences of interaction so that the couple as a unit will have an appreciation of the defensive dance in which they engage. This phase is not equivalent to the working-through phase (Masterson, 1976, 1981) of individual treatment. Although affectively charged historical material will come into the picture at intervals during this phase of treatment, the overriding emphasis of the work is on the here-

and-now adaptation of the couple. Let us return to Mr. and Mrs. A. to illustrate this phase of treatment.

One year into their couples therapy, Mr. and Mrs. A. reported that their relationship was dramatically different. They were now regularly active sexually. Also, the family sat down to dinners together and ate without the television on. Every night, Mr. and Mrs. A. made a point of talking with each other about what was going on. Also, collaboratively they had decided that Mr. A. needed to return to school (which he recently did). It was around the coordination of their schedules that they were having difficulties. Mr. A. rarely informed his wife of his schedule, and often told her of changes at the last minute. He did this with the expectation that she was always "on the same page" he was—that is, fused—and that if he moved in one direction, she would move in that same direction without hesitating. Mrs. A. felt enslaved, a second-class citizen whose wishes and needs would be ignored. She had recently withdrawn, both physically and emotionally, to get a feeling of safety.

In the first of this series of sessions, Mrs. A.'s distance was the primary focus. She spoke of being cut off and totally withdrawn, fearing mistreatment if she really expressed her needs. I interpreted that the prospect of taking a step toward her husband stimulated in her the fear of punishment and mistreatment, and so she settled for the safety of keeping her wishes to herself and remaining at a distance.

In the following session, Mrs. A., taking a step toward her husband, asserted that she wanted him to make some specific changes in his schedule and to treat her with consideration. Although Mr. A. was resistant initially, taking the position that she was asking for something that was "out of the question," Mrs. A. contained her defensive responses and persisted. Eventually, Mr. A. conceded, at which point Mrs. A. broke into tears, reporting that she literally had the feeling that she would be slapped, as she so often had been by her psychotic mother. Sobbing, she reported feeling that her needs and wishes were never considered before, and that while it felt good to be closer to her husband at this moment, "Closeness is scary."

In the next session, Mr. A. struggled to hold onto the feeling that his wife's request was legitimate and not to experience it as another item on her list of "things to do." At the end of the hour, he casually mentioned that he would not be able to make the next appointment, and since I was going to be on vacation for the following two weeks, we would not meet for a month. He added that we were going to need to change the day we met. The process in the room was mirroring the content of the sessions. He now was doing with me what he had been doing with his wife.

I took up this transference acting out with him in the next session. I interpreted that giving up his expectation that others would be on the same page as him put him in touch with feelings of not being good enough, which he dealt with by reestablishing the same-page mode of relating with me and his wife. This led Mr. A. to report spontaneously how this was interfering with his relationship with his daughter, whom he would not see for the next three days because of his schedule. Then, pausing, he began to sob for the first time. He reported how he had no memories of his own father, who had died when Mr. A. was eight years old, and that the reason there were no memories was that his father was never there. He said, "It's painful to recognize that others are separate because then you might lose them."

In the following session, Mr. A. announced happily that he had not thought about the last session all week and that he had no intention of doing so. He did not want to experience his feelings. I said I was surprised by that, and I summarized the content of the last session. It activated in him the harsh attacking unit, which he projected onto me. He fell silent, stated that he did not trust me and did not feel safe, and that he thought he might not return. Mrs. A. withdrew into the safety of her own silence. The last 30 minutes of the hour were occupied by silence.

In the following session, I reinterpreted the sequence of the last several sessions, adding that when Mr. A. had gotten in touch with his painful feelings of being rejected and not good enough, it made him feel very vulnerable to being attacked and hurt. I said that those feelings were hard for him to hold onto and contain within himself, and he put them out onto me as a way of getting them away from himself. Mr. A. responded positively, saying that he was aware intellectually that what I was saying was true, but that his emotions made it very difficult for him. He said that he was doing his best, that he would keep trying, and that he would persist despite these feelings. In essence, he was saying that he would continue on in his alliance with his wife to work things out.

Over the next few sessions, the couple's relationship came back into view, and a collaborative discussion about closeness and affection was begun. They joked about how things had improved sexually for them, recalling that when they had first seen me, there had been a debate about whether it had been seven months or a year since they had had sex. Now things were much better, but they needed to work out how to be close and affectionate and not always sexual.

This series of sessions illustrates the ebb and flow of the work in the working phase. Although the same defensive operations are apparent, they are much easier to contain. The couple evidences a collaborative spirit. The therapist feels that he or she has more of an alliance with the couple and can count on their enduring deeper and more disruptive affects without its posing a threat to the treatment.

TERMINATION

As the couple moves through the working phase of treatment a gradual shift begins to occur that signals the approach of termination. More and more frequently, the couple will report that problems came up during the week but were resolved successfully. Tension in the sessions continues to diminish. When problems do arise, they tend to be more of an individual nature, more appropriately taken up in individual therapy. The couple is more focused on the future than on the past. Generally, the couple evidences the capacity to contain their projections and maintain their alliance with each other through affective storms. Then, at some point, one or both partners initiate the idea of ending therapy, and eventually a termination date is set.

Case of Mr. and Mrs. D.

Mr. and Mrs. D. had initially sought couples therapy because of their concern about their daughter, who seemed to have few friends in school and a general lack of self-confidence. But although their concerns centered around their daughter, they did not wish to bring her to a consultation yet because they thought that perhaps her problems had something to do with their marriage. In fact, the daughter's problems were the direct result of their marital difficulties of insecurity and social isolation.

Over the course of a year and a half of couples therapy, the couple worked on Mr. D.'s withdrawal in his marriage and the world and on Mrs. D.'s difficulties with self-regulation. Repeatedly, they reviewed the sequence of Mrs. D.'s expectations that her husband would perfectly anticipate her need for a "deeper interest" in her feelings, which often arose when she suffered a deflating disappointment. Her devaluing attacks on him often reinforced his experience of her as a sadistic and hurtful object, from whom he would withdraw into days of silence. They had increasingly gained understanding and control of their interlocking projections and projective identifications. They reported a dramatic improvement in their daughter's behavior at school and at home, an improved sex life, and greater success in the world, as well as a deeper appreciation that the origins of many of their problems lay in their childhoods, and not in each other. Mrs. D. had returned to school. Mr. D. was finally doing well in his profession and getting along with colleagues.

Three months before the end of their treatment, Mr. and Mrs. D. reported a blowup while having sex. Mrs. D. said, "I felt like he was out of touch with me and everything he did felt wrong. When I told him about it, he got hurt and became silent." Mr. D. picked up the recital at that point and acknowledged his falling silent, but then talked about how he came back to his wife the next day. He asked, "Didn't I initiate a discussion the next day to sort things out?" She acknowledged that he had and that they had a constructive conversation. In the course of their conversation, they were able to see that, earlier in the day, Mr. D. had failed to tune into how overwhelmed Mrs. D. was feeling by her studies. This failure had started the ball rolling. They reported going on in their discussion to agree that Mrs. D. would begin intensive analytic therapy to "really get at the root of her insecurities."

Over the next month, they spoke of ending couples therapy, but said they were a bit hesitant because they were not sure if they could maintain their new footing without the sessions. Mrs. D. began an intensive course of analytic therapy. At that point, they agreed that they would stop their couples therapy. To Mrs. D. it felt like too much juggling of schedules to keep three individual sessions and a couples session going, with all the other demands on her time. She acknowledged the usefulness of the couples therapy but said she felt that her priorities were shifting and that her own work in individual therapy was far more important. Mr. D. said he felt good about stopping the couple sessions, but expressed concern that his wife's intensive treatment might stir things up in the relationship. He had just been made a partner at his firm and finally seemed to be doing well with his colleagues. He wanted assurance that my office door was open if they should need to return. In summary, both felt that the obstructions in their marriage were no longer interfering with the challenges of their lives.

CONCLUSION

The aim of this approach to couples therapy is to alter the couple's defensive operations sufficiently so that they are able to maintain a working alliance. It is hoped that this will serve as a platform upon which the couple can meet their changing needs within and outside the relationship. This therapy is not a substitute for individual treatment of the patient with a disorder of the self, but is an ancillary treatment that can be a prelude to individual treatment or a concurrent treatment.

REFERENCES

Bowen, M. (1976). Theory in the practice of psychotherapy. In P. Guerin (Ed.), *Family therapy: Theory and practice*. New York: Gardner Press.

Freud, S. (1913). On beginning treatment. (Further recommendations in the technique of psycho-analysis.) *Standard Edition*. London: Hogarth Press.

Freud, S. (1914). Remembering, repeating and working through. (Further recommendations in the technique of psycho-analysis, II.) *Standard Edition*. London: Hogarth Press.

Greenson, R. (1965). The working alliance and the transference neurosis. *Psychoanalytic Quarterly, 34*, 155–181.

Greenson, R. (1967). *The technique and practice of psychoanalysis*, Vol. 1. New York: International Universities Press.

Hoffman, L. (1981). *Foundations of family therapy: A conceptual framework for systems change*. New York: Basic Books.

Keeney, B., & Ross, J. (1985). *Mind in therapy: Constructing systemic family therapies*. New York: Basic Books.

Kerr, M., & Bowen, M. (1988). *Family evaluation: An approach based on Bowen theory*. New York: Norton.

Klein, R. (1989). Application to differential diagnosis. In J. Masterson & R. Klein (Eds.), *Psychotherapy of the disorders of the self: The Masterson approach*. New York: Brunner/Mazel.

Klein, R. (1993). Schizoid personality disorder. In J. Masterson, *The emerging self: A developmental, self, and object relations approach to the treatment of the closet narcissistic disorder*. New York: Brunner/Mazel.

Langs, R. (1974). *The technique of psychoanalytic psychotherapy*, Vols. 1 & 2. New York: Aaronson.

Levenson, E. (1983). *The ambiguity of change: An inquiry into the nature of psychoanalytic reality*. New York: Basic Books.

Masterson, J. (1976). *Psychotherapy of the borderline adult: A developmental approach*. New York: Brunner/Mazel.

Masterson, J. (1981). *Narcissistic and borderline disorders: An integrated developmental approach*. New York: Brunner/Mazel.

Masterson, J. (1993). *The emerging self*. New York: Brunner/Mazel.

Nichols, M. (1984). *Family therapy: Concepts and methods*. New York: Gardner Press.

Scharff, D., & Scharff, J. (1987). *Object relations family therapy*. Northvale, NJ: Aaronson.

Sluzki, C. E. (1975). The coalitionary process in initiating family therapy. *Family Process, 14*, 67–77.

Watzlawick, P., Beavin, J., & Jackson, D. (1967). *Pragmatics of human communication: A study of interactional patterns, pathologies, and paradoxes.* New York: Norton.

Watzlawick, P., Weakland, J., & Fisch, R. (1974). *Change: Principles of problem formation and problem resolution.* New York: Norton.

Zetzel, E. R. (1956). Current topics of transference. *International Journal of Psychoanalysis, 37,* 369–376.

CHAPTER 20

Working with the Collective Marital Self

Candace Orcutt, Ph.D.

The therapist who works toward strengthening the marital bond (or toward dissolving it) does not attend to a simple "one-plus-one" situation. Since the pioneering work of Nathan Ackerman in the 1950s, family therapy and marital therapy have been conceptualized in terms of an overall dynamic. In an important sense, it is the family as a whole, or the marriage as an entity (a collective "impaired self") that is the patient.

Focusing on the marriage as an entity with its own dynamic takes the pressure of blame off the individual patient, and the burden of partiality off the therapist. The marital interaction is central, and the therapist becomes an impartial observer, whose job it is to assess what impedes the interaction, to clarify the impasse, and so to open the way to a more desirable outcome. The authority of the therapist is based on the therapist's skill combined with the couple's motivation for finding a better way of being together. This authority eventually is claimed by the couple, as they understand their situation and assume a new level of mutual responsibility based on that understanding.

Unfortunately, working with the overall dynamic does not absolve the therapist from having to understand the individual dynamics of the partners. A diagnostic assessment of the individual partners is critical for a sound collective approach. If the therapist is in luck, both partners have the same type of disorder of the self, so that a uniform intervention can be used. If both partners are borderline, confrontation can be used consistently to address the couple (that is: "You tell me how much you want your marriage to work, but I notice each of you is looking to the other to take responsibility"). Or, if both are narcissistic, mirroring interpretation can be used (that is: "I believe each of you is so sensitive to feeling at fault, that you protect yourselves by seeing what you can correct in your partner"). Very often, however, the pair has different styles (the complementarity appealed to them when they first met), and to deal with this requires some technical agility.

ADAPTIVE WORK WITH A COUPLE WITH TWO DIFFERENT DISORDERS OF THE SELF

Mr. and Mrs. A., a sophisticated, well-to-do couple in their later middle age, came to treatment for help in managing their arrogant adolescent son. The son was seen by an associate (Fischer, 1989), while I worked with the couple. Issues of managing an adolescent rapidly shifted to issues of managing the parental, marital situation.

The marital therapy was complicated from the outset because the wife suffered from a borderline disorder of the self, while the husband demonstrated the characteristics of a manifest narcissist.

While I had the luxury of working with a motivated couple who had no intention of dissolving their union, I had the problem of dealing with two people who communicated in two very different ways. I had to be able to acknowledge each individual's own style as a prelude to speaking to their combined marital self.

Mrs. A. was volatile, engaging, and a caretaker. In her real-self capacity, she was able to appeal to others, and to act altruistically and with much practical effectiveness. Within the family, she tended to be compliant, in a self-defeating borderline way, and was given to hysterical outbursts and frightening flights into illness to coerce or manipulate others.

Mr. A. was a man who had achieved substantial professional status, which he carried with authority and a certain charm. However, he managed his family situation by assuming that there would be automatic harmony in his presence, and by retreating into his work when his narcissistic expectation was not mirrored.

To communicate with both partners, I had to shift my interventions from confrontation (while addressing her) to mirroring interpretation (while addressing him). This fancy footwork was required primarily in the beginning, when defenses were running high, and at stressful times in the process, when there would be a resurgence of resistance.

I might say to Mrs. A.: "You tell me your health is being ruined by your son's refusal to take responsibility, yet you tell me that, once again, you made his bed and picked up his room on a morning when you were running a fever and needed to rest."

Or I would shift gears and say to Mr. A.: "Telling your son to get his act together spoils your picture of the good father–son relationship, so you shelter this ideal by not disciplining him."

When both were in a fairly receptive mode, I could then address their collective self with a here-and-now interpretation. For instance: "Mr. A, when you act as the head of the household, you command respect—your son falls in line and your wife feels supported. Mrs. A, when you stop doing everything for everyone and back your husband's authority, you see your goals met without becoming frantic and sick. And both of you have the satisfaction of working together effectively instead of each feeling so alone and unappreciated."

Technique, basically, is finding a way to talk to a patient in defense. When the correct technique has been used to lower the anxiety level of each partner, then the couple can be addressed collectively, still on the level of the ego.

Because of this couple's strong motivation, I could move relatively easily into work with the collective marital self. I focused on calling the observing part of the ego into play especially, to encourage awareness of patterns of interaction. I also encouraged them to notice the effect of their communication.

Mr. and Mrs. A. tended to hurl accusations at each other. I deliberately interrupted this process, saying, in her case, that I did not see how she hoped to have control in the situation when she placed responsibility on her partner. In his case, I said I believed it was less painful for him to assess her difficulties than to assess his own, but that the marriage required that he use his analytical skills on his own behalf, also.

Then I tracked their communication closely to show them how they subverted their own needs through the ways they had been using to meet those needs.

For example, Mr. A. had come home to find his wife in a rage at their son. When his attempt to intervene was rebuffed, he retired to the company of his computer (which also allowed him to avoid facing his son). His wife, feeling unsupported, then became hysterical, and both father and son became compliant in order to placate her. A pseudo-calm had been established, but everyone was distraught.

THERAPIST: Mrs. A., what did you want from your husband when he came home?

SHE: I wanted him to tell Joey to take his sneakers off the table, but he just went to his computer as if nothing else was important.

THERAPIST: I don't know. I see why you might make that assumption, but why not find out from him? Mr. A.—what took you to your computer just then?

HE: There was nothing I could do. My presence just seemed to upset her.

SHE: No matter how loudly I say it, you just don't hear how I need you to help.

THERAPIST: But I think that's the point—the way you ask for help, Mrs. A., has the opposite effect of what you hope for. When you are so upset, he doesn't know what to do, and you defeat your own purpose. Mr. A., am I reflecting your position accurately?

HE: Yes. If she would explain what she wants me to do, I'll do it. I don't want her to get sick.

In time, Mrs. A. was able to enlist her husband's support by directly stating her needs instead of dramatizing them. Mr. A. was able, then, to understand clearly what she wanted, and was provided space in which to help her. In addition, he no longer could use her upset as an excuse for avoiding his family responsibilities. Mr. A. listened to his wife, the son listened to Mr. A., the sneakers were put away, and Mrs. A. felt supported. The household grew genuinely calmer, and some of the barriers set up by miscommunication came down.

It should be mentioned again that work with communication and mutual observation is roughly analogous to the ego work in individual treatment that precedes the dynamic work of the inner world and its projections. Just as the maladaptive defenses of the individual are made observable and more adaptive, the defensive communication within the marriage is brought under scrutiny and repaired.

It was in the 1950s that the family therapy theoreticians—Bateson and Ruesch (1987), in particular—stressed the fundamental importance of communication in assessing and working with the family system. Communications theory is highly complex, and many techniques have been evolved for its clinical application. But, in brief, one might say that working with family communications provides a neutral approach (once one learns to speak the family's "language"). This approach strengthens the observing, containing, and adaptive functions of the collective ego.

In psychotherapy, as well as in a great many areas of thinking about people, the viewpoint has shifted from the linear model to a more systemic pattern of interrelationship. The field is having a difficult time creating a synthesis of these two perspectives, and has tended to dichotomize them.*

Family systems theory would define marriage as an interactive whole in which each person is seen as both affected and affecting in a continuous, cybernetic process. This control process tends to support health when it is adaptively self-correcting, and tends to promote dysfunction when it is rigidly repetitive.

In object relations theory, a linear model, the relationship with the mother of infancy is internalized as the paradigm for meaningful attachment, and is subsequently projected onto all future significant relationships. If the internalization is adaptive and flexible, its later projections support healthy attachments. If the internalization is defensive and rigid, its later projections lead to repetitive, self-defeating connections with others. In the latter case, the person projects onto the other old, unchanging behavior that is neither comprehended nor clearly remembered. In the therapy situation, this is identified as transference acting out, where the patient is condemned to repeat the past until the behavior is interrupted, opening a possibility for understanding.

If systems theory and object relations theory are combined, the result is something like the following: The husband, at emotionally sensitive times, reacts to his wife as if she were his mother. This, in turn, reminds his wife of *her* mother, and she responds accordingly. Since both partners come from households that were not open to questioning or clarification of emotionally intense situations, the couple keeps automatically reacting to each other's misperceptions, and the gulf between them widens as their hurt and anger escalate.

Ken Seider, of the Masterson Institute's faculty, has used the term "interlocking projections" to describe this phenomenon (see Chapter 19). The term elegantly sums up the systemic/dynamic nature of the problem.

INITIATING CHANGE WITH AN ADAPTIVE COUPLE

Mr. and Mrs. X. are a quick-minded and motivated couple, prone to idealization and hypersensitive to any nuance of disapproval. They customarily withdraw to manage their grievances. They both show the characteris-

---

*Fortunately, a common ground is now being established by therapists such as Samuel Slipp (1984) and David and Jill Scharff (1991), who demonstrate the compatibility of object relations theory and family therapy.

tics of the hidden, or "closet," narcissist, with distancing, schizoid features. In their case, it is possible to use the same basic "language" when intervening: I mirror their vulnerability and acknowledge their need for self-protection and validation.

Here is a sample of the work with their interlocking projections.

HE: Sometimes I know something is on her mind, so I ask her to tell me what it is, but she says nothing is wrong, or she doesn't know, so I give up.

SHE: He's so insistent, so excited, I can't think. Then he won't talk to me, so I don't *want* to talk to him.

THERAPIST: (Addressing the couple) There's something here about Mr. X. feeling turned away and isolated, so he first works hard to make his point, then pulls back protectively. Then something else comes in, where Mrs. X. steps back from his level of energy—that, also, sounds self-protective to me.

HE: You said a word that touched something in me. "Isolated." When I was a kid, a car hit me and I was hospitalized a long time. Whenever I feel that isolated hospital feeling, I give up.

THERAPIST: So you're saying something profound. Isolated situations make you feel like the kid in the hospital, and you go into your shell.

HE: Yeah. It's like I'm back there.

THERAPIST: You're describing what is often the problem—an important person in your life touches off a child state, and you find yourself protecting yourself as you did when you were a vulnerable child. (Turning to wife.) Is it possible that something similar happens to you? You say you can't think when he gets excited, insistent.

SHE: In my family, there was always a lot of noise. They drank a lot and yelled at each other. So I tune out loud talk—it doesn't mean a thing to me.

THERAPIST: Then you've learned to tune out when the voice level goes up?

SHE: Right. To me, loud voices always mean "lie low."

THERAPIST: Mr. X., this seems to answer part of your question. When you are concerned about your wife, and ask her what's on her mind, something gets in the way of her hearing your concern. You don't realize it, but the intensity of your voice sets off an old reaction in her, and she tunes you out without thinking.

HE: But why can't she *tell* me?

SHE: The more you insist and insist, the less I *want* to tell you.

THERAPIST: O.K. This is where you were both wise to seek out a third party. I don't think either of you was aware of how old reactions can be set off unintentionally by someone close to you. You felt hurt, but didn't really know why.

SHE: (Calmer) So it's not really him I'm reacting to. His intensity puts me back where they were yelling and I stayed out of the way. That's why I feel like a child at those times.

THERAPIST: And that's when you pull away and unintentionally trigger a child state in him. He feels isolated the way he did in the hospital.

HE: And then I don't talk to *her*, either.

THERAPIST: You both pull back to protect yourselves, just as you did when you felt isolated or threatened as children.

SHE: So we bring all these other people along with us when we think it's just him and me.

THERAPIST: Just so. You have to slow down and find your husband in the crowd!

Mr. and Mrs. X. experienced a sense of revelation during this session, and this feeling continues, although, as Mr. X. says, this exploration of old business has touched "a deep well of anger." As transference acting out is understood, the neglect and abuse of childhood emerge in feeling and memory, and are no longer lost in uncomprehending reenactment.

The working through, in marital therapy as in individual therapy, consists of tracing the acting-out transference projections to their beginnings in the early relationships that froze the child's capacity for healthy, self-expression, for empathy and interpersonal regulation. Perhaps the larger part of this task in the working-through phase lies in the individual treatment that ideally should support intensive marital therapy.

WORKING THROUGH THE INTERLOCKING PROJECTIONS

I would like to close by describing a liberating moment of truth from the marital therapy of Mr. and Mrs. Q., whose progress through the adaptive phase was traced in *Psychotherapy of the Disorders of the Self* (Masterson & Orcutt, 1989). The interlocking projections of this couple had been especially intractable, despite a number of years of individual and marital therapy.

Mrs. Q. is a sensitive, creative woman with a powerful need to idealize those she cares about. When that expectation is disappointed, she becomes ferociously defensive to the point of panic. Her idealization defends her from painful memories of an abusive childhood.

Mr. Q. is an emotionally isolated man who disguises his vulnerability behind a blustery façade, or absents himself into a world of books. His bluster is his learned reaction to a mother who expected him to counteract her depression and fulfill her ambitions by showing no "defeatist" feelings, and by offering constant solutions buoyed by positive expectations. When he could not meet these expectations, the mother probably canceled him out emotionally, since he withdraws in present time when he cannot counteract an upsetting situation. At such times, he automatically gives up the expectation of interpersonal comfort and seeks the intellectual comfort he can be sure of because it is (in his words) self-generated.

Mr. Q. is a manifest narcissist who can show no weakness. Mrs. Q. is a closet narcissist with a demanding need to have her feelings validated. He must feel appreciated; she must feel understood and protected.

However, when she needed his support, he would respond as he might to his mother—proclaiming that the problem was not a problem, and even joking about it. She would be enraged and hurt—perceiving him as if he were her abusive father mocking her, or her distracted mother disregarding her. She would turn on him defensively, like the embattled child, and he would withdraw, like the child who had failed. The cycle would build viciously on itself, and escalate into a crisis.

Although they came to grasp this pattern intellectually, understanding was lost again and again under the onslaught of emotional reaction.

Recently, however, a family upset gave them a glimpse of each other's real self. Their much-loved family dog had been nursed devotedly through a series of illnesses by the wife. It finally became clear that the dog would have to be put to sleep, although it was young, and together they took it to the veterinarian. Mrs. Q. embraced the dog as it was given a lethal shot, and, after it died, looked to her husband for consolation. He walked away, facing the corner of the room, then left without saying a word while she stayed near the animal.

In the session, she reproached him for his coldness. He took a chance, and for once expressed his vulnerability: he said that he had been overwhelmed by a sense of sorrow and helplessness. She looked at him as if she had never seen him before: "Is that why you turned away?" He replied that he had been immobilized: "I didn't know what to do." For the first time in the sessions, she saw him in pain and needing her comfort, and reached out to him spontaneously. He, in turn, realized then that his vulnerability could make him more sympathetic and approachable. On that day, the shadow of the past did not separate them, and they found each other on a new level of understanding.

A couple may approach with high motivation or in stubborn defense; they may be in the adaptive phase of treatment or the working through; and they may have dramatically different personal styles. However, just as the goal of marital therapy is the healing of the relationship shared by the two, so the treatment addresses itself to the couple as a collective self, defined by its own characteristics, values, goals, and internal balances.

REFERENCES

Ackerman, N. W. (1956). Interlocking pathology in family relationships. In S. Rado & C. Daniels (Eds.), *Changing concepts of psychoanalytic medicine*, pp. 135–150. New York: Grune & Stratton.

Ackerman, N. W. (1958). *The psychodynamics of family life*. New York: Basic Books.

Bateson, G., & Ruesch, J. (1987). *Communication: The social matrix of society*. New York: Norton.

Fischer, R. (1989). Psychotherapy of the narcissistic personality disorder. In J. F. Masterson & R. Klein (Eds.), *Psychotherapy of the disorders of the self*, pp. 79–85. New York: Brunner/Mazel.

Masterson, J. F., & Orcutt, C. (1989). Marital co-therapy of a narcissistic couple. In J. F. Masterson & R. Klein (Eds.), *Psychotherapy of the disorders of the self*, pp. 197–210. New York: Brunner/Mazel.

Scharff, D., & Scharff, J. (1991). *Object relations couple therapy*. New York: Aronson.

Scharff, J. (Ed.) (1991). *Foundations of object relations family therapy*. New York: Aronson.

Slipp, S. (1984). *Object relations: A dynamic bridge between individual and family treatment*. New York: Aronson.

CHAPTER 21

Antidepressants in Psychotherapy: Use and Abuse

David Grubb, M.D.

She took no medication at all on these mornings, and would arrive feeling pretty ill, but always by the end of the session felt much better and found that a "person" was better than a "pill," a highly important discovery for her, for she had been under heavy medication for years.

Harry Guntrip, 1969 (pp. 362–363)

INTRODUCTION

This chapter discusses the use and abuse of antidepressants with new patients who request them and with the patient who develops a severe abandonment depression in psychotherapy.

I will define antidepressants as those medications that inhibit the reuptake of norepinephrine and serotonin in the central nervous system, including tricyclic antidepressants, such as Tofranil (imipramine) and Elavil (amitriptyline) and second- and third-generation antidepressants, such as Ludiomil (maprotiline), Asendin (amoxapine), and Prozac (fluoxetine). Monomine oxidase (MAO) inhibitors would be included as antidepressants, but I am excluding lithium; antipsychotic agents, such as phenothiazines; and benzodiazepines, including Xanax (alprazolam).

The most common problem with prescribing antidepressants to patients with borderline personality disorder is that of resonating with the rewarding unit projection by making medication response the issue rather than the patient's need to face and deal with emotional problems. This phenomenon became clear to me before I was introduced to Masterson's work, but I did not understand the psychodynamics. While working at various community mental health centers, I became aware that despite my best efforts at education, I was persistently asked by staff to see patients and to prescribe medication in situations that I thought they would have understood were inappropriate. Generally, these were situations of an acute nature with complaints of suicidal ideation caused by separation experiences.

These requests were usually inappropriate because antidepressants are most effective for what have been called endogenous depressions. Examples are the depressive phase of bipolar disorder and recurrent unipolar depressive illnesses.

These disorders cause symptoms that are described in the fouth edition of *Diagnostic and Statistical Manual of Mental Disorders* (DSM-IV) as criteria for major depressive disorder. Antidepressants, although they may affect such symptoms as insomnia quickly, take several weeks to be effective for endogenous depression. Beyond that, summaries of research studies of patients admitted to psychiatric hospitals with the diagnosis of depression show that only 40 percent of those patients are helped by antidepressants. Furthermore, those patients are at risk for suicide attempts, and an antidepressant overdose can be fatal. A very common reason for admission to a psychiatric hospital is the actual overdose or the threat of overdose by a borderline patient who has been on antidepressants for some time, but is experiencing some type of separation crisis. I would now say that these persistent requests for medication evaluation stem from the powerful feelings generated by rescue fantasies on the part of the therapist and the patient's acting out of the WORU. My attempts at education were no match for these powerful emotions.

I also think antidepressants can contribute to the patient and therapist's colluding in the performance of ongoing pseudotherapy. Certainly, other factors, such as lack of knowledge on the therapist's part, can be involved. Nevertheless, antidepressants used in this way can reduce the affective motive for therapy and provide a ready focus for the externalization of problems. Medications are easier to blame than are people, and they do not talk back. They provide evidence of a concrete rewarding unit, with such ideas as, "Someone gave me these, I deserve this help from outside and the good feeling they are supposed to produce."

Here are two case examples of the misuse of antidepressants in borderline patients:

Ms. L. was a 50-year-old woman whom I was asked to see in the hospital intensive care unit after her second serious overdose with antidepressants. The first time, she angrily told me that she did not want to talk to me. The second time, she agreed to talk. She had had one hospitalization about 10 years earlier for depression. She had begun to take a maximum dose of Elavil, and had never decreased the dose or received any psychotherapy. It became clear that she took the medication to hide her marital unhappiness from herself and to help her cope with a job that required her to work different shifts on an erratic basis. Her children had grown, leaving her with no external reason to stay with her husband, whom she seemed to despise. She was using the antidepressants to stifle her feelings and thoughts.

However, this pathological defense was losing its effectiveness and becoming dangerous. A few office interviews confirmed the diagnosis of borderline personality disorder. I confronted her use of antidepressants and told the well-meaning family physician, who had been prescribing the medications for years, about the possibility of further misuse if she continued to take them. This did not go over well with her, but the family practitioner seemed to understand and began to decrease the dose. She stopped seeing me after a few nasty telephone calls to me about the situation. I believe she took further overdoses. I lost follow-up, but she remained an egregious example of the defensive use of antidepressants.

It is not easy for a physician to deny requests for such seemingly powerful and available helpful agents. The busy practitioners with 10 minutes to deal with a distressed, "depressed," patient will quite likely prescribe medication for depression if requested. Far more antidepressants are prescribed by nonpsychiatrists than by psychiatrists (Beardsley et al., 1988).

Talk of suicidal ideation can be powerful and can move systems to provide reassurance at the cost of infantilizing the patient. An example was a 15-year-old boy who presented with a very clear case of an identity crisis, anxiety, suicidal ideation, and a borderline personality structure. He was in the hospital for several weeks; the diagnosis was clearly established. His parents left the area for a two-week vacation, which proved a good thing in this case. I myself went to a conference out of town for a week. When I left, he was improving satisfactorily. When I returned, he was on constant observation, being checked every 15 minutes, and was on antidepressant medication. I immediately stopped both. He had not developed an endogenous depression while I was gone, but he had had some increase in suicidal ideation and the staff and doctor covering for me responded with close observation and antidepressants. They thought they were helping him, but instead they gave him the false notion that he should receive medication and have someone check on him, rather than explore his own thoughts and feelings. They put him on close observation to allay their own anxiety.

Does this mean that it is always wrong to prescribe antidepressants in a crisis, or to any borderline patient? Life is not that simple. The patient who presents acutely "depressed," agitated, or with suicidal ideation often is demanding and acting out. The hospital environment, however, can provide a frame of safety during which a therapeutic alliance may be built. When dealing with patients initially as outpatients, however, no such frame is available. To refuse medication may be appropriate, but may also result in the projection of any negative part object representation, and in the loss of the patient. If the medication is offered and held as a constant while the patient's psychic structure is being understood, it may provide some symptom relief and keep the patient in therapy while a therapeutic alliance is being built. If someone else will hold the medication constant, so much the better. However, the therapist who can prescribe cannot avoid the issue easily. The counterargument may be that one cannot worry about keeping patients if they will leave if not given medication; that may or may not be unfortunate, but it is their business. This is true, but I offer the following consideration from Hippocrates.

> Life is short
> Art is long
> The occasion instant
> Experiments perilous
> Decisions difficult.

ANTIDEPRESSANTS WHILE BEGINNING PSYCHOTHERAPY

My experience has been that antidepressants combined with psychotherapy, when properly used, can help psychotherapy rather than hinder it, but it is not always so easy to decide when it will be a help. There are no blood tests to aid in deciding; the decisions must be clinical. Antidepressants are expensive, provide no feelings of euphoria, often have unpleasant side effects, and are by no means eagerly embraced by all patients. Here are some examples of psychotherapy combined with antidepressants.

The patient, Mr. C., was a 55-year-old white man, a successful executive who had been married and divorced twice. He presented with a complaint of depression, poor concentration, lack of interest in work, an empty lonely feeling, and persistent psychosomatic complaints and problems that were limiting his life and of which he could not rid himself despite the reassurance of his internist. He felt that he was having a recurrence of a depression for which he had been treated twice previously. The first of these depressive episodes had occurred during the separation–individuation crisis of marrying, establishing a career, and having children. The second had occurred after the second divorce, when he decided to give up his idea of moving to another city with a much younger girlfriend, and to stay to support his children. He had been in once-weekly psychotherapy during these previous episodes, with benefit from both therapy and medication. At his request, after the end of the first hour, I prescribed an antidepressant and scheduled him for ongoing psychotherapy.

It turned out that my task in the ensuing meetings was to explore his prominent defense of psychosomatic preoccupation. It became clear that this was a defense he used to avoid painful affect. He reported symptom relief over the next month. The issue that he was again faced with was a separation and individuation crisis. With two older children graduating from college, he now had the prospect of travel and a career change as real possibilities.

He had always felt that his real interests lay in travel and mechanics, rather than in business, but now that fulfillment of these fantasies was possible, he found himself developing psychosomatic symptoms that kept him at home. He began to want to reduce the medication and to understand himself more. It became evident that he had a narcissistic personality structure.

One might expect, therefore, that medication could be seen as magical and powerful and as enforcing the fantasy of imperviousness to stress, unpleasant feelings, and so on, or as a hideous marker of defectiveness, an unpleasant outside influence or the like. I think my patient felt entitled to medications, but the interpretation of narcissistic vulnerability and the protective mechanism of psychosomatic symptoms that were generally ego dystonic to him kept this need for medication open for exploration.

All cases, however, do not proceed so smoothly. Mr. E. was a 33-year-old, single white man who had never lived away from his parents for more than a month or two; they "needed" him. He presented with complaints of headache, crying, decreased sleep, being too emotional, having little energy, and having suicidal thoughts. His symptoms began after he fractured his leg in a bicycling accident and was required to use crutches to prevent aseptic necrosis of the head of the femur. He wanted medication and was quite willing to come in weekly, although he did not want to commit to psychotherapy.

He was the third of four children, with sisters five years and seven years older, and one sister seven years younger. He liked to be by himself, he stated, and had not caused problems as a child, being neither disciplined nor rewarded. He had no problems in grade school, but dropped out of high school when the family moved from the Midwest to California. He had generally kept himself very busy working with his parents; buying, fixing up, and renting houses; doing specialized appliance repair; reading; watching television; and learning about computers.

His experience with women had been extremely limited. He described episodes of depression at the age of seven or eight, at the age of 17, and two years prior to his presentation with me. He related this last depression to his mother's paying attention to his youngest sister rather than to him. He described feeling like dying, not eating or sleeping, and having a psychosomatic reaction, which he thought was a heart attack. After the psychosomatic "heart attack," his father paid more attention to him, but he was quite clear in saying that he improved when his younger sister moved out of the house.

My diagnosis was that he had a schizoid personality, based on his history; prominent schizoid defenses of intellectualization, isolation, and fantasy; and my feelings of being unable to connect with him in the interview. He thought of himself as rarely angry, although it appeared that he was quite an intense and emotional person. When asked about his emotions, he denied what appeared to be obvious feelings. I initially gave him a prescription for Ludiomil, 50 mg, one to three at night. He worked himself up to 150 mg and stated that he felt better right away, which implied a placebo effect. That is, although he might be feeling better, the degree of mood improvement he reported was not consistent with the known pharmocological action of the medication. This well-known clinical phenomenon has been confirmed by studies (Quitken et al., 1993a, 1993b). Nevertheless, he reported he could not sleep and wanted to try a more sedating antidepressant. I gave him some Elavil. The next week he reported that he had taken up to 150 mg of Elavil at night, slept better, but had a dry mouth and did not feel as well as he had on Ludiomil. I continued to try to understand his history and assess his object relations. Although generally cooperative in giving history, he was reluctant to describe anything emotional and rejected any idea of connection between his mood and events in his life.

Dissatisfied with Elavil, he asked for Prozac, which I gave him. He said he felt a very positive effect, but also had increased feelings of jitteriness and some obsessive thoughts. Still attempting to understand him psychologically but to accommodate his demand for antidepressants, I gave him

Pamelor (nortriptyline). Against my advice, he continued on Prozac for a few days, but then began to feel intrusive suicidal thoughts.* I again told him to stop the Prozac and to take some Ativan (lorazepam) for the jitteriness.

It became clear that he did not follow my prescription directions. His schizoid compromise with me was as follows: He found connection and safety by seeing me regularly and fantasizing that I could relieve his symptoms by prescribing the right medication. However, to follow my directions would be to be enslaved, and to consult with and report openly to me about the medication effects in a timely manner would be frightening and would engender feelings of powerlessness. Therefore, he told me about himself, but denied the psychological significance of it all, and took as much control of the medications from me as he could.

The weekend following an appointment, he was admitted to the hospital after a small overdose of Prozac, Ativan, and some alcohol. It had become clear to me during the preceding five sessions that the precipitant for his depression was a combination of inactivity due to his fractured hip, which interfered with his usual defensive mode of business, and repeated rejection by a woman whom he had been pursuing. Although she had not spoken to him until 14 months after they became neighbors, he was convinced on their first meeting that she was interested in him. He joined a bicycle club and invited her on a bicycle ride. After falling and breaking his hip, he continued to ride for a while in a stoic attempt to avoid disappointing her. She had been quite clear from the beginning of the relationship that she was not interested in a romance, but she did not reject him completely. After the accident, probably motivated by guilt and concern, she visited him several times in the hospital, which rekindled his romantic fantasies about her. There was a continued cycle of advances and rebuffs. The incident precipitating the overdose was another rebuff when she asked him not to invite her out on dates, but said that they could be friends.

In one hospital interview, he revealed to me new material of intense loneliness, concern about his failure to move out of his parents' house, despair about finding an appropriate career, and continued romantic fantasies about this woman. She had said, "If we were to meet by accident, we could say 'Hi.' " His interpretation was that she meant that he could call her and renew the relationship. The next day, however, he denied all significance of

---

*In my opinion there is no evidence that Prozac directly causes violence of any type. However, a person who experiences agitating side effects, but no benefit, from any antidepressant would be suffering additional stress, which could lead to suicidal ideation or even action.

the events and insisted, again, that his problem was biochemical and unrelated to what we had discussed on the preceding day.

His parents bustled in to see him one morning while I was on the ward. I went in to introduce myself and found that they did not want to deal with me at all. His father seemed concerned, anxious, and shy. His mother was avoidant of eye contact with me and busied herself making the patient's bed, hanging up his clothes, and otherwise infantilizing him. She seemed to be a domineering and intrusive person. They assured me that they had no questions about any of the events preceding this hospitalization or the hospitalization itself. I thought that these family dynamics were consistent with my diagnostic formulation. He was discharged without suicidal ideation after five days. He did not follow up with me. The woman he had been pursuing called me and confirmed my impression that his description of the relationship had been highly distorted by his fantasies.

In this case, attempting to meet the patient's demand for antidepressants bought some time and understanding of his psychodynamics, but did not lead to a therapeutic alliance. His use of antidepressants for the overdose gesture was also very uncomfortable. I do not think I harmed the patient, but I fear that my perilous experiment brought me more knowledge than it did him. Articles by Marcus (1990) and Brockman (1990) illustrate the value of an accurate psychodynamic formulation before making a decision to begin or withhold medication. Obtaining such a formulation first, however, is not always easy, as this case illustrates.

Patients are not always so demanding of medication. Those who are fearful of intrusion or external control may try, but reject, antidepressants, convinced that they are having side effects. Those side effects are generally not related to the medication and are experienced on very low doses. They may be presented very vaguely and with the affect of hopelessness. This is not a good prognostic sign for psychotherapy or medication, as it can be part of a paranoid presentation. I have wondered if, in these cases, prescribing medication has been an act that resonated with a negatively tinged part object representation and contributed to the patient's leaving therapy.

My hypothesis is that antidepressants and psychotherapy can be complementary ways of dealing with abandonment depression. I agree with Dr. Masterson's statement that medication does not build psychic structure, but I think that used properly it may aid ego repair.

For a comment on this situation, I refer again to Guntrip (1969).

> Environmental factors over which we have no control can in this
> way greatly complicate the handling of the inner problems, which

may themselves be greater than the patient can face. One may well feel that, in spite of advances in understanding, it may often be a practical impossibility to secure the conditions in which radical psychotherapy can be carried to a successful issue. Given a fair chance, some can win through and some cannot, but we must go on to explore this problem as thoroughly as possible. (p. 321)

My literature search did not find any references to antidepressants and abandonment depression, although I found one fascinating case in Guntrip (1969, pp. 111–114). The patient had improved in a psychoanalysis by Guntrip after being hospitalized, but remained vulnerable to abandonment depression with psychosomatic symptoms and an ongoing need to antidepressants. Guntrip does not pursue this theme to a conclusion.

ANTIDEPRESSANTS IN ONGOING PSYCHOTHERAPY

Ms. G. was a 35-year-old white woman who had been married three times and divorced twice. She was taking 50 mg of Sinequan (doxepin) when she first came, but still had complaints of suicidal ideation, hopelessness, and an inability to carry on the activities of daily life quite compatible with a major depressive disorder. Her depression related to her borderline personality structure and life circumstances, and a family history of major mental illness and drug abuse made a genetic predisposition toward depression possible. Her father had been a distant, explosive, and physically abusive man. Her mother was very emotionally abusive and intrusive. The only positive figure in her childhood had been an older sister, whom she idealized. This sister, who was supportive to her as an adult as well, developed cancer and died three years prior to Ms. G.'s first seeing me.

The patient had completed high school and had done some clerical and day-care work. Her first two husbands (she had her only child by the first) were angry, abusive men. Her third husband was described as an overweight teddy-bear sort of man. Sex was not important in their relationship. The husband also developed cancer, while the patient's sister was battling hers. Although he survived treatment, he became emaciated, as the cancer involved his gastrointestinal tract, and his personality changed under the stress of his illness. He became controlling, angry, and emotionally unavailable.

Ms. G. had a borderline personality disorder with an RORU consisting of a warm caretaking and infantilizing part object whom she could "trust 100 percent" and the affect of feeling good and being taken care of connected to a part self representation of being a cared for child. This RORU, however, was heavily tinged with merger fears. Her WORU consisted of a part object representation that was extremely angry, demeaning, and powerful, with the affects of hopeless and helpless despair, guilt, and rage connected to a part self representation as an angry, bad, worthless, and defective person.

Psychotherapy proceeded with the confrontation of prominent acting-out defenses of helplessness, hopelessness, projection of aggression, silences, attempts to turn the tables and interview me, distractions, and trouble with concentrating. Although there were some stormy sessions, therapy proceeded satisfactorily and a therapeutic alliance was built.

The initial issue was her rebellious teenage daughter, who was unhappy at home. As she dealt with this daughter more effectively, stood up for herself, and identified her own thoughts and feelings in therapy, the focus gradually shifted to her problems with her mother and her husband, and the activation of her real self through enrollment in college. The disorder-of-the-self triad figured prominently, as each expression of her real self was followed by abandonment depression. Over the next two years, she did very well in school. Her relationship with her husband, however, continued to degenerate as he moved out of the bedroom, and finally out of the house. Although his move seemed unavoidable, her ability to activate herself to study and go to school declined markedly when he left.

Up until this time, her antidepressant level had remained fairly constant. Suggestions for medication dose changes were infrequent and usually were generated by her. She had tried several times to reduce her medication, but was not able to function if the dose were reduced too much. When she was on a reasonable dose of medication, she was able to carry on, but was not as aware of how she felt. On lower doses, she found herself constantly tearful and unable to function. Her performance in school was a clear marker of her ability to activate her real self. In the month after her husband left, her abandonment depression increased and her adaptive defenses decreased despite continued confrontation. Finally, it became clear that she was in danger of not passing her courses. This would have severe effects on her future, as she was in school on grants and loans, and hoped eventually to be able to support herself and her daughter in a reasonably well-paying job. This was, I thought, her only opportunity to acquire a higher education, and it became necessary for me to point out to her signs and symptoms that she had reported but ignored despite confrontation, and to suggest first an increase in the Sinequan and then a change to a much higher dose of Desyrel (trazodone). This seemed to be quite effective, and she was able to salvage her academic career and future.

I had stepped into her rewarding unit projections by being directive. She asked me how I had known to tell her to increase the medication and then to change it. I pointed out that I had merely done that which she had not been doing; that is, paying attention to her thoughts and feelings. The reiteration of this theme served to add to the therapeutic alliance and to establish a more neutral way of seeing my actions. The main issue became her conduct in school and her process of exploring new ways of relating to people. Her psychotherapy has continued and she has done well, but the task of dealing with the antidepressants remains. The responsibility for decreasing the medication, reporting and understanding her thoughts and feelings, and assessing her overall functioning must become hers. If she can do this, my medication management could then become a parameter, in the psychoanalytic sense—that is, a necessary temporary departure from standard technique, dispensable, and leading to insight (Kantor, 1990).

ROLE OF COUNTERTRANSFERENCE

I have made errors both in prescribing and in not prescribing. Most commonly, the errors have been in the context of repeatedly having patients complain of depression and demand antidepressants, and project the withdrawing unit on me while I search for objective signs and symptoms of depression and the real stressors that led to their hospitalization. The first illustration is of an obvious (in retrospect) unconscious countertransference error as an example of countertransference interference with the process of deciding whether or not to use medications.

A 25-year-old married white woman came to the hospital after a fairly serious suicide attempt. She had had only a little psychotherapy and had not been on any medications and was not eager to try them. Although she functioned fairly well in the hospital, she persistently reported feelings of hopelessness and helplessness and a black mood. Her psychic structure seemed to be that of a borderline personality. She had remained enmeshed with her family of origin, as had her husband with his. It was easy to hypothesize a severe depression based on anger turned inward. Her true self was not activated; she was stifled and frustrated. She also wanted to have a child, but her husband was against it.

She did improve somewhat during the hospital stay, but a couple of weeks after discharge, she wrote me a letter informing me that she had found a psychiatrist who had prescribed Sinequan for her and that she felt vastly improved. I thanked her for the letter, and realized what the problem had been. On several occasions, I had treated her mother with electroconvulsant therapy for a recurrent unipolar depressive illness that she had had since the patient was a child, if not before. The mother's illness fed into the patient's engulfment in the family. Her father seemed passive and unable to deal with the situation. She, of course, desperately wanted to deny that she was developing the same illness as her mother had, and early in the hospital course, she stated that she did not have that illness. Unfortunately, I agreed, as I did not want to think of her prognosis if she did. The clue in this case should have been the strong family history and the persistent black mood that this patient presented.

I allowed myself to be fooled because she did not always report feeling miserable and acted quite differently with other people at other times, as is frequently the case with depressed borderline patients in situational depressions. Put differently, I allowed those facts to enforce my rationalization that she did not have her mother's illness, because she said that she did not, and my awareness of evidence that she did have it was denied.

The second case involves another patient well into therapy who developed increasing depression for reasons obscured by the depression itself, her trouble with revealing herself, and my countertransference.

Ms. M.L. was a 45-year-old woman who had been married for some 23 years and had two children. Her older son, who had moved out of the home, was not particularly successful. Her husband was an administrator. Her beloved and beautiful daughter had developed severe anorexia nervosa with a decrease in school performance, rudeness, depression, anger, drinking, and sexual acting out. The patient came in recognizing her own unhappiness, her difficulty with separation from her daughter, and her difficulty in dealing with her daughter's abusive behavior and her husband's dominance. I made the diagnosis of borderline personality disorder, and was able to help her make some headway, seeing her mostly twice a week. Quite capable of being angry at times, she stood up to her daughter and husband and allowed her daughter more freedom to navigate her troubled psychological seas on her own.

One prominent piece of transference acting out persisted, however, seemingly impervious to all my attempts at confrontation and understanding. She would become extremely fearful and anxious, and experience an intense urge to bolt from the room and stop therapy. In other areas, therapy proceeded and I learned more about her childhood as memories emerged.

Her childhood was remarkable for her position in the family and the emotional, physical, and sexual abuse she had suffered. Her recall of this, however, was very sporadic and she had tremendous feelings of disloyalty and badness when she did talk about it. She was the family scapegoat and her mother's main assistant. Her father was largely absent. Eventually, I understood that she was much better conceptualized as having a schizoid personality disorder and began to treat her more appropriately with interpretations relevant to the schizoid personality's specific conflicts and defenses about emotional closeness and distance. Her desires to bolt diminished markedly, her memories deepened, and exploration of material related to her mother provided strong affect. She was able to deal with her still emotionally abusive and intrusive mother and various aspects of upsetting behavior by her siblings, to whom she was still attached, in a better manner.

She had originally been on 50 mg of Elavil, prescribed by her general practitioner to relieve her insomnia and nightmares. She asked for additional sleeping medication, which I refused, and continued to take Elavil. She ran out of the medication on one or two occasions after some months of therapy, and because of the fear of me engendered by the master/slave projections that needing to ask me for something caused, did not let me know. I noticed that she showed more tearful anguish and depression, which led me to ask her if she had renewed her prescription. The insomnia and nightmares had reappeared when she did not have Elavil. My willingness to prescribe the medication and my lack of desire to see her suffer for the sake of fruitless intrapsychic exploration were clarified. It took a great deal of thinking and of observing her responses to my therapeutic interventions, as well as consultation, before I could estimate where the line could be drawn between fruitless and productive. The medication dose remained constant—evidence that her mood changes were psychological, not biochemical, in origin.

Soon after, her daughter went overseas for a year in a student exchange program. The patient anticipated this, recognized that it would be good for her daughter, and supported her as best as she could, and then talked about her loss when her daughter left. Nevertheless, a slow decline in her mood began to be noted. She related this to her relationship with her mother and agreed to come in twice a week, instead of once a week, as she had been doing for several months. It was very difficult for her to reveal her inner thoughts and feelings about herself, but a confused image of herself and her mother became apparent.

With great difficulty and shame, she revealed that her true thoughts were that everything that had happened to her had happened because she was a bad person, and that her feeling of discontent only proved that she was as worthless as her mother had always told her she was. She expressed hopelessness about change and psychotherapy and intense suicidal thoughts. Attempts to understand more about the origin of the depression only led to further suicidal ideation and thoughts compatible with the self-in-exile unit. It seemed she had worked through the defense of idealization of her mother (part of the master/slave unit) and had begun to recognize her rage, as well as her fear of abandonment. She then seemed to experience the introject of her sadistic mother to recover her (another part of the master–slave unit). However, her self representation became that of a horrible little girl who deserved her mother's criticism and was despised and hated, or ignored, by her part objects because she had not complied with them.

I wondered if this were not a partial fusion, the double refusion of self and object in ego and superego described by Kernberg (1985, pp. 90–95) in writing about Jacobson. She lost some reality testing as well as she projected aggression on me, distorting neutral comments into attacks and confirmations of her badness. Fortunately, my process notes were available to support my therapeutic neutrality and reality testing about what was actually said in the sessions.

Not clear myself about the origins of her depression, I was especially hesitant to tell her what to do or take over because of her schizoid personality structure. I did not want to prescribe medication if it would keep her from recovering and experiencing affects, thoughts, and memories that could be integrated into her conscious in an adaptive way.

However, there were a number of factors that indicated that she did not have sufficient ego capacity to integrate the material. They included her repetitive desires to stop treatment and her lack of integration of confrontations and interpretations about transference acting out and increased projection of aggression on me. There was a weakening of the therapeutic alliance. She had increased suicidal ideation, which, although reported as ego dystonic, she did not feel confident about controlling, and she reported decreased functioning at home and work. She said that she would cry unexpectedly while at work, and that on some days she simply did not go to work.

I thought she would proceed beyond a point of no return if she stopped treatment, would attempt suicide, or would quit or lose her job and so have to stop treatment. I then asked her to increase the Elavil in several steps. This produced some relief, but it proved to be temporary and psychotherapy continued to be an anguished struggle for her.

I changed her antidepressant to Desyrel. She said that she felt much better within a week. With fewer side effects, she could tolerate a higher dose of the medication, and she reported a much better mood. However, the black mood began to creep into the picture again within a few weeks, but this time she was better able to discuss herself with me. The result was a more adaptive ego and a therapeutic alliance.

Although I had felt that part of her depression had to do with her daughter's distance from her, I had waited for material from her to confirm this, as her capacity to hear questions as neutral rather than intrusive was so limited.

Now she revealed that she felt that her loneliness and feelings about her daughter were bad in that they were clinging. Clarification of those feelings showed they were the bad mothering for which she condemned herself. As it turned out, her daughter had been writing every week and telephoning frequently until the fall holidays, when she had stopped abruptly—and that was the precipitant for Ms. M.L.'s increasing depression. The meaning of the decrease in contact with her daughter, and the resultant pathological self and object representations, however, were as described. Now, since that had been explored, her mood continued to improve, her therapeutic alliance strengthened, and she began to move on to other areas. In this case, the use of medication, as well as knowledge of objects relations theory and supervision, were all necessary.

Some of my countertransference had to do with feelings of inadequacy in that her psychological state was not being improved by psychotherapy alone. My sense of defectiveness must have resonated with hers. I think that my own feelings about adjusting the distance and becoming intrusive, my fears that clarifications were directive, and my feelings about being responsible for the intensity of her emotions and her life had been a part of the problem as well.

Getting a perspective on my countertransference allowed better psychotherapy, as well as better pharmacotherapy. Did the pharmacotherapy undo the pathological refusion? Perhaps it reduced the strength of the affective glue that pulled the part self and object relations together, thus allowing for better ego functioning, and, therefore, it salvaged the psychotherapy.

CONCLUSION

One might ask, why I did not avoid the entire issue by having someone else prescribe medication for these patients. An interesting discussion of the evolution of thought regarding the mixing of medications and psychotherapy appears in the textbook *Psychiatry* (Michels et al., 1990). Both prescribing medications and not prescribing them bear a cost. The advantage of being able to prescribe medications is that a person who is involved in both psychotherapy and the prescription of medication is in the best position to use data to adjust both. A coherent framework of psychotherapy and medication use can be formulated for each patient. Articles by Kandel (1979), Cooper (1985), and Goodman (1991) that address some well-known connections between mind and brain show the relevance of knowledge about each to patient care. The possibility that two people can coordinate this knowledge in an effective and practical way is severely limited. Nevertheless, it is common practice to have both a psychotherapist and a pharmacotherapist treating the same patient, particularly in a mental health clinic. A psychological understanding of these triadic relationships is essential to the success of such an arrangement (Bradley, 1990).

The appropriate use of medications depends on an understanding of both the pharmacological and psychological complexities involved. Often the temptation is to ignore one and pursue the other. This chapter illustrates both the difficulties with and the advantages of trying to maintain both perspectives. It further emphasizes the vital contribution of an understanding of the psychodynamics of the use of medications.

REFERENCES

Beardsley, R., et al. (1988). Prescribing of psychotropic medications by primary care physicians and psychiatrists. *Archives of General Psychiatry, 45,* 1117–1119.

Bradley, S. (1990). Nonphysician psychotherapist–physician pharmacotherapist: A new model for concurrent treatment. *Psychiatric Clinics of North America, 13*(2), 307–322.

Brockman, R. (1990). Medication and transference in psychoanalytically oriented psychotherapy of the borderline patient. *Psychiatric Clinics of North America, 13*(2), 287–295.

Cooper, A. (1985). Will neurobiology influence psychoanalysis? *American Journal of Psychiatry, 142*(12), 1345–1402.

Goodman, D. (1991). Organic unity theory: The mind–body problem revisited. *American Journal of Psychiatry, 148*(5), 553–563.

Guntrip, H. (1969). *Schizoid phenomena, object relations and the self.* New York: International Universities Press.

Harvard Medical Society (1989). *Harvard Medical Society Health Letter,* December, p. 8.

Kandell, E. (1979). Psychotherapy and the single synapse. *New England Journal of Medicine, 301*(19), 1028–1037.

Kantor, S. (1990). Depression: When is psychotherapy not enough? *Psychiatric Clinics of North America, 13*(2), 244.

Kernberg, O. (1985). *Internal world and external reality.* London: Jason Aronson.

Marcus, E. (1990). Integrating psychopharmacotherapy, psychotherapy and mental structure. The treatment of patients with personality disorders and depression. *Psychiatric Clinics of North America, 13*(2), 255–263.

Michels, R., et al. (1990). *Psychiatry* (Chap. 13). Philadelphia: Lippincott.

Quitkin, F., et al. (1993a). Loss of drug effects during continuation therapy. *American Journal of Psychiatry, 150*(4), 562–565.

Quitkin, F., et al. (1993b). Further evidence that a placebo response to antidepressants can be identified. *American Journal of Psychiatry, 150*(4), 566–570.

CHAPTER 22

Three Bipolar Women: The Boundary Between Bipolar Disorders and Disorders of the Self

David Grubb, M.D.

In those patients who have prolonged free intervals between their manic or depressive attacks, psychoanalysis should be begun during that free period. The advantage is obvious, for analysis cannot be carried out on severely inhibited melancholic patients or on inattentive maniacal ones.

Karl Abraham, 1911

Patients with bipolar disorder are likely also to have a narcissistic disorder of the self. The recognition of that fact can be very important in their treatment, particularly in the essential area of medication compliance. The specific psychotherapeutic techniques for this disorder of the self can be extremely helpful to them in their struggle with a chronic mental illness.

The point of this chapter is to discuss aspects of psychotherapy that can help the patient with bipolar disorder ameliorate the cost and course of the illness. Effective psychotherapy can be a vital matter to those afflicted with bipolar disorder, as the natural history of the mood disorders is to worsen with time, the cost and inconvenience of hospitalizations are considerable (Coryell et al., 1993), and stress can bring on attacks of the illness. One of my case examples will illustrate the psychodynamics of a patient who brings on a manic attack herself, in response to worry about her husband. As has been pointed out (Michaels et al., 1992), both the biochemical and psychodynamic approaches to mental illness are aimed at dealing with symptoms rather than with causes. However, the descriptions of psychotherapy as an adjunct to treating bipolar disorder are extremely limited as compared with the material available on lithium. Of what use is lithium when the patient will not take it?

This chapter focuses on the psychotherapy of patients on lithium, in a euthymic state. There is literature (Cohen et al., 1954) about the psychotherapy of bipolar patients before the discovery of the usefulness of lithium in Australia by Cade in 1959. Janowsky et al. (1970) comment on the psychodynamics of the manic patient, but do not address the goal of psychotherapy between manic states. My experience has been that even in the free interval, psychotherapy is very difficult to administer, and the patient is rarely interested in it.

A discussion of the place of psychotherapy must be put into the context of a broad question: What is the relation between bipolar disorder and disorders of the self? More specifically, what is the relation between treatment of a bipolar disorder with medication and of a disorder of the self with psychotherapy? In my experience, the patient's disorder of the self is the biggest obstacle to treatment with medication. If bipolar disorder is considered to be genetically based and biochemically mediated, it may not be relevant to talk of psychotherapy. Indeed, the pessimism displayed toward a purely psychodynamic approach to the patient with bipolar illness is consistent with this view. However, the biochemical and verbal must interface, and there are a few landmark articles that speculate about this area (Cooper, 1985; Kandell, 1970; Kantor, 1970). Cloniger (1987) has written an extremely thought-provoking article linking the three major brain neurotransmitters (dopamine, serotonin, and norephinephrine) with three personality dimensions (reward dependence, novelty seeking, and harm avoidance) and the personality disorder schema in the third edition of *Diagnostic and Statistical Manual of Mental Disorders* (DSM-III). Seiver and Davis (1991) propose a model of personality based on dimensions of cognitive-perceptual organization, impulsivity/aggression, affective instability, and anxiety/inhibition. A critique of the psychoanalytic concepts of the area between neurosis and psychosis, where the psychological and biochemical can be most clearly seen to overlap (the borderline disorders, in the broad sense) has been advanced by Martin Willick (1990). Post's (1992) paper explains the hypothesis connecting specific psychological life stressors and the biochemical and genetic underpinnings of bipolar illness. Hobson and Mcfarley (1977) show how research on a cellular level casts a new light on the hallowed area of dream analysis by locating the origin of dreams in random neuronal firing, rather than in the unconscious. Freud's expectation of a neurological basis for psychoanalysis is continuing to prove reasonable.

The patient brings symptoms to the clinicians that they must treat. Clinicians need to be able to use both psychotherapy and medication, to the best of their ability, as numerous writers have pointed out (Ducherty et al., 1977; Karasu, 1982; Rounsaville, 1981). This is an extremely complex subject, and I recommend the June 1990 *The Psychiatric Clinics of North America, Combined Treatment: Psychotherapy and Medication* (Marcus, 1990) for the breadth and accessibility of its selections.

I am interested in exploring methods of psychodynamic psychotherapy that produce intrapsychic change, rather than in educational or supportive efforts to help with medication compliance. That is not to say that medication compliance should not be a goal with either supportive or insight-oriented therapy. However, I think a psychodynamic approach may produce permanent psychological and biochemical benefits for the patient with bipolar illness beyond better medication compliance.

Structural change could be the end point for both psychotherapy and medication as shown in Figure 1, which is a schematic model illustrating the interaction between the physical and the interpersonal. That is, psychotherapy, which is a verbal and interpersonal relationship, should be approachable in terms of neurophysiology, if we are to grapple with the mind–body dichotomy. If psychotherapy leads to medication compliance, this process (the introduction of lithium into the physical-events side of the psyche) can be described in psychodynamic terms with great benefit, as all the knowledge regarding psychotherapy can be brought to bear in this area. Furthermore, the loop from lithium back to psychotherapy via emotions and thoughts shows the synergistic potential of psychotherapy and lithium. Although the exact mechanism of lithium is not understood, it is known to affect neurotransmitters.

I am also interested in the possibility of establishing a psychodynamic formulation of the typical personality characteristics of the bipolar patient. Specifically, in my experience, every patient with bipolar illness had what had seemed to be, superficially at least, a narcissistic disorder of the self. By this I mean a personality with a pathologically grandiose self representation, the prominent use of defenses of anger and devaluation, an extreme sensitivity to other people's opinions, and self-esteem as the central psychodynamic issue. I refer to psychodynamic formulations as described by Masterson (Masterson, 1981; Masterson & Klein, 1989) or Kernberg (1975), rather than to the DSM-IV description of the narcissistic personality dis-

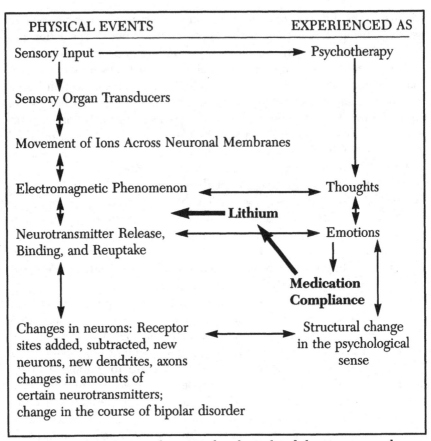

Figure 1. Interaction between the physical and the interpersonal.

order. The DSM-IV can be used as a starting point for psychodynamic diagnosis. Its Axis II descriptive diagnoses can be organized from a psychodynamic viewpoint per Masterson and Klein (1989, p. 5), and most DSM-IV narcissistic personalities would be diagnosed as narcissistic disorders of the self from a psychodynamic viewpoint as well.

The need for pathological narcissistic defenses to support a stable sense of the self, in my experience, has made acceptance of their diagnosis and medication very difficult for patients with bipolar disorder. In addition, appropriate continuous medical follow-up is eschewed by those patients for the same reasons. That is, seeing a physician for lithium levels and prescriptions, let alone psychotherapy, seems to be a narcissistic wound that is so severe to these persons that they typically deny the existence of their illness and put off the need for treatment until a manic or depressive episode has begun.

Theoretically, if one were to say that bipolar disorder is an inherited trait and that personality comes from environmental influence (the character of the ego is a precipitate of abandoned object cathexes [Freud, 1985], there would be no reason to say that a person with bipolar disorder could not have any particular disorder of the self, per Klein (Masterson & Klein, 1989, chap. 22). His article contains a number of clinical examples of differentiating Axis I from Axis II disorders. However, there is a large genetic component to personality in the general sense, or temperament in the specific (Thomas & Chess, 1977; Turecki & Tonner, 1985). There could be as-yet-undiscovered relationships between temperament and Axis I disorders. To complicate matters further, there can be very important psychological differences among people who may fit the DSM-IV criteria for a given personality disorder. Many patients whom I have seen in the Washington State penitentiary at Walla Walla are diagnosed as having mood or bipolar disorders and antisocial personalities. They do fit the antisocial personality disorder of DSM-IV in a descriptive manner. However, I do not think that the examination of their psychodynamics would lead to the same diagnosis. The importance of understanding the lives and psychodynamics of sociopaths, and the importance of doing so, rather than dismissing them as untreatable, have been described by George Vaillaint (1975). The significance of this has to do with the use of specific psychotherapeutic techniques for dealing with different disorders of the self. In particular, sensitivity to self-esteem issues and the interpretation of interpersonal vulnerability for those with a narcissistic disorder of the self, rather than confrontation of maladaptive defenses for those with a borderline disorder or neither for the antisocial disordered individual, are called for.

All three patients in the following cases had clinical evidence of a bipolar disorder. Two are examples of patients who do not fit the textbook or DSM-III-R description of bipolar disorder, and yet benefited from psychiatric medication. They were at the boundaries (Blacker et al., 1992) of more than one disorder.

CASE OF MS. A.

Ms. A. was a 37-year-old married white woman, whom I had seen for some years, first at a mental health center and then in private practice. Her mother also had bipolar disorder, although she had not received treatment or taken lithium until after her daughter had done so. Ms. A.'s bipolar disorder began when she was 24 years old and on a long trip to another country. She traveled a good deal and took risks, but fortunately did not encounter any danger. On her return home, she began to experience feelings of inferiority, guilt, and depression, and the symptom of social isolation. She quit working and stayed at her mother's home. Her mother did not notice the symptoms, undoubtedly out of the need to minimize her own psychiatric illness. My patient took a serious overdose of alcohol and pills and was hospitalized. After this depressive period, she married a man who seemed to give her direction, but was somewhat domineering. She was treated first with an antidepressant and then with lithium. She had had a manic episode with marked paranoid features when I first became acquainted with her. She responded to lithium and a short course of phenothiazines. I did not see her again for three years. Meanwhile, she had had another psychiatric hospitalization, having stopped her lithium. She continued to see me, but at long and erratic intervals—letting a year elapse between the first two appointments and then coming back about every six months after that. She remained married and employed during this time and progressed to better and better jobs. It became clear that she had a bipolar disorder with cycles of several years. Some hints of serious marriage problems then arose. She was disappointed that she and her husband had decided not to have children, and it became clear that he was an alcoholic. Although she had talked to him about it, there was no change. She continued to do well in her career.

She then had another manic episode and psychiatric hospitalization after going off her lithium again. It appeared that the stress was her husband's hospitalization for a serious illness. She responded well to lithium and phenothiazines, which were necessary for three to four weeks. However, she had to take time off from work and was not able to support her husband during much of his serious illness. On discharge from the hospital, she agreed to see me every six months rather than once a year so as to remind her to stay on the lithium and to resist the temptation to change the lithium dose on her own. Six months later, she returned. She had a therapeutic serum lithium level, but was upset, tearful, and concerned about her last manic episode and hospitalization. I pointed out to her that there was a difference between her self and her mental illness, and suggested that there could be psychological factors other than her bipolar disorder that had led to her decision to stop her lithium. Specifically, I thought that the stress of her husband's drinking and then his illness had been the factors she had tried to deal with in a self-destructive manner—by discontinuing her lithium.

She agreed to explore this area, saying that if she had been more assertive with her husband about his drinking and had better self-esteem, she might have been able to deal with the situation in a more adaptive method. She then began to come in weekly.

She spent a good deal of time giving me new background history. Themes of abandonment by her biological father and her mother were prominent. She had clung to her mother and wanted to be a perfect little girl because she was afraid that her mother would leave. I wondered if her psychotic break had not been precipitated by her stopping her lithium as a manic defense against her fear of desertion by her husband because she was afraid of his illness and possible death. In this sense, one can use the term "manic defense" both in the literal sense of developing the manic phase of a bipolar disorder and in the Kleinian sense, with actions to produce feelings of contempt, control, and triumph when guilt and loss cannot be borne (Segal, 1988, p. 90).

She continued to explore her relationship with her mother and described several incidents during which she had disagreed with her and had stood up to her mother's inappropriate responses. She generally controlled against tears in psychotherapy by fairly obvious maneuvers, such as abruptly talking about someone else. She was very concerned about offending me, and avoided affect-laden material when she thought my viewpoint might be different than hers. For instance, when she talked about Catholicism, she became very concerned about whether or not I was Catholic. Gentle confrontation of these defenses—that is, clarifying them or pointing out that they would keep her from following her own trend of thoughts and feelings—seemed to be sufficient.

This led to understanding that what had appeared to be tearful sadness was actually anger and feelings of powerlessness. She questioned whether her manic behavior, rather than being a disease, might not have been learned from her mother's example. She described seeing her mother less often as a result of the psychotherapy, but also became angry at me when she thought that I implied that it was a good thing. (I thought that the exploration of this issue, and clarification that whether or not she saw her mother was up to her, was understood, but it turned out that this was not so.) However, she continued to explore her feelings about her mother.

She became aware that she might have stopped her medication to overcome inhibitions against saying what she really thought to her mother and her husband. She continued to talk about separating herself from her mother but defended against the ensuing tears by turning to me or rationalizing. However, she responded to mild confrontations about her avoidance of affect and feelings of abandonment.

She attributed some of her lack of direction and her difficulty in applying herself in school as a child to the fact that her mother was not there to guide or encourage her. She continued to explore this theme, and stated that it was better to be physically abused than to be emotionally abused by a mentally ill mother, but that she had always coped by putting on a cheerful face and accentuating the positive. She displayed those same defenses throughout the interview, but again mild confrontation led to tears.

She missed a couple of appointments, and then spent the next interview talking about a party at which her husband had gotten drunk. She said that she had challenged him about it and felt quite satisfied. However, the treatment fell apart in the next interview.

She spent the time talking about very superficial topics. When I asked why, she said that she had a meeting after the appointment and did not want to look as though she had been crying. I pointed out to her that she had spent the hour and her money on being more concerned about what others thought than on what she thought. She became extremely angry and began to cry, and as she cried, she became angrier. She accused me of manipulating her. I attempted to clarify this, but she stormed out of the office and canceled all further sessions.

What had gone wrong? In this case, I think, the problem was a diagnostic mistake on my part and, therefore, the use of the wrong technique. I had thought that she had a borderline disorder of the self separate from her bipolar disorder. She seemed to describe clinging to her husband as a father figure who knew more than she did and to look to me in a helpless way as if she could not find the answers herself. Furthermore, she had seemed to respond well, without undue sensitivity, to mild confrontation on my part of her intellectualization and the subject changes that took her off herself and her own feelings.

However, I think the events proved that what I saw as a response was really a false compliance with what she saw as a powerful but dangerous figure. What might have been a longed-for benevolent father in the transference was really a dangerous, treacherous, demeaning, vicious, and psychotic mother figure. Furthermore, her self-esteem was much more fragile than I thought, and once she began to cry, perhaps in anger, feelings of humiliation and rage overtook her and wiped out any sense of therapeutic alliance she had with me.

Her disorder of the self could best be described as narcissistic, and I should have used interpretations of narcissistic vulnerability. She returned a year later in order to continue lithium, but not for further psychotherapy. She reported integration of some of the insights she had obtained.

CASE OF MS. B.

Ms. B. came to see me on referral from a psychologist who had an employee-assistance contract for brief therapy. A 39-year-old woman who had been married twice and divorced once, she lived with her 40-year-old husband, her 15-year-old son by her first marriage, her 12-year-old niece (her older sister's daughter), and her six-year-old daughter, fathered by a man whom she had never married.

She described recurrent patterns of depression that would come on slowly and were characterized by sad feelings, suicidal ideation, irritability, retreat from social situations, and decreased activity and energy. She also described episodes when she was very busy, felt energetic and happy, and slept very little. Both types of episodes seemed to be increasing in frequency and intensity over the years. When she felt depressed, she felt helpless and unable to help herself or others. The family history that she gave at that time was positive for drug and alcohol abuse and dysfunction, but not for psychiatric hospitalization, though she herself had had a brief psychiatric hospitalization years earlier. She said that she was particularly troubled by what she recognized as angry paranoid feelings that were not based in reality during times when she was not sleeping much. I discussed antidepressants and lithium with her, but did not prescribe anything during the first interview. She returned about two months later and said that she wanted to try lithium as she had thought more about her times of being frightened and paranoid. I wrote a prescription for lithium, which she continued to use until three months before the end of therapy, two years later.

She was very concerned about her relationships with her family of origin and wanted to try psychotherapy to help her deal with her mother and siblings. Although she came once a week for the first month or so, she settled down to coming about twice a month, feeling that this was adequate and as much as she could afford beyond her insurance coverage. She began to tell me about her horrifying experiences of poverty and psychological and physical abuse in her early childhood. She described her mother's taking diet pills, ranting and raving, and humiliating and beating her. Her maternal step-grandfather had molested her sexually and taken pictures of her and her sister in the nude when she was young. She described feeling suicidal at the age of 12, and hating her life and her home, which she wanted to shovel out as it was so filthy. She thought of suicide every day until she became pregnant at the age of 15.

Her transference acting out required that I say little, except to clarify my understanding of her emotions, when necessary, to enable her to continue to talk. She told me that she was extremely sensitive to my comments. She was able to describe herself, and was psychologically minded (Akhtar, 1992, pp. 292–296). I did not use confrontation, but rather made some interpretations of her vulnerability, and clarifying comments and simple statements of understanding about what seemed to be constructive actions on her part. Although I was eventually able to say some frank things about my concern that she drank too much when she was under stress, I had to ignore some very inappropriate things she did to and said about her children. There was no abuse involved, but she seemed to have to deny or distort her children's reactions to the turmoil in their lives caused by her instability, episodic drinking and drug abuse, and emotional dyscontrol. At one time, she was able to stop using the benzodiazapine for which she had an open-ended prescription (from her family doctor) by taking an antidepressant I prescribed. However, she said that she did not like the feeling it gave her, and discontinued it.

Her main task in the next two years of therapy was separating from her family of origin, and then from her husband. She tended, she said, to see men as sexual predators, and herself as having grave difficulty in getting close to anyone. She described herself as a satellite circling a planet. That is, although relationships with people were important and she was dependent on them, she could only circle them and never get very close. She occasionally made mildly disparaging comments about my lack of overt reaction to her, but she also said that I seemed to maintain what I would interpret as a part of therapeutic neutrality: walking a thin line between saying too much and not saying enough.

I thought that she had a narcissistic disorder of the self, with prominent defenses of humorous rage at times, and frank rage at others, devaluation, distancing, acting out, and episodic substance abuse. Prominent defenses of splitting were seen in that although she might spend a series of interviews talking about fears of closeness or the need to separate, there was very little continuity from session to session on those important themes. Exploration of that issue led nowhere. She did respond to my interpretations about vulnerability with increasing affect and continuity of material.

Her niece eventually ran away to a temporary social services shelter for adolescents, and expressed the wish to reside with my patient's mother. Ms. B. was extremely upset and angry in response, feeling hurt and devalued by her niece's attitude. I pointed out that she had done all she could for the niece and that her feelings were understandable. She was troubled by the shelter's request for a family meeting and at having to expose herself to others' scrutiny. The meeting and separation went well, however, and, her life at home was calmer without her niece there.

Other major events occurred during Ms. B.'s psychotherapy. She was able to establish a distance from her family of origin. For a number of months, she did not see them. She was then able to visit them without becoming reengulfed in a destructive relationship with them.

Life became very turbulent for her when she started a sexual relationship with a woman at work, and she suffered tremendous conflict between her feelings about the woman and her feelings about her husband. This sexual attraction was extremely powerful and came as a surprise to her. She said that she found the initial attraction and subsequent sexual relationship more exciting than sex with any man had been, as well as more intimate and orgasmic. She struggled with this for some months, but then separated from her husband and moved into a different house with her children.

She continued to work, but it was difficult for her because of her fear of exposure and her projection of hostility onto her co-workers. She was able to take a short leave of absence, during which she saw me more often and reconstituted her self. Although she continued the relationship with the woman, she did not ask her to move in with her, but maintained a reasonable distance between them. She was able to see her lover as having some good and some bad points and to view her fairly realistically. She began to feel safe and accepted by her, and yet was fearful of the relationship. A stormy divorce from her husband followed that resulted in a resurgence of her substance abuse. However, she was finally able to stop all substance abuse in her new, safer environment, and several months later stopped taking lithium. I followed her for several more months and did not see any evidence of bipolar disorder in that time. She had lost much of her insurance coverage due to the divorce, but she felt she was able to discontinue therapy in any event, except on an occasional basis. She said that the lithium had enabled her to survive for two years without acting out destructive rage or suicidal depression, and so had been helpful to her, but she no longer needed it.

CASE OF MS. C.

Ms. C. was a 39-year-old white woman who had been married three times and divorced twice. She worked in a professional capacity, having recently obtained a master's degree. She had seen a psychiatrist intermittently since 1988, after the death of her mother, which had been inordinately upsetting for her. She described herself as lacking self-confidence, feeling as if she fell apart at times, and was not connected to herself or anyone else. She was taking lithium carbonate, 300 mg three times a day, which had been started about six months before I saw her by her previous psychiatrist, who had left our area. She had made a serious suicide attempt about a year before I saw her, but had had only one day of psychiatric hospitalization. She denied any other suicide attempts, but she described frequent depressive periods of short duration, and also periods in which she needed little sleep and was very busy. The latter never lasted more than a week or so. She had difficulty sleeping in general, which was reasonably treated by 0.5 mg of Xanax, and she tended to keep rather erratic hours. At times she would stay up until 4 A.M. and wake up after four hours of sleep, but not be drowsy. She thought her previous psychiatrist had put her on the lithium because of those symptoms, and because she went to see him one day talking a "mile a minute." Her family history was negative for inheritable psychiatric illnesses, as far as she knew. However, she did have a deceased older brother who had been violent and alcoholic and had had one psychiatric hospitalization.

She had one child, from her first marriage, a son with whom she seemed overly close, and who had recently left home to join the military. She articulated difficulties with most people, feeling as though she always needed to do what others wanted, and she complained of severe difficulties with her third marriage, although it had lasted 15 years. She described her present husband, an engineer, as emotionally distant, controlling, and rigid, and obsessed by his version of logic. However, he was also a "rock," which had attracted her to him.

She had grown up in a southern coal-mining area until she was 16 years old. Her father was mostly absent and shunned her when she became an adolescent. She saw him as an old man who was alcoholic, but her siblings described him as distant and cold. There were 20 years between her and the youngest of her six older siblings. Her maternal grandmother, described as a verbally demeaning and demanding woman, lived with them. The family atmosphere, according to my patient, was one of repression, with a false happy facade maintained at her mother's insistence. Her childhood theme was that she had to find out what was required to be with someone in order to be safe. When she was involved in disagreements with people, she usually felt very shamed and guilty, as if she had done something wrong. She remembered times when, as a child, she felt that her outside body was a shell and that her real self was inside and could not be touched by anything that was outside. She felt that she was used as a go-between, manipulated by her family members, including her older sisters, who had a partial parenting role.

She said that when she talked about things that would be assertive in the true sense of the word, she knew it would lead to her perception of herself as stupid, weak, dumb, and powerless. She felt she was like her mother, who was passive.

Ms. C. responded quite well to a confrontation of helplessness and hopelessness as avoidance of focusing on herself and taking action. Although she often vigorously protested against my confrontations, continued confrontations to help her focus on her own experience and not to give in to her intellectualized and psychologized protestations of helplessness and hopelessness were quite effective.

She was aware of her struggle with various introjects as "voices." There was some acting out in therapy, such as her pretending to feel better and do better, but she did do well. For instance, she described having difficulty with friendships as she was always too self-revealing. Examining this allowed her to realize that she did not have to be so revealing and that she could modulate relationships and set boundaries, and she was able to act on this insight.

She found a good job and was much more assertive with her husband about money. But she had troubles on the job, she would project angry feelings onto her co-workers and her husband and assume the role of feeling helpless and trapped, as if she had no choice but to suffer in silence. Confrontation of the fact that it was not necessary for her to work and that she could do what she wanted generally produced good results.

She dropped out of therapy after getting another good job and doing well in it. Her termination was also triggered by a technical mistake I had made in dealing with her anger that was related to my questioning of her symbiotic relationship with her son. By this time, she had been off of the lithium for several months. I was concerned about whether she might be experiencing some type of manic episode. I saw her four or five months later on an emergency basis when she again had had difficulty with ego boundaries at work and had been overly aggressive, and then had felt guilty and suicidal afterwards. She had not restarted the lithium.

It seemed clear that she had a borderline, rather than narcissistic, disorder of the self. She had erratic mood swings that related to feelings of guilt and success, and were expressions of severe demeaning or idealizing superego precursors (Kernberg, 1975, pp. 317–322). She tolerated depression and responded to confrontation of pathological defenses. Although able to use her intellect and knowledge of psychological terms to criticize people, she was not generally cold, demeaning, or devaluing, but rather was involved in fairly constant chaotic interpersonal relationships in the confines of her family and work, all of which are more typical of those with borderline rather than narcissistic disorders of the self. Although some of her self-description made me wonder about a schizoid disorder of the self, she described enough material consistent with the good, taken-care of feelings typical of a RORU to support a borderline diagnosis.

CONCLUSIONS

These cases illustrate the difficulty of dealing with patients with a mixture of disorders of the self and affective symptoms. It took the crucible of psychotherapy and experience to sort out what role, if any, medications had in their management. In hindsight, I would say that although all three women presented taking lithium and seeming to benefit from it, and with some symptoms compatible with bipolar disorder, only one patient actually suffered from that disorder.

With Ms. A., the lithium was necessary. Her diagnosis of bipolar disorder was confirmed by her family history and her repeated manic episodes without lithium. I hope that the psychotherapy, besides helping her deal with her family, will prevent further self-induced manic episodes—by stopping lithium to deal with problems.

With Ms. B., it appeared that lithium was an entry point for psychotherapy and helped her negotiate a crucial time in her life for the better. However, she did not appear to have bipolar disorder, needing neither lithium nor an antidepressant to carry on. In addition to the narcissistic disorder of the self, she probably could be diagnosed as having a cyclothymic disorder, which appears clinically as an attenuated form of bipolar disorder.

In Ms. C.'s case, the lithium turned out to be unnecessary. She did not need it; she never reported any benefit while taking it. Her patterns of sleep, impulsiveness, and relationships were the same with or without it. Occam's razor (the rule that the simplest of competing theories be preferred to the more complex) would limit her diagnoses to those of borderline disorder of the self and marital disorder.

I hope that these cases illustrate the fact that whether or not the medications are vital, it is important to help patients manage their feelings about medications and to work with them rather than insist that they do or do not take a medication a certain way. The regulation of affect by medication may allow psychotherapy and, therefore, change in psychic structure. Medication by itself does not produce permanent intrapsychic changes. However, it may allow the environment (psychotherapy) to produce intrapsychic, and perhaps neurophysiological, changes as hypothesized in

Figure 1. The neuroanatomy of such interactions among temperament, self-awareness, and medication has been proposed (Cloninger, Svrakic, & Przybeck, 1993).

As for my second hypothesis (that people with bipolar disorder have a narcissistic disorder of the self), the three cases bear out my experience. The patient with true bipolar disorder had a narcissistic personality. Of the other two, both seeming to show clinical evidence of benefit from lithium by their initial self-reports, one was borderline and one was narcissistic. The patient with a narcissistic disorder of the self (Ms. B.) seemed to benefit the most from lithium. The patient who clearly had a borderline disorder of the self (Ms. C.), in spite of taking a serious overdose and having very erratic sleep patterns, was not bipolar. Three cases do not prove a hypothesis, but they do illustrate an approach to it that may prove useful.

I entertained the possibility of a bipolar disorder in all three patients, and treated them with lithium and psychotherapy. Without the instrument of a psychoanalytic understanding of the three women, I do not think I would have had much to offer them. However, through the therapeutic alliance forged by psychotherapy, I was able to be confident that Ms. C. did not need lithium (no small matter), and I was able to help Ms. A. learn some things about herself that may prevent further psychiatric hospitalizations. The judicious use of lithium and a knowledge of the psychodynamics of the narcissistic disorder of the self enabled me to work effectively with Ms. B. in a time that was very difficult for her.

I hope that this chapter will provide some useful ideas for other clinicians and encourage them to add their experiences to the clinical literature.

REFERENCES

Abraham, K. (1985). Notes on the psycho-analytical investigation and treatment of manic-depressive insanity and allied conditions. In J. Coyne (Ed.), *Essential papers on depression*. New York: New York University Press.

Akhtar, S. (1992). *Broken structures: Severe personality disorders and their treatment*. New York: Jason Aronson.

Blacker, D., et al. (1992). Contested boundaries of bipolar disorder and the limits of categorical diagnosis in psychiatry. *American Journal of Psychiatry, 149*, 1473–1483.

Cloninger, C. R. (1987). A systematic method for clinical description and classification of personality variants. *Archives of General Psychiatry, 44*, 573–588.

Cloninger, C. R., Svrakic, D. M., & Przybeck, T. R. (1993). A psychobiological model of temperament and character. *Archives of General Psychiatry, 50*, 975–990.

Cohen, M., et al. (1954). An intensive study of twelve cases of manic-depressive psychosis. *Psychiatry, 17*, 103–137.

Cooper, A. (1985). Will neurobiology influence psychoanalysis? *American Journal of Psychiatry, 142*(12), 1345–1402.

Coryell, W., et al. (1993). The enduring psychosocial consequences of mania and depression. *American Journal of Psychiatry, 150*(5), 720–727.

Docherty, J., et al. (1977). Psychotherapy and pharmacotherapy: Conceptual issues. *American Journal of Psychiatry, 134*, 529–533.

Freud, S. (1985). *The ego and the id.* New York: Norton.

Hobson, J. A., & Mcfarley, R. (1977). The brain as a dream state generator: An activation-synthesis hypothesis of the dream process. *American Journal of Psychiatry, 134*, 1335–1348.

Janowsky, D., et al. (1970). Playing the manic game: Interpersonal maneuvers of the acutely manic patient. *Archives of General Psychiatry, 22*, 252–261.

Kandell, E. (1970). Psychotherapy and the single synapse. *New England Journal of Medicine, 301*(19), 1028–1037.

Kantor, S. (1990). Depression: When is psychotherapy not enough? *Psychiatric Clinics of North America, 13*, 241–254.

Karasu, T. (1982). Psychotherapy and pharmacotherapy: Toward an integrative model. *American Journal of Psychiatry, 139*, 1102–1113.

Kernberg, O. (1975). *Borderline conditions and pathological narcissism.* New York: Science House.

Marcus, E. (Ed.) (1990). *Psychiatric Clinics of North America, 13*(2).

Masterson, J. (1981). *The narcissistic and borderline disorders: An integrated developmental approach.* New York: Brunner/Mazel.

Masterson, J., & Klein, R. (Eds.) (1989). *Psychotherapy of the disorders of the self: The Masterson approach.* New York: Brunner/Mazel.

Michels, R., et al. (1992). *Psychiatry* (Chap. 61). Philadelphia: Lippincott.

Post, R. M. (1992). Transduction of psychosocial stress into the neurobiology of recurrent affective disorder. *American Journal of Psychiatry, 149*(81), 999–1010.

Rounsaville, B. (1981). Do psychotherapy and pharmacotherapy for depression conflict? *Psychiatry, 38*, 24–29.

Segal, H. (1988). *Introduction to the work of Melanie Klein.* London: Karnac Books.

Siever, L., & Davis, K. (1991). A psychobiological perspective on the personality disorders. *American Journal of Psychiatry, 148*, 1647–1658.

Thomas, A., & Chess, S. (1977). *Temperament and development.* New York: Brunner/Mazel.

Turecki, S., & Tonner, L. (1985). *The difficult child.* New York: Bantam Books.

Vaillant, G. (1975). Sociopathy as a human process. *Archives of General Psychiatry, 32*, 178–183.

Willick, M. (1990). Psychoanalytic concepts of the etiology of severe mental illness. *Journal of the American Psychoanalytic Association, 38*, 1049–1082.

Name Index

Subject Index

429

Printed in the United States
by Baker & Taylor Publisher Services